*Topics in Down Syndrome*

*Second Edition*

# Gross Motor Skills for Children with Down Syndrome

## A Guide for Parents and Professionals

Patricia C. Winders, PT

Woodbine House ■ 2014

Originally published as *Gross Motor Skills in Children with Down Syndrome,* ©1997, Woodbine House

All rights reserved. Published in the United States of America by Woodbine House, Inc., 6510 Bells Mill Road, Bethesda, MD 20817. 800-843-7323. www.woodbinehouse.com

Library of Congress Cataloging-in-Publication Data

Winders, Patricia C.
  [Gross motor skills in children with Down syndrome]
 Gross motor skills for children with Down syndrome : a guide for parents and profession-als / by Patricia C. Winders. -- Second edition.
     pages cm
 Revision of: Gross motor skills in children with Down syndrome.) 1997.
 Includes index.
 ISBN 978-1-60613-009-4
 1.  Down syndrome. 2.  Motor learning. 3.  Motor ability in children.  I. Title.
 RJ506.D68W56 2013
 618.92'858842--dc23

                                                                    2013029966

Manufactured in the United States of America

10 9  8  7  6  5  4  3  2  1

*This book is dedicated to all parents
of children with Down syndrome.*

*Your commitment and hard work to help your children
reach their full potential are an inspiration
to all of us who know you.*

# Table of Contents

## Appendix: Evaluation and Treatment Worksheets

# Acknowledgements

*Until one is committed, there is hesitancy, the chance to draw
back, always ineffectiveness. Concerning all acts of initiative
(and Creation), there is one elementary truth the ignorance of
which kills countless ideas and splendid plans: that the moment
one definitely commits oneself, then Providence moves too. All
sorts of things occur to help one that would never otherwise
have occurred. A whole stream of events issues from the decision
raising in one's favour all manner of unforeseen incidents and
meetings and material assistance which no man could have
dreamed would have come his way.*
—W. H. Murray *(The Scottish Himalayan Expedition)*

This book is the result of the contributions of many people who gener-
ously gave their time, their experience, and their knowledge and insights. I
wish to thank:

- Children with Down syndrome and their families: for contribut-
  ing countless hours of hard work, your understanding and insight, and especially your perspective as a family on the impor-
  tance of focusing on the lifespan from infancy to adulthood;
- Fran Hickey, M.D., and the team at the Anna & John J. Sie Center for Down Syndrome, Children's Hospital Colorado: for your
  commitment to provide the best care for people with Down
  syndrome, your expertise, collaboration and teamwork, passion,
  and sense of urgency;
- The Global Down Syndrome Foundation with Michelle Whitten,
  Executive Director, and her team: for your unwavering commitment and vision to lead and to do what's next to create new ini-
  tiatives and opportunities for people with Down syndrome;

- Anna and John J. Sie: for your love for Sophia and your passion and generosity to create the best future for her and everyone with Down syndrome;
- Tia Brayman, photographer, Children's Hospital Colorado: for capturing the joyful moments of children with Down syndrome;
- Bernie Veldman, orthotist: for creating SureStep orthoses, which provide critical foot support for children with Down syndrome;
- Mickey Cassella, PT, Children's Hospital Boston, and the Adaptive Dance Program at Boston Ballet: for having the vision to create this model program so that this extraordinary dance experience is a possibility for children and young adults with Down syndrome;
- Colorado Ballet and the Be Beautiful Be Yourself Dance Program: for collaborating to create a wonderful dance experience for children with Down syndrome in Colorado;
- Pat Oelwein, Educator: for your pioneering work on methods for teaching children with Down syndrome and for our special collaborative work at the Saut Education and Training Center for Down Syndrome;
- Fatima Malak, CEO of Saut: The Voice of Down Syndrome, the Board of Directors, and the training center staff of Saut Education and Training Center for Down Syndrome, Riyadh, Saudi Arabia: for the opportunity to collaborate with you and assist you in your mission to meet the needs of children with Down syndrome and their families
- Susan Stokes: for your expertise, decisiveness, guidance, and patience during the writing process and bringing the book to completion;
- Jim & Elizabeth Winders: for your love and support, ability to help me see the whole picture, your willingness to do whatever was needed, and your patience from start to finish.

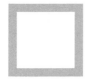

# Introduction

**A**s parents of a child with Down syndrome, you have the same job that every parent has. You are embarking on a lifelong partnership with your child where the job is to teach him what he needs to know to be successful in life. The first challenge that every child faces is the development of gross motor skills; for example, learning to roll, sit, crawl, stand, and walk. The opportunity in tackling this challenge together is for you to learn how your child learns so you can be an effective partner with him throughout his life. The key will be to understand your child's unique learning style. Knowing how to facilitate your child's learning will be critical to your success in collaborating with him throughout his lifetime.

Children with Down syndrome have tremendous potential in the area of gross motor development. Gross motor skills will be one of your child's strengths and an arena that also builds confidence, pride, and self-esteem. He will be excited to learn to run, jump, ride a tricycle and bicycle, and be active with his siblings and friends. As he grows up, he will develop his own areas of interest, such as dancing, swimming, horseback riding, karate, jogging, weight lifting, skiing, or sports. With ongoing practice within his areas of interest, he will experience joy in his achievements and develop a strong and fit body.

The purpose of this book is to teach your child gross motor skills in a fun, effective way, based on his learning style. The book will show you how to teach each skill in a way that develops a body that can run, jump, and engage in athletic activities.

It will teach you how to build the motor skills that he will need as an adolescent and adult. It will answer your questions about *what* to teach, *why*, *when*, and *how*. It will give you the tools you need to understand your child and to read his cues, and it will provide you with methods to practice skills. Once you know what to focus on and how to teach the skills, you can challenge your child so that he learns how to use his body and gains confidence in his own physical abilities.

This introduction will discuss:
1. the goal of physical therapy;
2. the factors influencing gross motor development, both physical and learning;
3. an overview of gross motor skill development in children with Down syndrome, how to provide strategic support, and the crucial role of parents and siblings;
4. the critical times for physical therapy intervention;
5. the learning style of children with Down syndrome.

# Goal of Physical Therapy—The Big Picture

Many parents and professionals assume that the goal of physical therapy in children with Down syndrome is to accelerate gross motor development—to help them acquire gross motor skills at a rate closer to that of typical children. In the short term, this goal seems to make sense. But if you consider the child's motor functioning throughout his life, there is no evidence that accelerating the rate of gross motor development makes a difference. Having a child walk at 20 months rather than 24 months has not been shown to result in any qualitative difference in his motor abilities 10 or 20 years from now.

Based on many years of clinical experience working with children with Down syndrome, I have concluded that what does make a difference in the long run is to focus on the goal of developing a body that is functional throughout an individual's life. It won't be important that he learned to walk early, if as an adult he has developed a walking pattern that is so inefficient and painful that he is unable to walk for more than very short distances.

There are certain crucial results that need to be accomplished early in your child's development so that he will have a body that is fit and functional throughout his life. I refer to them as the *four critical results,* and they are:
1. to walk with an efficient pattern with his knees and feet pointing straight ahead, a narrow base, a long stride length, and toe push off (see fig. 0.1 )
2. to have optimal alignment of his hips, knees, and ankles to support this walking pattern
3. to have a strong, upright trunk with balanced strength between his back muscles and abdominal muscles
4. to have strong arms and shoulders, with balanced strength between the front and back shoulder muscles, so the shoulders and arms fall in the middle of the side view, not tilting forward (see fig. 0.2)

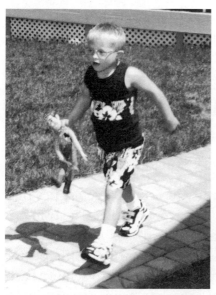

(fig. 0.1)

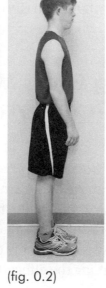

(fig. 0.2)

If your child achieves these four results, he will develop a body with a solid foundation to support exercise and fitness activities throughout his life.

A typical child develops that body without any special intervention. But the process is more complicated for a child with Down syndrome. He *can* develop that body, but it does not automatically occur in the process of achieving gross motor milestones. Because of his physical problems, he is prone to develop compensations, which are ways he adapts to make up for the physical problems. Some of these compensations, if allowed to persist, will eventually result in inefficient and painful movement patterns that will compromise his function as an adult.

Let me illustrate what I mean with an example of a compensation that can result in a long-term loss of function. When learning to stand, the physical problems of ligamentous laxity and hypotonia (discussed under Physical Factors) will cause him to feel unstable. Most children with Down syndrome compensate for this instability by broadening their base, locking their knees, and turning their feet outward. If this posture is allowed to persist, it will be transferred to his walking pattern, and he will learn to walk with a wide base, knees and feet turned outward, and weight bearing on the flat arches of his feet. If this becomes his habitual walking pattern as an adult, he will tire easily, find walking painful, and be limited to walking for short distances. Neither walking nor running will be functional abilities in his lifetime.

It is important to understand the purpose for which the book is designed and how to use it. The goal of the book is not to have children with Down achieve gross motor skills more quickly. The goal is to have your child achieve his maximum physical potential and to build a body that is fit and functional throughout his life. The way to do this is by minimizing compensations that, in the long run, lead to impairment of optimal motor functioning.

The goal of physical therapy is to produce the four critical results listed above, so your child has the posture, strength, and movement patterns that he will need as an adolescent and an adult. This is the **big picture** to always keep in mind. The focus will be on *how* and *what* your child learns, not how fast. If physical therapy focuses on this long-term perspective, then PT services can make a lifelong contribution to the quality of your child's life.

# Factors Influencing Gross Motor Development in Children with Down Syndrome

## A. *Physical Factors*

Children with Down syndrome have several physical characteristics that affect how they spontaneously move and learn gross motor skills. The primary physical factors are: hypotonia, ligamentous laxity, decreased strength, short arms and legs, and medical problems. The influence of each factor is different for each child. Each child needs to figure out how to move his body to achieve each gross motor skill, while overcoming the effects that each factor exerts on him.

### Hypotonia

Children with Down syndrome have low muscle tone, which is also called hypotonia. Muscle tone is different than muscle strength. Muscle tone is described as the resting tension of the muscle when it is relaxed, and it is controlled by the brain. It is evaluated subjectively by feeling the muscles and limbs and measuring the resistance or stiffness or tension when passively moved. In hypotonia, there is *decreased* resistance or stiffness. Hypotonia is most noticeable in children with Down syndrome when they are infants. When you pick up a baby with Down syndrome, you will notice that he feels "floppy" in his neck, trunk, arms, and legs. When he is lying on his back, his arms and legs will fall away from his body and feel floppy when resting on a surface. This floppiness is due to reduced muscle tone.

You and your physical therapist can observe the **degree** of hypotonia that your child has, **where** it is less and where it is greater, and if there is a **difference from one side of the body to the other**. The degree of hypotonia can be mild, moderate, or severe. It can vary from one area of the body to another, and from the right side to the left side. In general, hypotonia is usually more pronounced in the arms and abdomen. Understanding your child's pattern of hypotonia will help you understand how it is affecting your child's ability to learn certain gross motor skills. Hypotonia in a particular area affects the development of skills that require the use of that area. For example, hypotonia in the arms makes it harder to learn to combat crawl. More hypotonia in the abdomen makes it harder to move onto hands and knees and creep. Your child's muscle tone will improve over time, and when he is school age, you may only see subtle remnants of it.

At first, you may not be able to tell the degree of hypotonia that your child has or whether some areas are more affected than others. As you practice gross motor skills with him, you will begin to recognize movement patterns that are difficult for him. For instance, you may notice that he has trouble with, and tends to avoid, activities that require the use of his arms. He may not like to prop on his stomach or pull with his arms. These skills may be difficult due to hypotonia. Even though he has hypotonia, he can develop strength in his arms, and he will learn to do the gross motor skills with practice.

### Increased Flexibility in Joints or Ligamentous Laxity

Children with Down syndrome have ligamentous laxity, which causes increased flexibility in their joints. The ligaments that hold the bones together have more slack or are easily stretched, which allows excessive movement in the joints. You will notice the ligamentous laxity in your baby's hips as he lies on his back on the floor. His legs will be wide apart with his knees straight or his knees will be bent and wide apart, resting on the floor with the soles of his feet close together (like the "frog leg" posture). When he begins practicing pulling to sit, you will feel the excessive flexibility in his shoulders. You may notice or feel "popping" in his joints. Another area to watch is his neck, since children with Down syndrome are at risk for atlantoaxial and atlanto-occipital instability (see page 313).

You and your physical therapist can observe the *degree* of laxity that your child has and *which joints* are most affected. Then you can teach your child gross motor skills customized to his body make-up. You will not be able to lessen the laxity, but you can prevent further stretching of his ligaments. You can be proactive to avoid injury. For example, avoid lifting your child by his arms, since this could dislocate his shoulder. You can also strengthen the muscles around the joints by focusing on building strength with the desired movements.

The increased flexibility will cause decreased stability in the joints. You will need to provide the right support for your child to feel stable practicing a new skill until he has developed the strength in the muscles surrounding the joint, and he knows the right way to position his body. For example, learning to stand will be difficult since his hips, knees, and ankles may be unstable and wobbly due to laxity in the ligaments. You will need to stand him in the right position and teach him to strengthen his hip, knee, and ankle muscles to feel stable in standing.

The excessive flexibility of the joints can also make it difficult to learn certain gross motor skills. For example, moving out of sitting may be blocked by excessive hip mobility. When he tries to move from sitting down to the floor by moving over his side, his wide base may block moving out of sitting. These kinds of difficulties will be addressed in each chapter under the "Tendencies" sections.

## Decreased Strength

Children with Down syndrome have decreased muscle strength, but your child's strength will improve with repetition and practice of the desired movements. Muscle strength is defined as the force exerted to overcome resistance. For example, when your baby is lying on his back on the floor, he uses arm strength to lift his arms and move his hands to his chest or mouth. He also uses arm strength to pull his body forward when he is combat crawling with his belly on the floor. As your child is learning gross motor skills, the focus needs to be on developing strength in the desired movements. On his own, he may develop compensatory movement patterns and strengthen muscles that will cause faulty mechanics and become problematic later. For example, he may choose to stand by holding his knees very stiff and straight, which would affect standing balance and walking and may cause future knee problems due to overstretching of the joints.

He also needs to develop a balance between opposing movements, rather than overdeveloping one movement. As an infant, the muscles on his back will be stronger and cause him to arch his head and trunk. To balance out the arching, he will need to learn to activate the muscles on the front of his neck, chest, and abdomen, to tuck his chin and abdomen. When he learns to straighten his hips and knees to stand with support, he also needs to learn to bend them to lower to sitting on the floor. In the following chapters, you will learn which movements to strengthen (**components to develop**) and which movements to avoid (**tendencies**).

You and your physical therapist can work together to observe what muscle groups are weak or inefficient and need to be strengthened. Sometimes, your child will have the strength but not understand how to use it to do a skill. To help your child achieve each gross motor skill, you will need to learn the desired movements to focus on and the best strategies for activating and strengthening the muscles needed. By practicing often in a strategic way, your child will develop the strength to do the skill.

## Short Arms and Legs

Children with Down syndrome have short arms and legs relative to the length of their trunks. Having short arms makes it more difficult to learn sitting because the baby cannot prop his hands forward on the floor without bending his trunk too far forward. It is also difficult to catch himself when he falls to the side or backwards, because he will fall farther before he is able to prop on his hand. (See Stage 3.) Having short legs makes it harder to learn to climb onto the sofa, climb stairs, and to walk up and down curbs and stairs. The combination of short arms and legs also makes pedaling and steering a tricycle more difficult. When practicing these skills, you may need to wait for increased growth before he will be successful. Another strategy is to use equipment better proportioned to his arm and leg size. For example, when your child is ready to learn to walk up and down stairs, it is best to practice on toddler size stairs at a playground for toddlers.

Children with Down syndrome also tend to have short fingers and small, broad hands. When your child is an infant, you will need to select rattles and balls that are small enough for him to hold. When he is ready to pull to stand and wants to hold onto the edge of a surface, he needs a surface that is thin enough for him to grip. To be successful walking up and down stairs by himself, he will need a railing that is small enough in diameter for him to safely grip it.

## Medical Problems

Many children with Down syndrome have medical conditions that affect their ability to learn and practice gross motor skills. These can include heart defects, stomach or intestinal problems, obstructive sleep apnea, chronic upper respiratory infections, seizures, and ear infections. The medical issues are the first priority, and while they are being managed, simple positioning strategies may be helpful. When your child's health is compromised, he needs to focus on recuperating. When he is sick, his strength will be diminished, he will fatigue easily, and he will be frustrated and upset if asked to practice challenging gross motor skills. It is counterproductive to stress him with practicing new gross motor skills when he is not healthy. If you wait until he has the strength and stamina to practice the skills, you will set him up to be successful, and he will show you his best performance.

For more detailed information on the medical concerns and health issues of children with Down syndrome, refer to Dr. Len Leshin's chapter in *Babies with Down Syndrome: A New Parents' Guide* (Woodbine House, 2008), *A Parent's Guide to Down Syndrome: Toward a Brighter Future* by Dr. Sigfried Pueschel (Paul Brookes, 2001), and the clinical report on "Health Supervision for Children with Down Syndrome" published in *Pediatrics* by the American Academy of Pediatrics (Bull, 2011).

Each child with Down syndrome has a unique combination of physical factors. Because of these differences in physical make-up, children with Down syndrome do not develop gross motor skills in the same way that the typical child does. The order in which your child learns skills will be similar, but how he learns to do the skills may be different. Because of his hypotonia and ligamentous laxity, he will find ways to achieve each skill employing compensations that help him overcome these factors. These compensations are necessary and functional adaptations for him to learn the skill. It is not our goal to totally eliminate them. The goal is to minimize the compensations that, if allowed to persist, would prevent him from reaching his full potential.

## B. Learning Style in Children with Down Syndrome

When teaching your child gross motor skills, it is crucial to understand how children with Down syndrome tend to learn in general, and in particular, how they learn gross motor skills. With this framework, you can begin to study the unique way that your child learns and have that knowledge guide *how* you teach each skill. This section of the book will give you valuable insights into teaching your child gross motor skills. You may wish to reread it several times during the birth to walking and post walking periods of development.

When teaching a child with Down syndrome a new skill, you tend to get one of two outcomes: a successful learning experience, or a frustrated, unhappy child. If he is taught according to his learning style and is set up to be successful, then you will be partners, and the learning experience will be fun. However, if his learning style is not understood and mastery of the skill becomes more important than the child's experience, the child may feel imposed upon and may resist and avoid learning. Jennifer Wishart, a psychologist who has done extensive research on the learning style of children with Down syndrome at the Edinburgh Centre for Research in Child Development (Department of Psychology, University of Edinburgh, Edinburgh, Scotland), writes:

> *"The need to reach a better understanding of the nature of developmental processes in DS is therefore pressing. Our attempts at facilitative intervention are severely handicapped as long as our understanding of how learning progresses in children with DS is incomplete. Intervening in developmental processes that are not fully understood can at best hope to meet with limited success; at worst, **adoption of inappropriate teaching methods could run the risk of changing slow but willing learners into reluctant, avoidant learners**" (1995, p. 62).*

This quote highlights how crucial it is for parents, therapists, and educators to understand the learning style of children with Down syndrome so they gain proficiency in how to facilitate their learning.

Through years of clinical experience, I have learned to customize my approach to each child and accommodate his learning style to elicit his best performance. In the next two sections, I will share some of the things that I have learned and that guide my approach to teaching each child new gross motor skills.

### Learning Behaviors

***Children with Down syndrome tend to underperform and use avoidance routines.*** Jennifer Wishart (1991) writes:

> *"Infants with DS consistently showed evidence of underperforming, with avoidance routines being produced on many of the tasks presented, regardless of whether these were above or below the infant's current developmental level."*

When practicing new gross motor skills, the aim is for your child to perform, and, if possible, to provide his best performance. You will need to elicit your child's cooperation and participation by finding ways to motivate him. You will need to get his attention and cause him to move. You will need to be creative with the toys you use, and save the best motivators for the more challenging skills. Your child's success and enjoyment will depend on how you play, the toys you use, and where you place the toys.

Since children with Down syndrome tend to use avoidance routines, you need to learn to recognize the types that may be used. Examples of possible avoidance routines are:

- To cry, fuss, or "holler" at you in order to protest
- To refuse to pay attention to you and the skill you are trying to entice him to do
- To make no attempt to do the skill
- To abandon the task prematurely
- To make a minimal attempt and not his best attempt
- To charm you to divert your attention by smiling, clapping, dancing, or playing gesture games

You will notice the avoidance routines most when you are challenging your child with learning new skills. When you see these reactions, you can decide how to respond to them. By understanding his intent in using these avoidance routines, you can come up with a new plan when you practice the skill again.

***Children with Down syndrome need to learn to consolidate skills.*** According to Jennifer Wishart (1991):

> *"New skills, even once mastered, proved to be inadequately consolidated, often disappearing from the infant's repertoire in subsequent months."*

When teaching a new skill, you will need to provide a structured approach to help your child organize what he needs to learn. By practicing with a specific setup, in a consistent way, he will learn the new game. With each practice, he will become familiar with the beginning, middle, and end of the activity. Once the routine is familiar, he will feel in control and know what to anticipate, and this will make him happy. To keep him focused on the skill, you need to limit distractions, so it is best to do it in a familiar environment by yourselves. When he is learning the new skill, he will learn best if his full attention is directed toward it.

With repetition and practice through his home program, he will learn to consolidate the skill into his repertoire. After he learns the skill, you can set him up to practice in a variety of settings. When he consistently initiates the skill, then you will know that he has consolidated it.

***Follow your child's lead and practice what he is motivated to do.*** He will do his best if the skill is valuable and functional for him. Try to understand how your child is thinking. When you notice that he likes to do certain skills, then build new skills from those skills. For example, if he likes being on his belly and can reach, teach him the progression of skills beginning with pivoting, then combat crawling, then climbing. If he is motivated to sit and is able to sit independently, then teach him how to move into sitting. Children with Down syndrome often are motivated to learn skills in a different order, so practice what he is ready and willing to learn.

If he resists a new skill you are introducing, stop the activity and plan a new strategy for a future practice. If you impose, he will only learn to resist you and the activity more. The more you practice it against his resistance, the more you set him up to be an avoidant learner. This will damage your collaborative learning partnership.

***Set your child up to succeed.*** Each new skill is a challenge for him. To help him be successful, it is important to follow these steps:

1. Only practice ***what*** he is ready to learn.
2. Practice ***when*** he is at his physical best so he has the strength, concentration, and patience to perform at his best.
3. Use the ***best*** motivators.
4. Know ***when to quit*** by being attentive to his cues.

It is counterproductive to practice new skills if he is tired, hungry, or not interested. He will become frustrated and quit. He may remember the unpleasant experience or failure and avoid the skill the next time.

***Understand your child's temperament and teach new skills based on how he reacts to learning new skills.*** Temperament is defined as a person's characteristic manner of thinking, behaving, and reacting. My definition for our purposes in this context is: the child's way of thinking, behaving, and reacting when learning ***new*** gross motor skills. It is my observation that children with Down syndrome fall into two main categories, the ***observer*** type and the ***motor-driven*** type.

You will be able to distinguish which temperament your child has by observing whether he tends to be careful (observer) or risky (motor-driven) when learning new skills. Is he cautious with new movements or does he like being moved? Does he want to practice new skills for a couple of repetitions or does he like doing many repetitions? Does he fatigue after practicing a couple of new skills and become overwhelmed, or can he do many without any reaction? Does he do better in a quiet environment or tolerate a stimulating environment? Is he detail-oriented and attentive, or does he just move and make adjustments when needed? You

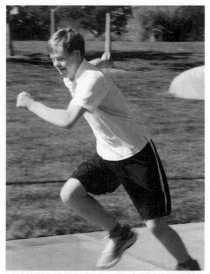
(fig. 0.3)

can begin to observe these behaviors when your child is six months or older (after he is able to roll and when he is working on sitting). You will continue to notice them when he is practicing new post-walking skills. Once he masters

## Motor-Driven v. Observers

**Children Who Are Motor-Driven:**
1. tolerate new positions and movements and take risks
2. want to move from one place to another and spend limited time in one position
3. prefer to be moving and exploring rather than being held
4. love to move fast
5. like gross motor skills such as rolling, crawling, creeping, moving in and out of positions, climbing, pulling to stand, and walking
6. resist stationary positions such as sitting, kneeling, and standing

**Children Who Are Observers:**
1. are cautious, careful, and easily frightened by new movements and positions, and want to be in control
2. like to stay in one position and are content to watch, socialize, and play with toys that are available; they need to have a reason to move
3. love to be held and tolerate it for long periods of time
4. prefer to move at a slower speed so they can feel balanced and in control
5. like to learn gross motor skills such as sitting, kneeling, and standing
6. initially may resist crawling, creeping, moving in and out of positions, and walking

the post-walking skills and is confident in his performance, these tendencies will be less noticeable.

After children learn to combat crawl or creep, parents often think all children now have the motor-driven temperament. However, if your child has the observer type of temperament, when he is ready to learn to take independent steps, you will see his carefulness reemerge. He will prefer support to walk, and he may be upset when he falls. He will be cautious and only take steps after he can balance in standing. The child who is motor-driven will take risks to take independent steps and will not be upset if he falls.

By understanding your child's temperament and his behavior when learning new skills, you can better plan how to set him up to be successful. Knowing this will give you insights into what skills are easier or harder, how to provide support, how to pace him when practicing the skills, and how to motivate him. You can begin with new skills that he will like and then alternate with a more challenging new skill using the best motivator.

### Learning in the Area of Gross Motor Skills

The guidelines discussed in this section have been described in the literature or are from my clinical experience practicing gross motor skills with children with Down syndrome. By paying attention to these areas, you will better understand the learning style of your child—specifically, his learning style when learning *new* gross motor skills.

*Anticipate this four-step learning process when teaching your child new gross motor skills.* To learn each skill, he will need to go through a gradual, step-by-step, systematic process. Apply this process to *new* gross motor skills that he is ready to learn and treat each skill as a new game to play together. *If you gradually introduce the movements for the new gross motor skill, he will learn it.*

1. *Introduce the new skill slowly and carefully*, focusing on having your child feel it and tolerate the movement. In this step, he will experience the extent of the skill and learn the beginning, middle, and end.
2. *Allow the new skill to become familiar with practice,* until you see that he understands the game, is accustomed to it, and anticipates it.
3. *Encourage him to collaborate and participate with executing the skill.* Practice together so he builds strength and learns how to do the skill, and decrease your support as tolerated.
4. *Build mastery of the skill and independence* so he can do it on his own. Once he can do it, look for him to own it and use it spontaneously. When he self-initiates it, then you know that he

has consolidated the skill and it is in his repertoire. In this step, you will generalize the skill to a variety of settings.

During this four-step process, you need to pay attention to ***how you support*** your child and the ***quality of the movements*** he uses while learning to do the skill.

***Provide support strategically.*** Your child needs to actively participate in the skill to learn it. If he is fully supported and is passive when practicing a skill, he will "go for the ride" but will not learn the skill. In each step you will provide a different level of support. In step 1, you will provide full support so he can relax, feel, and tolerate the movement. When he is familiar with the skill, you will lessen your support in step 2 so he is alert and participating. In step 3, you will progress to providing the least support possible to specific points of his body so he does more and more of the skill. In step 4, you will provide intermittent support so he is successful, until he can do the skill consistently by himself.

During this four-step process, you will give support to teach the skill, but decrease your support as soon as possible. Children with Down syndrome tend to quickly become dependent on support; if you give too much, they will take it, expect it, and depend on it. When you provide support, you will need to know what the most strategic support is for his body and that skill, place him in that position, and *wait* for his action. When you set your child up using this method of strategic support, the setup will also provoke the action you want him to do.

Providing strategic support will give your child the opportunity to do what he wants to do and is ready to learn, but cannot do on his own, due to his physical problems. This book will explain how to provide the support your child needs so that he is successful, and then he will be motivated to do it again. Through repetition of these movements, he will begin to develop strength so that he requires less support. Eventually, he will be able to do the skill with no support at all.

***He will learn skills grossly at first, and later he will refine them.*** In steps 1 and 2, you want him to fully experience the gross movement of each skill, so you will not worry about the quality of the movement. In steps 3 and 4, you will look at the quality of the movements and shape them if needed so he will be successful. For example, you will teach him to move out of sitting onto his belly by *falling* over one side. After he learns this gross movement, he will practice it and learn to do it with control. When your child first learns to do a skill, he will use compensations, due to the stress of learning the new activity and learning how to do it with his unique physical make-up. When he is motivated to do the skill, the practices will help him gain proficiency in doing the motions more smoothly and with control. When the skill is established and is in his repertoire, you can help him refine it, if needed.

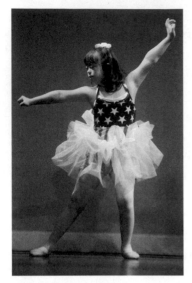

(fig. 0.4)

If you nag your child by providing too much intervention or correction while he is learning a skill, he either will become passive, depending on your support, or he will lose interest in the skill. For example, when he is learning to walk, if you support him to walk perfectly, he will resist the support and the activity, and lift his legs to move to the floor to creep where he wants to go. There are two skills that are exceptions to this guideline of learning the skills grossly and later refining them: 1) learning to sit, and 2) learning to stand. For sitting and standing, you need to teach the optimal postures from the beginning (see Stage 3).

*Teach your child using bite-size pieces, by breaking down the skills into smaller parts.* When you practice each new skill, you need to teach your child each part and then show him how to put the pieces together. For example, consider the skill of moving into sitting by himself. First, he will need to learn to push up with his arms from lying on his side. Second, he will need to learn to weight shift his pelvis over one side, and he can practice this part by moving from kneeling to sitting. Once he has learned these parts, you will practice both parts by moving to sit from his stomach or hands and knees. As you practice the parts, you need to watch his participation and reactions. The focus is to facilitate learning the new skill, so if he is being passive or avoiding it, try another strategy or motivator. *If it seems like your child is not making progress, or is at a plateau, it means he needs the skill broken down further or a new way to practice.* The challenge is to keep creating new ways to practice the skill to elicit his participation and success. Keep innovating new approaches until you *find the way in.* Sometimes, it may seem as if your child is not strong enough to do a skill, when in fact, he has the strength but does not know how to use his strength for that skill.

*Wait for your child to respond when learning a new skill, due to a delayed or slow reaction time.* Reaction time is the interval from the onset of a stimulus to the initiation of the movement response. Children with Down syndrome take more time to initiate a response to a stimulus (Anson, 1992), meaning they have a longer reaction time. They also take more time to complete a motor task, giving them a longer movement time (Latash, 1992). Because of the longer reaction time, when your child is learning a new skill, you will need to set him up with strategic support and then wait 5 to 10 seconds to give him time to respond. Giving him sufficient time to respond is critical. If you do not wait long enough, you prevent him from participating and teach him to depend on your support rather than to initiate the movement. Since it takes him longer to respond, you and his therapist may think he cannot do the skill, when, in fact, he could, if just given enough time.

*Your child will have difficulty generalizing a new skill to different settings, so keep this in mind when practicing gross motor skills.* When your child is learning a new skill, it is best to teach the skill in the specific setting where he will use it on his own. For example, if you want him to learn to move out of sitting to his stomach, practice with him sitting on the carpet. To master the skill, he will need to learn to self-initiate the motion of weight shifting to one side and landing on his stomach. By practicing on this surface, he will also learn to do it with control.

Once he learns a new skill, he needs to practice the skill in each new setting. For example, if he learns to walk up and down your stairs at home, he will need to practice on the stairs at school to develop proficiency on them. Each setting will have different details to adjust to, and he will need time and practice and to figure out new methods for each setting. If you understand and anticipate this, you can provide the strategic support he needs to be successful.

*Children with Down syndrome have patterns of muscle activation characterized by higher levels of* **co-contraction** *(Latash, 2000).* Co-contraction is the simultaneous activation of muscle pairs acting at a joint in opposite directions. By activating his muscles in this way, your child stiffens the joint and then cannot move it in either direction. I have observed this particularly when a child is learning a new skill or when stressed. For example, he may do this when he is learning the alternating leg pedaling movement on a tricycle. He will stiffen one or both legs, with co-contraction of the muscles of his knee(s), and then his knee(s) will become "stuck" in that position, and he will not be able to pedal.

*Your child will learn best if given visual and tactile cues.* Many children with Down syndrome are visual learners, so seeing a skill or having a model to watch can motivate them to imitate the skill. They are also responsive to tactile cueing. If they feel it, they will imitate it. For example, if you practice running with hand support, your child will feel the speed of running and the way his body moves, and then he will try to do it on his own. When giving tactile cues, you want to exaggerate the movements to engage his attention and make sure he feels it. If you give subtle tactile cues, he will not be aware of what you are trying to teach him. It is generally more difficult for children with Down syndrome to process verbal instructions, so if you give them, make sure they are brief and to the point.

*Progress to the next skill at the right time or else the current skill will become so automatic that he may be unwilling to do the new skill.* When your child is able to use rolling to move where he wants to go, he may not be interested in learning to pivot sideways to toys, or later to combat crawl. By knowing the progression of gross motor skills, you can be proactive in teaching the next one in a timely way. If you delay teaching the next skill, your child will resist you more because he is so efficient with the current skill. This is particularly important when your child is ready to learn to walk. If you do not teach him the stepping pattern at the right time, he may prefer to crawl or creep to get around. This is also true of progressing him from walking with two-hand support to one-hand support. You need to know what the next skill is and when to teach it, and then figure out a way to interest him in learning the new skill.

*When practicing new skills, be* **strategic** *in how you set up his body and the equipment you use so he is successful.* You want to find what makes the new skill easiest to learn. When teaching a skill, always practice over both sides to test which way is easier. For example, if he can roll better over the right side, let him learn to roll this way until he is successful and can consistently roll where he wants to go. It will be confusing for him to practice rolling both directions when he is just beginning to learn to roll. Let him master the easier direction and then move on to the other.

Also experiment with equipment and furniture and figure out what works best for your child for that new skill. Check whether the skill is easier with a higher or lower surface. If the surface is lower, he may be able to pull to kneel or cruise better. If the surface has an edge, he may be able to pull to stand. If you are teaching him to combat crawl, it may be easier to use a slippery surface and dress him in a onesie. The easier you can make the skill, with the least amount of support, the more willing he will be to do it, and then he will assimilate it into his repertoire. (These types of tips will be provided in later chapters with each skill.)

*Be attentive to how many repetitions your child will do when practicing each new skill.* How many is he comfortable doing? Also notice whether he learns skills better if he focuses on two or three skills and repeats them several times a day, or if he prefers to do many skills for a few repetitions each. If you notice these details and adapt how you practice the new skills, his cooperation will improve, and he will be open to practicing the new skills. Ultimately, the repetitions will improve his performance by increasing his strength, speed, coordination, accuracy, and his timing and sequencing of movements.

*Practice as* **long** *as your child is performing at his best. The* **quality** *of time practiced is more important than the quantity.* Watch how long your child will practice new skills with you. If you know he will practice for 5 minutes, you will plan differently than if you know you have 15 minutes. You need to work within his timeframe. It is better to stop early than to go one minute or one repetition too many. If your child understands the new skill and is practicing it well, you can continue. When he starts to lose interest,

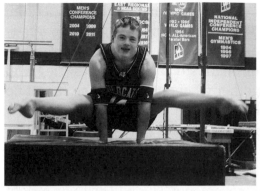

(fig. 0.5)

move on to another skill. If given a break, he may want to do it again later. You want to end the practice with a happy and successful experience, not with him upset or overtired.

*When practicing new motor skills, sequence the practice time strategically.* Practicing a new skill takes more effort and concentration, so he will fatigue faster. He will do best if you plan out what you are going to practice and start with the harder skill first. Then you can alternate with practicing an easier skill so he recovers. In between practicing skills, give him a play break, and then he will be ready to practice again. When he is tired or disinterested in a skill, stop. Watch the pace of the practice time and customize it to him, with a combination of hard and easy skills and breaks. Then decide what to repeat with new motivators.

*Do not interfere with a skill that your child has learned to do independently.* If you interfere, your child will be mad and will become aggravated with how you are interfering with his movements. You will not succeed in introducing change in his movements during this skill, but you can practice desired movements in higher level skills. For example, if your child creeps on both hands, one knee, and one foot, he will be upset if you follow him around and help him practice moving on both knees. It is better to wait until he is learning to climb up stairs and then you can practice moving on both knees during that skill.

*When learning new skills, the fewer steps the better.* If there is any way to lessen the steps when learning a new skill, your child will be more attentive. For example, if he is ready to learn to move to stand from kneeling, he needs an easy way to see that he can move from one position to the other. You can set him up kneeling at a low surface, and then lean his trunk over the surface so he pops up to standing. Once he knows the connection between the positions, he will experiment with how to move to standing and later will learn the more advanced methods.

*Provide only as much hands-on support as your child needs.* Some children are distracted by too much handling, or resist it because they feel like you are controlling them. When your child is in Steps 3 and 4 of the learning process, you want your handling to be minimal, intermittent, timely, and given precisely where it is needed for your child to be successful.

*Look for variety in your child's movements, and a balance between opposite movement patterns.* You can help your child use the movement components you want him to learn. When he is moving on his own, let him move the way he chooses. You want him to learn to spontaneously use a variety of movements, and alternate between opposite movements. For example, if he moves his legs wide apart when lying on his stomach or when sitting, you would also like him to move his legs together when kneeling. If he can sit up tall, it is acceptable if he also slouches at times.

*Practice the gross motor skills yourself so you really understand and feel the movements and steps involved in doing them.* When you do the skill, you see how your body wants to do it. To understand it from your child's perspective, observe his body and imitate his movements. This will give you insight into what he needs to do to learn the skill. If he is having difficulty, do it the way that he tries to do it and see what is blocking him from mastering the skill.

You can also study his body parts and proportions and see if some skills are harder due to his physical make-up. For example, if his trunk is very long, it will probably take him longer to learn to sit independently due to the strength needed to hold his long trunk up straight. Or, if your child has significant ligamentous laxity in his hips, knees, and feet, learning to stand will be more difficult. By observing your child's unique body, you will understand how it affects his development of certain gross motor skills, and you can customize how you practice the skills so he is successful.

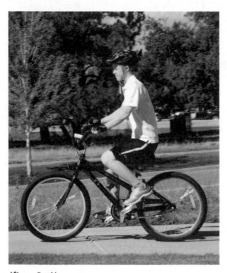

(fig. 0.6)

*Individualize.* As you practice the new gross motor skills that your child is ready to learn, be sure to use strategies based on his learning style to guide *how* you teach and *what* you teach. Focus on *"finding the way in"* to teach the new skill. If you can *introduce it* so that he understands what to do, then he can figure out how to do it with his physical make-up. You will give him ideas for strategies, but he will need to *find his own way* to do it. The hardest part for him will be the beginning, when he tries to initiate the beginning movements of the skill on his own. However, once he starts, is successful, and then repeats the movements, he will be on his way. If you can teach him a method that matches his movement patterns, rather than making him conform to the "typical way," you will be more effective in guiding him to find the best method for his body. You will have your way to teach, and you will need to watch his way of practicing, and then you both will collaborate to help him *find his way* to do it. *If you can find the right way in, he will do it.* Once he can initiate the beginning movements, he will work at it until he can do it consistently. As he is working on it, you will provide intermittent and timely strategic support so he is successful. If you can be partners in this way, you will both enjoy the experience of learning gross motor skills together.

# Timing: Critical Times for Physical Therapy Intervention

This book covers two periods of gross motor development: ***Birth to Walking*** (Part 1) and ***Post Walking*** (Part 2). Physical therapy services are critical during both of these periods to develop the essential movement components and the postural foundation needed to build a body that is fit and functional throughout his life.

As your child learns a particular skill, you will not only focus on the skill itself but also the movement components that make up that skill. You will need to ensure the development of those specific movement components. They will not happen automatically as a result of achieving the gross motor skill. As you read the ***Tendencies*** sections for the gross motor skills, you will get an idea of what will automatically happen. The ***Components*** sections will tell you what you want to teach. When you know what components to develop as you practice each skill, you can anticipate the tendencies (compensations) and develop the components needed to learn the skill properly.

In the ***birth to walking period***, you will focus on teaching your child the following movement components and building strength in them:

- Head: to lift and hold his head erect and in the midline
- Trunk: to hold his trunk up straight and be able to activate his abdominal muscles, so his back and abdominal muscles are evenly balanced
- Arms: to prop, reach, pull, hold on, and push
- Legs: to position his knees and feet pointing straight ahead (neutral hip rotation), feet in line with hips (narrow base), and use mild knee bending (unlocked knees) when standing.
- Weight shifting skills: to roll, reach (when lying on belly), move into and out of sitting, combat crawl (belly on the floor) and creep (on hands and knees), pull to stand, cruise, and walk.

In the ***post-walking period***, the primary focus is on refining your child's walking pattern. This will be accomplished by practicing the nine post-walking skills and by using effective foot management. He will develop an efficient walking pattern and be independent and proficient with walking for long distances in the community, walking on uneven surfaces, and walking up and down inclines, curbs, and stairs. He will also learn gross motor skills, including kicking a ball, running, jumping, riding a tricycle, and balance beam skills.

By the end of the post-walking period, your child will be on the path to achieve the goal of physical therapy and the four critical results. Not only will he have learned to walk with a refined and efficient pattern, he will have also developed the posture and movement components that he will need as an adolescent and adult. With this strong foundation, he will be able to choose his areas of interest to continue improving strength, coordination, speed, endurance, and balance.

## Progressing through the Book

Each chapter in *Part 1* addresses one of the five stages of development in the birth to walking period. Each *stage* consists of a cluster of *skills* that tend to develop at about the same time. Certain skills are prerequisites for the development of skills in the next stage. Skills build on top of one another—what you develop in one skill gives essential components for the next skill. Many skills also develop the strength needed to do the next level gross motor skill.

You will learn to recognize the signs of readiness, and know what prerequisite movements are needed. It is not helpful to teach your child skills that are too advanced. *When your child learns a skill* will depend on a number of factors coming together. He will need to be physically ready, be familiar with how to do the skill, and persevere to figure out how he can do the skill. He will need to have the necessary strength, stamina, motor planning, coordination, motivation, and temperament.

In general, you should complete most of the skills in one stage before moving on to the next stage. However, if your child has achieved the goals of the stage in one position, then you can move on to the next stage to work on the next goal for that position. For example, if your child is progressing well with skills on his belly and can pivot on his belly easily (goal for Stage 3), then you can begin practicing the next goal for that position in Stage 4, which is combat crawling.

*Part 2* describes the gross motor skills to learn after your child walks, and you will practice all nine of these skills simultaneously. Chapter 6 provides an overview of the post-walking period of development and will give you detailed guidelines for helping your child develop post-walking skills. Foot management strategies will also be covered.

# How the Chapters are Organized

For each *skill,* I will discuss:

- the *skill:* the qualitative criteria, for example, pivoting in stom-ach-lying means to use the arms to pull the body sideways to move to a toy
- the *goal:* what the child must achieve to accomplish the skill; for example, the goal of pivoting in stomach-lying is to pivot in a full circle, in each direction
- the *components:* the specific movements you want your child to develop when doing the skill
- the *tendencies:* the alternate or compensatory patterns that children with Down syndrome are prone to develop
- *how to teach* the skill *(Setup for Learning)*
- *guidelines* specific for each stage and skill: tips for how to practice
- *temperament:* how the observer and motor-driven child tend to behave and react when learning that particular skill
- *step-by-step instructions* and *home program activities* for practicing each skill

Your child will learn gross motor skills best through daily practice and doing the skills for many repetitions throughout the day. This is the best way to build strength and familiarity with how to do the skill. *Parents and siblings play a crucial role in implementation of the home program.* Rather than thinking about it as extra work, or worrying that you need to plan exercise times, think about it as it as *being creative* with your play times together. If you and his siblings practice the skills with him in a fun, motivating way, then he will see them as games to play with you.

You will need to know what skills to focus on and how to practice them. Your physical therapist will help you with this. During the session with the physical therapist, the PT will:

1. figure out what your child is ready to learn
2. test how to practice the skill based on your child's physical make-up, how he prefers to move, his learning style, and developmental trends of children with Down syndrome
3. determine the best strategy and setup to practice the skill, and then practice for a few repetitions so your child is familiar with the "game"
4. teach you how to practice the skill, and have you do it until you are comfortable with carrying it out at home
5. make a home program for your child and prioritize the home program activities

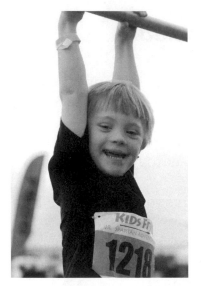

(fig. 0.7)

Once you have the home program, you can figure out how to do it in a way that works with your lifestyle and your child's schedule. Use your time effectively and practice the skills that require your support. When possible, build the activities into your daily routine. For example, after changing your child's diaper, have him hold your fingers and practice pulling up to sit before you pick him up. Through practicing the home program activities, you will have fun together while teaching him new gross motor games. Your time together will help you understand how your child learns and how to read his cues. This opportunity will benefit all future learning experiences.

At the end of each chapter, there is a ***checklist*** so you can keep track of the progress your child is making, and what steps are next. The book covers the major gross motor milestones and all of the details in between. If you know the major milestones and the intermediate steps, you can track each detail of your child's progress, will know what to focus on, and will see the progress he is making.

In both Parts 1 and 2, you will notice that masculine and feminine pronouns are used alternately by chapter when referring to children with Down syndrome. That is, I used "he" and "his" in the even-numbered chapters, and "she" and "her" in the old-numbered chapters. The only exceptions occur when I am referring to real children with Down syndrome I have known. In these instances, I used their actual names and genders.

# PART ONE:
## Infancy through Walking

# 1

# Stage 1:
# Head, Hands, and Legs
# in Midline

## Introduction

These first few months of your baby's life are the time for you to get to know each other. She will spend many hours out of the day eating and sleeping, so your free time together while your child is awake will be limited and therefore precious. In this stage, while you are holding your baby, you can give support in a strategic way to help organize her movements and then she can better pay attention, interact, and relate with you and toys. If she does not have this type of support, her movements will be more random and will distract her attention and she will not be able to focus her energy on you or on touching toys. When provided with the right support, your child will show you what she is interested in doing, like batting at a toy in side-lying or bringing her hand to her mouth.

The joy of this stage is discovering what your child can do and what she is interested in doing if she is given the right support. For example, in the section on back-lying, you will learn the best way to support her when you are holding her so that her body is calm and organized and then she can focus all of her attention on your face and respond to you with her eyes and mouth.

She will learn to look at you when you talk to her. Her eyes will brighten and she will smile or make faces in response to yours. She will engage with you and then look away. This is her way of saying: "I've had enough for now. I need a break." After a break of a few minutes you can talk to her to get her attention again or she may look at you to get your attention. You will learn to read her messages: "I'm tired"; "I'm hungry"; "I'm tuned in and ready to go"; or "I've dropped out." When she is tuned in, talk to her and play with her.

When she is tired, hungry, or tuned out, give her what she needs and hold her with the support she needs.

## Motor Skills and Components

The motor skills and components to focus on in this first stage of development are:

1. head control with her head in the center (looking straight ahead, not turned to either side), tucking her chin, and neck strength to begin lifting her head
2. moving her arms and hands to midline and beginning propping on elbows
3. moving her legs together to the midline

Your child will learn these skills using the positions of side-lying, back-lying, supported sitting, stomach-lying, supported kneeling, and rolling from side-lying to stomach.

## Tendencies

During this stage, the tendencies are:

1. to arch her head and trunk and pull her arms back (pinching shoulder blades together)
2. to turn her head to one side and keep it there
3. to keep her arms inactive because her legs are stronger and so active
4. to hold her legs in the "frog leg" position, with hips and knees bent and knees turned out

By providing strategic support, you will help your child learn head control and use of her arms while supporting and calming down the leg movements.

This chapter is organized differently than the other chapters in the book. While the other chapters provide instruction proceeding from one skill to the next, this chapter is easier to understand if we proceed from position to position. The easier positions are side-lying and back-lying, and you will start with these positions. When your child is ready, you can add supported sitting. Stomach-lying will be the hardest, and it may be easier for your child to start with supported kneeling. When moving from back to stomach, your child can assist by practicing rolling with your support.

## Guidelines

*Use only the positions your baby is ready to use.* She will initially tolerate the positions briefly, but her tolerance will improve as she understands what to do and gets stronger in each position. When she is tired and fussy, hold her and calm her down. Try to stop practicing before she is overtired.

***Watch to see when she is comfortable in a position and when she wants to move out of it.*** When she is finished with one position, move her to another.

***Alternate harder positions, such as supported sitting and stomach-lying, with easier positions, such as side-lying and back-lying.*** If she is feeling strong, you can start with harder positions and then she can recover using the easier position.

***Your baby will have alert and active periods for 20-30 minutes.*** The time you have to practice skills with her will be limited, so do the most important activities first. She will probably practice a position for five minutes and then want to change. After an active exercise period, she may become hungry or sleepy.

***When carrying or holding her, support her legs together.*** Then she will learn to move her legs with her knees in line with her hips rather than wide apart.

***For the first couple of months, your baby will be most interested in seeing your face.*** Over time, she will become interested in brightly colored toys and musical toys. At first, she will prefer toys that have contrasting colors like black and white and toys that have faces.

# Side-lying

Side-lying is an easy position for your child to use and she will be calm and organized with your support. She can look at you or at toys, maintain her focus, and initiate moving her arm to reach or bat at your face or a toy in front of her. It is the easiest position for your baby because her head is looking straight ahead, her hands are together and she can see them, and her legs are together. Gravity assists the position of her head, arms, and legs.

## Components

When your baby is on her side, the components to focus on are:
1. head in midline and tucking her chin
2. hands in the midline, moving them to her mouth or chest, or reaching toward toys and batting at them
3. legs together and calmed down with hips and knees bent

## Tendencies

The tendencies are:
1. to arch (stiffening and straightening) her head, trunk, and legs, throwing her head back, and then she will not be able to use controlled movements of her head and arms
2. to need support to maintain the side-lying position because she will arch or roll to her back

## Setup for Learning

To prevent the arch, you will need to maximally support her top knee against her abdomen with one hand and your other hand will be on her back or buttocks, to pat it and calm her in the position. With this support, she will be ready to look at toys placed in front of her shoulder. She will tuck her chin to gaze downward at the toy and focus on it. When she is ready, she will reach out and touch the toy and will initiate the movements for many repetitions. She may also bring her hand to her mouth. She will choose what she wants to do, either being active with her arms or looking at a toy. While in this position, her legs will be supported to minimize movements so that she can focus on using her arms (see fig. 1.1).

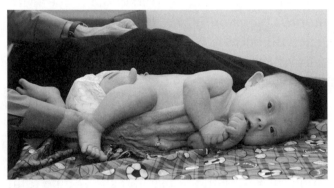

(fig. 1.1)

This position can only be used for a few months. In the beginning, your child will need maximal support to move to the position, and to use head control and activate her arms. Later, she will roll to her side by herself and play. Once your baby is able to roll, she will not use side-lying anymore. It is a good position for her during this stage and should be used as much as possible.

## Guidelines

*Motivate your baby by using toys that she can touch or watch.* They need to be large and stationary so they will not roll away. You don't want the toy to roll away when your baby touches it. Use toys that have bright colors and make sounds. Ideal toys include stuffed animals (Big Bird, Dalmatian puppy), fabric dolls or clowns with faces, rocking toys that have lights and make sounds (Happy Apple, Mickey Mouse, Fisher Price Sparkling Elephant), and musical toys (ring stack).

*Support her to prevent arching her head and trunk.* If this happens, bend her hip and knee and hold her knee against her abdomen. You can also give her more support by placing your leg behind her head and trunk. Make sure the toy is placed in front of her shoulders so her head is tilted down slightly. If the toy is placed above her head, she will automatically arch her neck to look upward at it.

## ACTIVITY #1: Supported Side-lying on the Floor

1. Place your child on her side and use one hand to hold her top knee against her abdomen.
2. Place your other hand on her back or buttocks and pat her to calm her.
3. If she needs more support, place your leg behind her head and trunk, if this support makes her feel more stable.
4. Place a toy at the level of her shoulder and she will tuck her chin to look down at it.
5. Watch to see what she wants to do—look at the toy or bat at it, or bring her hand to her mouth.
6. Repeat on her other side.

## ACTIVITY #2: Supported Side-lying on the Couch

1. Place your child in side-lying on the couch with her back against the back of the couch. Make sure her head and trunk are in a straight line and her hips and knees are bent.
2. Position yourself on the floor in front of her.
3. Hold her hips to support her in the position and keep her from rolling. If her legs are active, hold them to calm them down. This will enable her to move her arms more easily.
4. Place a toy at shoulder level in front of her hands. See if she will move her hand to the toy. If not, give a physical cue by holding her hand and touching the toy. Change the toy as needed to keep her interest.
5. Use the position as long as tolerated. Repeat by placing her on her other side.
6. If she becomes fussy, rock her hips gently and see if this calms her down.

# Back-lying

Children tend to prefer this position because they can socialize, watch people and toys, and play. When your infant is lying on her back, she is in the best position for face-to-face interaction with you. Your face can be close to hers and she can look at you and see you smile and talk to her. She will engage with you by looking at you and may make cooing sounds. She will probably give you her first smile while in this position.

## Components

When your baby is on her back, the components that you want her to develop are:

1. head in midline and tucking her chin
2. hands to her chest (midline) and beginning reaching to toys
3. legs supported together with hips and knees bent, feet on the floor, and knees together; also kicking movements

These movements will take time to develop and you will need to support her fully in the beginning. If she is supported in the right way, she can focus her attention on you and respond to you.

## Tendencies

Her tendencies will be:

1. to turn her head to one side and maintain her head there
2. to rest her arms on the surface and infrequently move them to the midline
3. to activate her legs since they are the strongest part; this will prevent arm movements because the young infant cannot move arms and legs at the same time
4. to position her legs in the "frog leg" posture (hips and knees bent and knees wide apart) when at rest, and to develop muscle tightness if she habitually uses this posture.
5. to use the arching pattern in the head, arms, and trunk, which inhibits chin tuck and moving the hands to the midline

If your baby is not supported, her head will be turned to one side, her arms and hands will rest on the surface, and her legs will be positioned with her hips and knees bent and her knees wide apart or she will do kicking movements. With the activity of her legs, she will not have the strength to move her head to the center to look at you or to lift her arms so she can bring her hands to her mouth and chest. With the tendency of arching, she will pinch her shoulder blades together and her upper chest will puff up and this will prevent chin tuck and moving her arms to the midline. She may also learn to stabilize her arms against the surface to be able to kick her legs more.

### Setup for Learning

The first position to try is laying your baby in your lap. If you support her head in the midline, her elbows higher than her shoulders (side view), and calm her legs, she will be able to focus on your face and bend her elbows to move her hands to her mouth or together in the midline (see fig. 1.2).

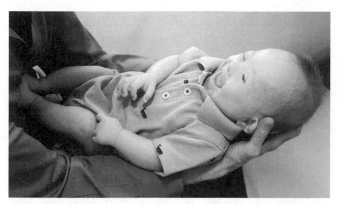

(fig. 1.2)

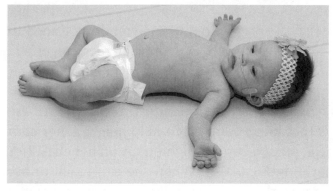

(fig. 1.3)

When she is familiar with holding her head in the center and moving her arms easily while lying in your lap, you can begin placing her on the floor with support. When she is placed on the floor, the best way to support her head and arms in the center is to use a "blanket roll." (See Activity #4 for instructions on how to make a blanket roll.) The blanket rolls (at head and shoulders) will minimize the arching pattern. If she still arches, you can gently place your hand above her breast bone and press down and toward her feet. This will lessen the arching and allow her to tuck her chin. You will need to support her legs together to calm them so she can practice head control and arm movements. She can move her legs while they are in between your legs and will strengthen the muscles that will move her legs toward neutral rotation and adduction (see definitions, below).

Your baby probably will have resistance to moving her knees together with hips and knees bent due to the habit of resting her legs in the "frog leg" posture (fig. 1.3). Hip mobility will need to be increased so she can move her hips to neutral rotation. Gentle stretching of the hips is recommended toward 5-10 degrees of internal rotation.

As your baby's head, arms, and legs become stronger with the desired movement components, support can be taken away. She will learn to hold her head in

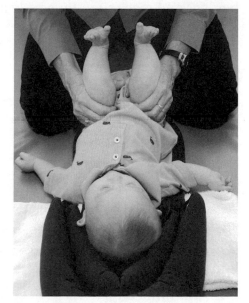

(fig. 1.4)

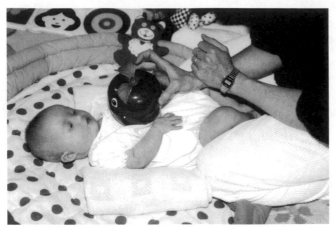

(fig. 1.5)

the center and then you can stop using the blanket roll at her head. When she is able to bring her hands to her chest and touch toys, and can do this for several repetitions, you can stop using the blanket roll under her arms (fig. 1.5). When she has gained head control and reaches often with her arms, you do not need to support her legs together.

## Guidelines

*Motivate your baby by using toys that she can interact with.* Use brightly colored toys and toys that make sounds. To help her tuck her chin and move her hands to her chest, place a large, weighted toy on her chest (for example, the Fisher Price Sparkling Elephant). When she can reach to her chest, you can hold a lightweight rattle above her hand/shoulder or suspend it from a play gym (so that it is almost touching her shoulder) and have her move her arm and hit it.

*If your baby's legs are active, hold them to calm them down.* You could also swaddle her legs together in a blanket. She will not be able to kick her legs and reach simultaneously at this stage.

---

### Definitions

- **Midline:** center or middle of the body
- **External rotation of hips:** turn the thigh bone outward from the midline (middle of the body)
- **Internal rotation of hips:** turn the thigh bone inward toward the midline (middle of the body)
- **Neutral rotation of hips:** turn the thigh bone so the knee is centered in the midline, for example, pointing up to the ceiling if the child is lying on her back
- **Hip adduction:** move the thigh inward toward the center of the body
- **Hip abduction:** move the thigh outward, away from the center of the body

## ACTIVITY #3: Back-lying in Your Lap (fig. 1.6)

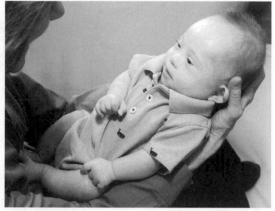

1. Place your baby in your lap as you sit on the couch or other comfortable chair with back support.
2. Place her with her head between your knees, her hips against your abdomen, and her legs supported against your chest.
3. Slide your hands along the sides of her body and under her arms until they

(fig. 1.6)

   are under her head. Hold her head in the center and tilt it upward so she sees you easily.
4. With this arm support, she will be able to bend her elbows and bring her hands to her chest or mouth.
5. Use your elbows to support her legs so that her knees are in line with her hips and not in a wide position.
6. Lean your head and trunk forward so that you can be close to her and you can see each other. Talk or sing to her and engage with her for as long as tolerated.

## ACTIVITY #4: Back-lying on the Floor (fig. 1.7 & fig. 1.8)

1. Make a blanket roll with a bath towel or a baby blanket. Fold it along its length so that it is 6-8 inches (15-20 cm) wide. Now roll each end toward the center until there is just enough space between the two rolled-up ends for your baby to lie in. Turn the blanket roll over so that the ends don't unroll and place it on the floor.
2. Place your baby on her back between the rolled-up ends of the blanket roll so that it is under her head and shoulders. The bottom edge of the blanket roll should be even with your baby's elbows. Your baby may need two blanket rolls, one under her head and one under her shoulders/elbows. You could also use an infant head support with an inner layer of padding for full head support in the midline.
3. Sit on your heels in front of her and use your thighs to support her legs with her knees in line with her hips. Use your legs as a boundary for her legs to move within.

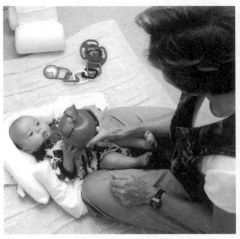

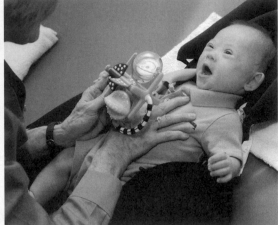

(fig. 1.7)                          (fig. 1.8)

4. With this support, lean your head and trunk forward and talk to her.
5. Place a toy on her chest and encourage her to look downward at the toy and bring her hands up to touch the toy. If needed, support her chest above her breastbone to allow her to tuck her chin.

## ACTIVITY #5: Back-lying on the Floor with a Play Gym over Her Chest

1. Place your child on the floor and place blanket rolls under her head and shoulders. Place her head in the center. (When she can maintain her head in the midline, then just use the arm roll.)
2. Place the play gym above her chest and add links/rings to the toys on the play gym so they dangle just above her shoulder or hand.
3. She will move her arms and hit the toys and will learn how to engage with them by hitting them.
4. When she is able to hit the toys repeatedly, eliminate the arm blanket roll.

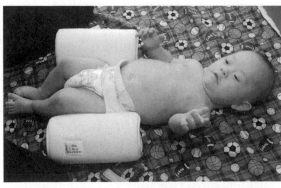

(fig. 1.9)

5. Watch her leg position and support her legs together if the leg activity inhibits her reaching. If she can reach well, does not need her legs calmed down, and holds her legs apart, you can support her legs together using a blanket roll or leg support (fig. 1.9). You can also swaddle her legs together with a blanket.

## ACTIVITY #6: Back-lying and Reaching Upward without Support (fig. 1.10)

1. Place your baby on the floor with her head looking straight ahead, not turned to either side.

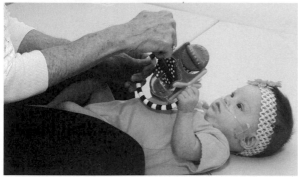

(fig. 1.10)

2. Position yourself sitting on your heels in front of her.
3. Place a large toy on her chest and have her reach and touch it with one or both hands.
4. If her legs are very active, support them to calm them down and then she will be better able to reach.
5. When she is able to consistently reach to her chest to play with the toy, hold it slightly above her chest so she needs to reach higher.
6. Watch her legs and support them if she holds them apart.

## ACTIVITY #7: Hip Stretch (fig. 1.11, 1.12)

1. Bend your baby's hips and knees to 90 degrees and hold the back of her thighs with the palms of your hands. Move her thighs gently toward neutral rotation (knees pointing up to the ceiling) and if you feel resistance, stop there and wait for her legs to relax. When she relaxes, move her thighs more until 5-10 degrees of internal rotation (knees turned slightly inward toward each other).

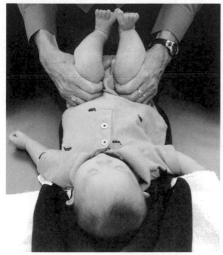

(fig. 1.11)

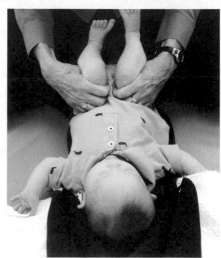

(fig. 1.12)

2. Talk to her and maintain the stretch for 1-2 minutes.

3. Practice 2-3 times a day and you will feel less stiffness each day.

4. When she can independently move her hips to neutral rotation and adduction (knees pointing up to the ceiling and knees together), then you can stop this exercise. See the section on "Bridging" in Chapter 2.

# Supported Sitting

When your baby is supported in the sitting position, she is able to look around and see the world from the vertical perspective and she will like this new orientation. In this position, she can be face to face with you or watch people around her. You can begin using this position at about two months of age if you give her the support she needs (fig. 1.13).

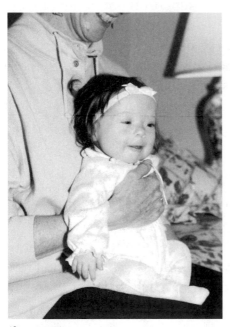

(fig. 1.13)

Learning head control is difficult for a baby with Down syndrome because her head is too heavy and her neck muscles are too weak to hold up this weight. In order for her to be able to lift her head, the rest of her body must be completely supported. With that support, she can focus on lifting her head up against gravity. She will need support behind her head to learn how far to lift her head and to be able to maintain it there once lifted. If she does not have support behind her head, she will lift it too far and it will fall back. As her neck muscles become stronger, she will be able to lift her head to the midline and maintain it there without losing control.

## Components

When your baby is supported in sitting, the components that you want to develop are:

1. head lifted to the midline, and maintained over time

2. trunk and pelvis supported fully erect

3. legs supported with thighs together and knees bent

## Tendencies

Her tendencies will be:

1. to sit with a slouched posture with her pelvis tilted back, trunk rounded, and head tilted back, resting on her neck and shoulders
2. to be supported with her legs too wide apart—for example, straddling both legs of the parent

## Set Up for Learning

Working on head control is the beginning of teaching your child to sit with the best posture. Therefore, her pelvis and trunk need to be supported fully upright so that she will learn to hold her head erect and in the midline. If her pelvis is allowed to tilt back, then her trunk will be rounded and her head will tilt back and rest on her neck and shoulders.

To support your baby in sitting, you can place her in your lap, facing away from you, or you can stand and carry her in this position. You can also place her on the couch or on a chair with her head, trunk, and pelvis supported upright against the back cushion (fig. 1.14). In either position, you will entertain her or talk to her to motivate her to lift her head up and hold it there. When she is tired and is leaning her head forward, it's time to quit.

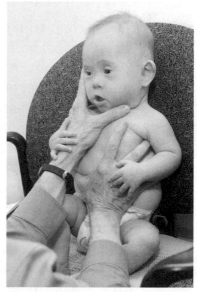

(fig. 1.14)

## Guidelines

*Use toys or people to motivate her to lift her head.* Use toys that she is interested in watching. You can talk and sing to her to encourage her to look at you. Make sure you or the toy are at eye level or slightly lower. If positioned above eye level, she will tilt her head back rather than lift it to the midline.

*When using these supported sitting positions, make sure that your baby's trunk and pelvis are up straight and not rounded or slouched.* If she is sitting in your lap, sit with your back straight because if you slouch, she will too. You will need to hold her pelvis with one hand and her chest with your other hand to make sure they are supported up straight. If her back and pelvis are rounded, she will not learn to lift her head properly. She will learn to lean her head back on her neck and shoulders. She can only lift her head properly in the midline if her back and pelvis are supported up straight.

*Use a reclining feeding chair or feeding seat for supported sitting positioning.* Place grip liner on the seat to keep her buttocks from sliding and to maintain her pelvis against the back of the seat. (Grip liner is a nonadhesive, nonslip product commonly used to line shelves or to keep rugs from sliding. It is sold in a roll and can be cut to any size. It has an open mesh structure and is washable.)

## ACTIVITY #8: Supported Sitting with Maximum Support in Your Lap

1. Sit in a chair with your back up straight (and even arched) and maintain that position.
2. Place your baby sitting in your lap so that she is facing away from you. Position her head against your chest; her trunk and pelvis against your abdomen.
3. Place one of your hands under her buttocks and use your thumb and fingers to hold her legs together. Hold her pelvis firmly against your abdomen.
4. Place your other hand across her upper chest and under her arms so her arms are free and forward. Support her trunk against you so it is up straight.
5. With this support, she can lift her head up against your chest.
6. Use toys or people to motivate her to lift her head. You can sit in front of a mirror or toys that she is interested in watching.
7. The goal of this position is to have her lift her head and hold it for as long as she can tolerate. As long as her head is against your

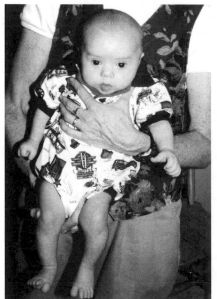

chest, she is actively lifting it. When her head leans forward, she is resting. This position can be used as long as she works on lifting her head.

8. If it is too difficult for her to lift her head with your trunk vertical, then recline your trunk slightly and have her practice holding her head against your chest in this position. When she is ready, move your trunk vertical and have her hold her head against your chest in this position.
9. You can also carry your baby in this position and walk around the house. The motion of walking will further stimulate her to lift her head (see fig. 1-15).

(fig. 1.15)

10. When she is able to lift her head up and hold it over time, provide support lower on her chest (around nipple level) and see if she can still lift her head.

### ACTIVITY 9: Supported Sitting with Maximum Support on a Couch or Chair (fig. 1-16)

1. Place your baby on the couch or chair with her pelvis and trunk up straight and supported against the back cushion. Place grip liner under her buttocks.
2. Kneel on the floor in front of her.
3. Place one of your hands at her pelvis to keep it from sliding forward and to hold it upright.
4. Place your other hand at her chest to support her trunk up straight.
5. Lean forward and talk to her with your face at eye level to her to encourage her to lift her head and hold it up as long as possible.

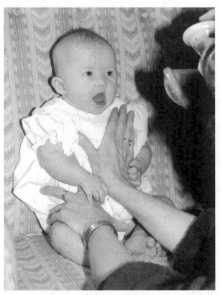

(fig. 1.16)

## Supported Kneeling

Supported kneeling at a 7-inch (18-cm) high cushion with full support is an easier alternative to using the stomach-lying position. With your baby's trunk placed diagonally, she will be able to see better with just a little head lift. When she can lift her head higher and maintain the lift longer, then she will be more successful in stomach-lying. Since this position is easier than stomach-lying, it can be used when your child needs more support—for example, if she has medical issues compromising her stamina, if she is tired, or if she needs more support to initially learn how to lift up her head. If this position helps your baby be more successful in learning to lift her head, then it is the best position to use.

### Components

When your baby is maximally supported in kneeling, the components that you want to develop are:

1. lifting her head in the midline and maintaining it
2. beginning weight bearing on her elbows

3. trunk supported up straight
4. stretching her hips to neutral rotation and beginning weight bearing on her legs

## Tendencies

Her tendencies will be:

1. to arch her head and trunk without control or bend into the surface
2. to lose head control suddenly and quickly fall into the surface
3. to not take weight on her elbows
4. to position her knees wide apart
5. to be fussy with taking weight on her knees and need a softer surface

## Setup for Learning

Your baby will need to be fully supported to use this position. You will support her knees together, support her trunk up straight, and support her elbows propping on the cushion. With her body stabilized, she can focus on lifting her head for brief periods (fig. 1.17). Using a soft surface like a sofa cushion (approximately 7 inches or 18 centimeters high) is necessary for her comfort and safety. Since she will be working on head control, she may lose control suddenly when she is tired and bump her face into the surface.

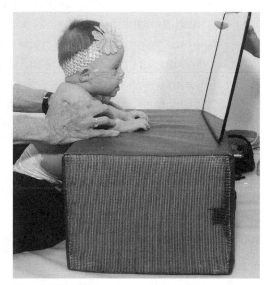

(fig. 1.17)

While the focus of this position is head control, your baby will also receive the benefits of taking weight on her elbows (with her elbows forward of her shoulders) and taking weight on her legs with her hips stretched to neutral rotation (by supporting her knees together and holding them there). She will also be supported with her trunk straight although leaned diagonally forward.

## Guidelines

*Use toys that she can look at since she will not be able to free her arms to touch the toy at first.* She will be propping on her elbows and we will be encouraging her to lift her head so use toys that have faces, music, and lights to entertain her. She will also be motivated if a sibling is in front of her, smiling and talking to her. She also will like a mirror or toys with black/white designs.

***Use a soft surface under her knees so your baby will be more comfortable.*** You can practice with her knees on a squishy mat or bed to start with. Then you can try a blanket or comforter. If she resists the position, it is usually because it is uncomfortable at her knees (pressure on boney surface) or ankles (because the front of her foot is stretched). Usually using a softer surface helps her tolerate the position.

## ACTIVITY #10: Supported Kneeling at a Sofa Cushion
(fig. 1.18, 1.19)

1. Select a soft surface to kneel on and then place a 7-inch (18 cm) sofa cushion on the surface in front of you. Sit on your heels and hold your baby sideways across your lap, facing away from you. Place one of your arms under her arms and your other hand will place her knees together with her hips and knees bent. (See fig. 1.18.)
2. Place her in kneeling with her knees together in between your knees and then snugly move your knees against hers to stabilize them together. Her buttocks will rest on your thighs so her pelvis is lifted a little (rather than resting on her heels).
3. Place her elbows on the sofa cushion and hold her upper trunk under her arms, and this will help her prop on her elbows, with her elbows forward of her shoulders (side view) and her elbows in line with her shoulders (fig. 1.19).
4. With her legs, trunk, and arms stabilized, place a toy (or person) in front of her and encourage her to lift her head. At first, she will lift

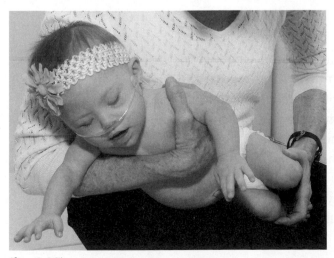

(fig. 1.18)

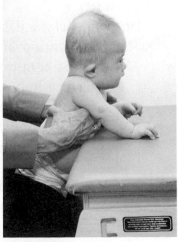

(fig. 1.19)

her head with bobbing movements, and as she gains strength, she will be able to lift her head and hold it, while looking at the motivator. If she lifts her head too far, then lean your trunk forward to prevent her from tilting her head back.

# Stomach-lying

Stomach-lying is the most physically challenging position for your baby. She has to move against gravity to lift her head and push up on her arms. This requires her to do two hard motor tasks at the same time. To make it even harder, her tendency will be to bend her hips and lift her pelvis up and this will cause her head and arms to collapse. Although this position is difficult, it is an important position to use to develop neck and arm strength. It is best to wait to use this position until your baby is ready. You can start with easier positions like placing your baby on your chest or on a ball, or use supported kneeling. It will be important to only practice this position while your child is strong enough to be active in it and while being entertained.

## Components

When your baby is on her stomach, the components that you want to develop are:

1. head lift in the center and looking forward toward the toy
2. propping on elbows with elbows forward of shoulders (side view)
3. pelvis flat on the surface
4. hips and knees straight, knees pointing into the surface, and legs together

## Tendencies

Her tendencies will be:

1. to position her legs in the frog-leg posture with hips and knees bent and pelvis lifted up off the surface, which will make it impossible to lift her head and prop on her arms
2. to use the arching pattern and position her arms with her elbows behind her shoulders, pinching her shoulder blades together; then she will not take weight on her elbows at all, or if she does, will not take weight effectively
3. to lift her head by arching her neck excessively and resting it back on her shoulders

### Setup for Learning

There are ways to prepare your baby to use stomach-lying so she begins to develop head control and propping on her arms. She can begin practicing lifting and controlling her head when you are carrying her with her head against your shoulder (see Activity 11). While you are carrying her, she will be able to lift her head for brief periods and then rest it back on your shoulder (fig. 1.20). You can also hold her against your chest while you are semi-reclined in a chair or on the sofa. With this support, she can lift her head and look at you while you support her arms. When she is tired, her head will rest against your chest.

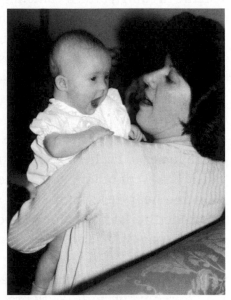

(fig. 1.20)

After she has practiced lifting her head in these easier positions and does it often, you can begin placing her on her stomach on a firm surface to test if she is ready to use the stomach-lying position. You will need to provide maximum leg and pelvic support, by first placing her hips and knees straight with her knees pointing down into the surface and with her legs together. With her legs in this position, her pelvis will be flat on the surface (fig. 1.21). She will need her pelvis and legs stabilized in this position and then her arms can be supported with her elbows forward of her shoulders. With this support, she can focus on lifting her head. If this position is still too difficult, then use the supported kneeling position.

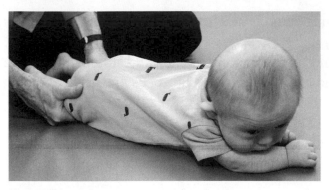

(fig. 1.21)

If you do not support your baby's pelvis and legs, her hips will bend and her pelvis will lift up off the surface. This will push her head and upper body downward and make it impossible for her to try to lift her head or prop on her arms. With this leg and pelvic support and as your baby learns to lift her head and chest higher and prop on her elbows, she will learn to straighten her legs and maintain her pelvis on the surface, and she will no longer need them supported.

Your baby's arms also need to be supported with her elbows placed forward of her shoulders (side view) and shoulder width apart. If her arms are positioned this way, she will be better able to lift her head, and she will learn the best position for propping on her elbows. Without arm support, she will use the arching pattern (pinching her shoulder blades together), and her elbows will be positioned behind her shoulders and wide apart, and she will not be able to prop effectively. With poor propping, it will be more difficult to lift her head and maintain the position. Arm support will be needed until she can maintain the position by herself consistently.

## Guidelines

*Use motivators that she is interested in watching.* You want to encourage her to lift her head to watch you, brightly colored toys, action toys, music boxes, or other people. She will also like to look at a shiny mylar balloon and hear the crinkly sound when it is touched. Change the motivators as needed to keep her interested in watching so she continues to lift her head as long as she can. Place the motivators at eye level to help her lift her head properly.

*Your baby will become tired easily in stomach-lying so use the position for short periods.* With practice, her strength will improve and she will be able to lift her head higher and stay in the position for longer periods.

 ## ACTIVITY #11: Lift Head When Placed on Your Shoulder

1. Place your baby against your chest with her head resting on your shoulder.
2. Place one of your hands across her upper back and stabilize her.
3. Place your other hand firmly against her buttocks and gently hold her legs straight and together.
4. Encourage her to lift her head.
5. This position can be done while sitting or when you are carrying her.
6. Watch her head position and support it if she loses control.

 ## ACTIVITY #12: Lift Head When Placed on Your Chest

1. Position yourself reclined 45 degrees on the couch or in a recliner chair.
2. Place your baby on your chest and support her legs straight and her pelvis flat against you.
3. Place her elbows forward of her shoulders so she can prop on them.
4. Talk to her and encourage her to lift her head to look at you.

5. As an alternative position, you could place your baby on her stomach on a large exercise ball. Place her so she is in this diagonal position and support her legs, pelvis, and elbows as described above. Encourage her to lift her head to look at someone in front of her.

 ## ACTIVITY #13: Stomach-lying with Full Support on the Floor (fig. 1-22)

1. Sitting on your heels, place your baby on her stomach on the floor in front of you, facing away from you.
2. Hold her thighs and rotate them until her knees point downward, then straighten her hips and knees and place them together. Make sure her pelvis is flat with her legs in this position. Then kneel over her and sit on your heels, and use your legs to support her legs and pelvis to anchor them in this position.

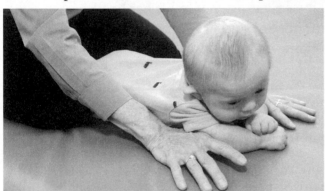

3. Lean forward and use your thumbs to support her elbows forward of her shoulders (and shoulder width apart) for propping.
4. Use a mirror, toy, or another person in front of her to motivate her to lift her head.

(fig. 1.22)

## ACTIVITY #14: Stomach-lying on an Elevated Surface

1. Place your baby on her stomach, facing you. Use an elevated surface like a bed or couch or padded table.
2. Position yourself on the floor at eye level to her.
3. Place her elbows forward of her shoulders (and shoulder width apart) for propping. Support her elbows to maintain the arm position if needed.
4. If her pelvis is lifted and her hips and knees are bent, place her legs straight and together and her pelvis flat and stabilize them.
5. Talk to her to encourage her to lift her head.
6. Have her hold her head up for as long as tolerated.

### ACTIVITY #15: Stomach-lying with Leg/Pelvic Support
(fig. 1.23)

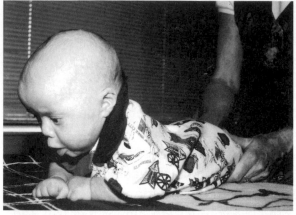

(fig. 1.23)

1. Place your baby on an elevated surface such as a bed, couch, or padded table. Place her on her stomach, with toys or a mirror in front of her.
2. Support her elbows forward of her shoulders and shoulder width apart.
3. Position yourself behind her supporting her pelvis and legs (as described above).
4. Use toys (or a sibling) to encourage her to lift her head.
5. When she is able to lift her head up well, let go of her legs and see if she can maintain propping on her elbows and lifting her head without the support.

# Rolling from Side-lying to Stomach-lying

Your baby will learn to roll by herself during Stage 2. In this stage, rolling from her side to her stomach is practiced to help her develop head control. Since you will be moving your baby from her back to her stomach, it is helpful to have her participate and have her practice the component of lifting her head.

## Components

When your baby is rolling from her side to her stomach, the components that you want to develop are:

1. lifting her head in side-lying and moving to her stomach
2. familiarity with lifting her arm so her elbow is above her shoulder
3. having her pelvis and legs anchored (and straight) so she can move her head and upper body to roll to her stomach

## Tendencies

Her tendencies will be:

1. to place her arm with her elbow bent and her elbow below her shoulder; this position will block the roll

2. to have tightness in her shoulder since she has not stretched her arm into this position before
3. to move her legs together with hips bent and knees bent or straight; this leg position will block the roll

### Set Up for Learning

When she is supported in the ideal position to encourage rolling from her side to her stomach, the key is to wait for her to choose when to move and to allow her to do it by herself. When in side-lying, with her arm placed up and her legs straight, and her pelvis anchored and pulled downward toward her feet, she will be led to lifting her head and rolling to her stomach. If we wait, she will be able to execute the movement (See figs. 1.24 and 1.25).

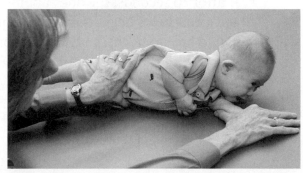

(fig. 1.24)

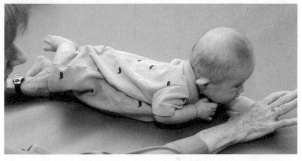

(fig. 1.25)

### Guidelines

*The key in using toys to encourage rolling is to pick toys your baby really wants and put them in the right place.* When encouraging her to roll from her side to her stomach, place the toy slightly above the level of her head and diagonally from her shoulder while in side-lying. When she is on her stomach, it will be right in front of her.

 ### ACTIVITY #16: Rolling from Side to Stomach with Full Support

1. Place your baby on her back on the floor.
2. Roll her to side-lying.
3. Place her underneath arm with her elbow above her shoulder and hold it there. Put your thumb below her elbow and use your palm and fingers to support her forearm. If her arm is stiff when you try to move it to this position, shake it gently to relax it and then it will move more easily.

4. Hold her pelvis with the palm of your hand and move it slightly past the side-lying position toward stomach-lying. Then pull downward (toward her feet) with gentle traction and wait for her to lift her head and roll to her stomach.

5. If after 10 seconds, she does not move, gently rock her pelvis and see if this helps begin the movement to her stomach. If she does not roll to her stomach, see if her arm or legs are blocking the movement. With the upward pull of her arm and the downward/forward pull on her pelvis, she will naturally follow with lifting her head and rolling to her stomach.

6. Repeat over her other side.

**MOTOR MILESTONE CHECKLIST**

### Side-lying
- ❏ When supported, she brings her hand to her mouth
- ❏ When supported, she looks at a toy and tucks her chin
- ❏ When supported, she touches a toy
- ❏ She stays in the side-lying position without support

### Back-lying
With maximum support in your lap:
- ❏ she looks at you and focuses on your face
- ❏ she brings her hand to her mouth or chest

On the floor with blanket rolls *under her head and arms* and her legs supported:
- ❏ she touches a large toy placed on her chest
- ❏ she brings her hand to her mouth
- ❏ she touches a rattle suspended from a play gym

On the floor with blanket roll *under her arms* and her legs supported:
- ❏ she moves her head to the center, tucks her chin, and holds it there
- ❏ she touches a large toy placed on her chest
- ❏ she brings her hand to her mouth
- ❏ she touches a rattle suspended from a play gym

On the floor with her legs supported:
- ❏ she holds her head in the center with chin tuck and she brings one or both hands to her chest to touch a large toy placed on her chest
- ❏ she holds her head in the center with chin tuck and touches a rattle suspended from a play gym

On the floor without support:
- ❏ she holds her head in the center with chin tuck and reaches for rattles suspended from a play gym for many repetitions
- ❏ her hips easily move to 5 degrees of internal rotation when stretched to this position

*(continued on next page)*

### Supported Sitting

When fully supported in sitting in your lap or on the couch,
she holds her head up for:

- ❑ 10 seconds
- ❑ 30 seconds
- ❑ 2-3 minutes
- ❑ When sitting in your lap or on the couch with support at nipple level and behind her head, she holds her head up for 5-10 minutes

### Stomach-lying

With maximal elbow, leg, and pelvic support, she holds head up for:

- ❑ 10-20 seconds
- ❑ 1 minute and longer
- ❑ With pelvic and leg support, she can hold her head up for 1-2 minutes with her elbows forward of her shoulders
- ❑ She can prop on elbows and hold her head up for 2-5 minutes with leg and pelvic support

### Supported Kneeling at 7-inch (18-cm) High Cushion

With maximal support at her legs, trunk, and arms:

- ❑ She will lift her head with bobbing movements
- ❑ She will lift her head and maintain it for 5-10 seconds
- ❑ She will lift her head and maintain it for 30 seconds or more

### Rolling

- ❑ In side-lying with underneath arm supported and pelvis and legs supported halfway between side-lying and stomach-lying, she lifts her head and rolls to stomach-lying
- ❑ In side-lying with underneath arm supported and pelvis and legs anchored, she lifts her head and rolls to stomach-lying

# 2

# Stage 2: Head Control, Reaching & Propping, Beginning Sitting, and Rolling

## Introduction

Now your baby is more alert and wants to move. He notices what is happening around him and wants to participate. He consistently smiles at you and everyone who talks to him. He makes faces and sounds to engage with you. He is motivated to interact with people and toys and initiates the interactions. He is awake for longer periods, and when awake, he loves attention and playing with people and toys.

He has gained strength in his head, arms, stomach, and legs so he is able to use his body more actively. He is able to move parts of his body but has not organized his movements to be able to play effectively. For example, he will be able to arch his head and trunk and move his legs but he will not be able to use his arms to reach for toys. He moves his body to look at what he chooses and is motivated to play, as long as it is close to him. He is learning how he can move and repeats the movements. He needs to learn how to use his strength to do the motor skills he is ready to learn.

### *Motor Skills*

The motor skills to focus on in this second stage of development are:
1. reaching, bridging (see below), and hand-to-foot play in back-lying
2. propping on elbows and hands, and reaching in stomach-lying
3. sitting with upper and middle trunk support

4. pulling to sit
5. supported kneeling and
6. rolling

## Components

The components to focus on are:
1. arm strength for reaching, propping, grasping toys to hold and shake them, and holding on and pulling to sit
2. head and upper and middle trunk control to learn to sit with the optimal posture with head and trunk erect (when supported)
3. abdominal strength through practicing hand-to-foot play
4. neutral hip rotation through practicing bridging, supported kneeling, and when stomach-lying
5. beginning weight shifting through practicing reaching when stomach-lying, and rolling

## Tendencies

During this stage, the tendencies are:
1. decreased use of the arms (and apparent weakness) due to overactive legs and underdeveloped strength because of lack of optimal support
2. sitting with a slouched posture
3. increased strength in back muscles resulting in overuse by arching, and lack of strength in abdominal muscles (to balance front and back muscles)
4. frog leg posture persists and resulting tightness in these hip muscles
5. resistance to weight shifting; for example to reach when in stomach-lying

## Guidelines

*Your baby will be able to use all the positions if you give him the support he needs.* He will initially prefer the back-lying position. He will be able to see you and easily play with toys. When he is able to prop well in stomach-lying, he will prefer that position. As his head control improves, it will be easier for him to pull to sit and use the supported sitting position. Supported kneeling can be used to practice propping and reaching, and it is also useful to develop head and trunk strength for supported sitting. Your baby will need to practice rolling with support until he is able to do it by himself.

*Watch to see which positions he prefers and which ones are harder for him.* What he chooses will depend on his tone, strength, and what he is interested in. Start with the harder positions and then alternate the easier positions with the harder ones. Use the activities as long as he tolerates them.

***Change the toys often to keep his interest and attention.*** If he is motivated to see or play with a toy, he will practice the activity longer.

***He will be able to be alert and active for 30-40 minutes.*** When he is tired, he needs a resting break to recover.

# Back-lying

Back-lying is your baby's preferred position in this stage because he can hold his head in the center and socialize with you, and reach, touch, and play with toys. He also can look around the room and see the people around him. During this stage, he will learn to reach for toys, move his legs together to the bridge position, and engage in hand-to-foot play.

## Motor Skills

When he is on his back, the motor skills to focus on are:
1. reaching above his chest and holding and shaking lightweight rattles
2. bridging, and moving his legs to neutral hip rotation
3. activating his abdominals to engage in hand-to-foot play

## Tendencies

Your baby's tendencies will be to:
1. move his legs rather than his arms, so reaching with his arms will need to be encouraged
2. position his legs in the frog leg posture and develop muscle tightness
3. arch his back and have difficulty learning to activate his abdominals to engage in hand-to-foot play
4. learn to engage in hand-to-foot play without using his abdominals and instead use the extra flexibility in his hips

# Reaching

Your baby will need to develop arm strength to reach, and leg movements will need to be limited to allow him to move his arms often with control. Parents frequently report that a child will kick his legs to play with toys on a play gym rather than use his arms. If we support the legs, then the child is able to use his arms to play. To gain strength, he will need to reach for many repetitions, and he will need support until he can do this on his own.

## Components

The components to focus on are:
1. chin tuck to look downward at toys on his chest
2. lifting arms off the surface to his chest or to a toy suspended at his shoulder and building the ability to do it for many repetitions
3. touching toys and maintaining the reaching position to play with the toys
4. grasping the toy, and holding and shaking it

## Tendencies

The tendencies are:
1. to constantly move the legs and this will limit arm movement
2. to arch the trunk, and with this arching pattern, the shoulder blades will pinch together, making it harder to lift the arms off the surface

## Setup for Learning

Your baby will begin reaching for toys placed on his chest or suspended just above his shoulder (using a play gym). If he uses any upward movement, he is participating with practicing this skill (fig. 2.1). He may prefer to reach with one hand. If so, this can be focused on, so he is successful with learning the skill. Once he learns the skill, he can also practice with his other hand. He may hold onto his clothes to keep his hands on his chest. He will let go with one hand to touch a toy while the other hand continues to hold on. By holding his clothes, he keeps his hands in a better position for play. As his strength improves, he will begin to reach above his chest. As his control increases, the toy can be raised higher. When he can reach with his elbows straight and maintain the reach while touching a toy, he will be ready to practice hand-to-foot play.

After he reaches for the toy, he will be able to hold it and shake it. The toy needs to be the right size to grasp with his small hands, and it needs to be lightweight. He will

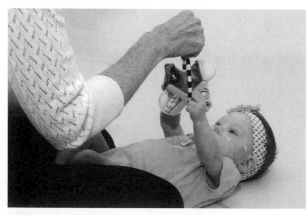

(fig. 2.1)

shake it back and forth, to and from his chest. He will bring it to his mouth and may lift it higher toward his head.

 ## ACTIVITY #1: Back-lying and Reaching above Chest

1. Place your baby on the floor with his head in the center.
2. Sit on your heels in front of him.
3. Place a toy 1-2 inches (2.5-5 cm) above his chest and have him reach and touch the toy. If this is difficult, place the toy just above his shoulder and see if he can touch it. Encourage him to reach with each hand by holding the toy to each side in turn.
4. Encourage him to reach and touch the toy as long as tolerated.
5. When he reaches well with the toy 1-2 inches above his chest, raise it to 3-4 inches (7.5-10 cm) above his chest. Continue to raise the toy until he is able to reach with his elbows straight.
6. Watch his leg position and support his legs together if he holds them apart. If needed, provide moderate support to his legs to calm them so he can focus on moving his arms.
7. This activity can also be done by positioning a play gym over his chest with the toys placed the proper distance above his chest/shoulder.

 ## ACTIVITY #2: Back-lying and Shaking Toys

1. Place your baby on a firm surface.
2. Sit on your heels in front of him.
3. Pick out a toy that is easy for him to hold onto and makes sounds when shaken.
4. Help him put his fingers around the toy so he can hold it.
5. Hold his hand and shake it while he holds the toy.
6. Let go and see if he will try to shake the toy.
7. Encourage him to hold, shake, and play with the toy as long as tolerated. You can also play tug-of-war playfully.
8. Use toys that are lightweight, easy to hold, and safe.

# Bridging

"Bridging" is the technical term for positioning his legs with his hips and knees bent, feet on the floor, and knees together. Your baby will only learn this skill if you teach him. Since Stage 1, you have stretched your baby's hips toward neutral hip rotation (with his knees in line with his hips) so he now has adequate mobility. The focus now is to have him activate his inner thigh muscles to move his hips to this position.

## Components

The components to focus on are:

1. rotating the hips to move the knees together with the knees pointing up to the ceiling rather than the knees turning outward to the sides
2. rubbing of the inner borders of the feet together

## Tendencies

The tendencies are:

1. to position the legs with the knees wide apart and turning outward (frog leg posture)
2. to have tightness in the hip muscles, which makes the frog leg posture persist since the child does not have adequate strength to move in the opposite direction (against the tightness), bringing his knees together

## Setup for Learning

The movement you want to see is moving his knees together when his hips and knees are bent and his feet are on the floor. After you stretch his hips, then you can try to activate the movement. As a warm up exercise, you can hold his lower legs and bang his feet into the floor playfully. Then you can intermittently tap the outsides of his knees, and then see if he will briefly hold his knees together (fig. 2.2). This is a good activity especially at diaper changes.

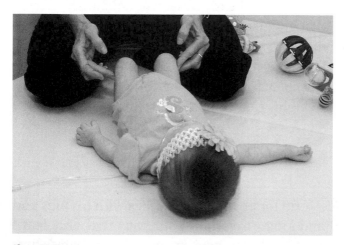

(fig. 2.2)

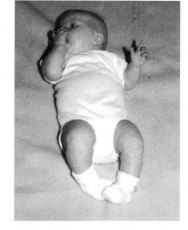

(fig. 2.3)

During this stage, your baby will learn to move his knees together (in line with his hips, with his knees pointing upward), and he frequently will do it as he rubs the inside borders of his feet together (fig. 2.3). This position will become part of his repertoire, and it will be further developed through positioning in supported kneeling and when stomach-lying. This movement is needed ultimately for an optimal walking pattern to promote knees and feet pointing straight ahead (rather than turned outward), with his knees in line with his hips (rather than a wide base).

 ## ACTIVITY #3: Bridging

1. Place your baby on his back on the floor.
2. Sit on your heels in front of him.
3. Do the hip stretch exercise.
4. Bend his hips and knees and place his feet on the floor.
5. Tap the outsides of his knees to try to cue him to move his thighs together (fig. 2.2). Do this 3 to 5 times. In between the taps, watch and see if he briefly holds his knees together.
6. With practice, he will begin to hold his thighs together. When he can do that, you can discontinue this exercise.

# Hand-to-Foot Play

You want to focus on this skill because it will strengthen your child's stomach muscles if practiced properly. (The back muscles tend to be stronger than the abdominal muscles so practicing this skill correctly will help to balance out the strength between the front and

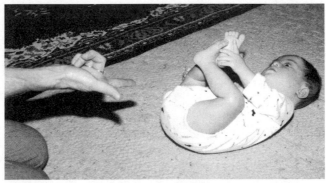

(fig. 2.4)

back muscles.) To engage in hand-to-foot play, your baby will need to be able to reach, kick his legs up, and lift his buttocks off the floor, and coordinate the kicking with the reaching so he can grab his feet at the right time (fig. 2.4). It takes time and practice to achieve this skill. If arching his back is the primary movement used, your child will need extra practice to learn hand-to-foot play.

## Components

The components to focus on are:

1. supporting his legs over his abdomen so he is interested in playing with his feet and is successful reaching for his knees or feet
2. stretching out his back and pelvic muscles (out of the arched position) so his trunk is rounded; with the trunk and pelvis in this position, the child will be able to activate his abdominal muscles
3. activating his abdominal muscles to assist with lifting his legs over his abdomen. Later, he will gain the strength to lift his pelvis up off the floor and hold it there while he plays with his feet
4. the ability to simultaneously reach with his arms while lifting his pelvis and legs over his abdomen

## Tendencies

The tendencies are:

1. to predominantly use the arching pattern when on his back so he resists this activity
2. to learn hand-to-foot play with his pelvis on the floor so he learns to do the skill by increasing hip flexibility rather than learning to use his abdominals

## Set Up for Learning

When he is able to reach above his chest, he can begin practicing reaching for his feet with his pelvis, legs, and feet supported. You will need to place his feet over his chest so he can see and touch them. You will need to make him aware of his feet and generate interest in his feet. You can rub or pat his feet together, or pat them against your face. By playing with his feet, you will motivate him to touch his feet. He will also be interested if you use colorful socks or place toys on his feet.

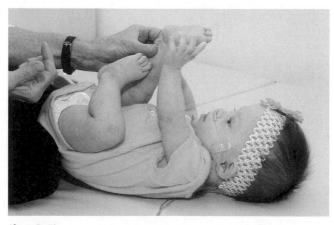

(fig. 2.5)

Your baby will need his pelvis supported and lifted so his back is rounded and not allowed to arch. With his trunk and pelvis in this position, he can activate his abdominals. In my experience, he will do best if his pelvis is on your thighs (or in between your thighs) (fig. 2.5) Then you can support his legs and feet over his chest and encourage him to reach for them. If he cannot reach them, you can move his foot to his hand and assist playful contact.

When his pelvis is supported, he will alternate between reaching and kicking his legs up. When he reaches, his legs may stiffen and straighten, moving away. When he kicks his legs up, you will notice horizontal wrinkles across his abdomen and activation of his abdominal muscles. While you are supporting his legs with his feet over his chest, he will feel where his legs need to be so he can touch his feet. He will work on kicking his legs upward until he has the strength to lift his buttocks off the floor. You will need to support his buttocks and legs so he can play with his feet until he is able to do it by himself. As tolerated, you can lessen the pelvic support and lower his pelvis. He will first be able to reach and touch his knees; later, when he can lift his buttocks off the floor, he will be able to touch his feet.

Your baby will work on the individual skills of reaching, kicking his legs up, and lifting his pelvis upward off the floor. When he is motivated to play with his feet and has developed the strength he needs, he will coordinate all of these actions to engage in hand-to-foot play.

 ## ACTIVITY #4: Back-lying and Kicking

1. Take your baby's shirt off and place him on the floor.
2. Tickle his belly or blow on it. Watch to see if he uses his stomach muscles and kicks his legs up. If he uses his stomach muscles, you will see wrinkles across his stomach.
3. If he does not kick his legs up, lift them up (to at least 90 degrees) and move them for a few seconds and then let go. After you let go, see if he tries to kick them up.
4. Also try this activity when you are changing his diaper. It will be easier for him to kick his legs up when his diaper and clothes are off.
5. When he is able to kick, he may like to kick rattles suspended from a mobile.

 ## ACTIVITY #5: Back-lying/Hand-to-Foot Play with Support (fig. 2.6)

1. Place your baby on the floor with his head in the center.
2. Sit on your heels in front of him at his feet.
3. Place his buttocks on your knees (or in between your knees) and support his legs over his abdomen so he can see his feet.
4. Play with his feet by patting and rubbing the soles together and placing them against your face.

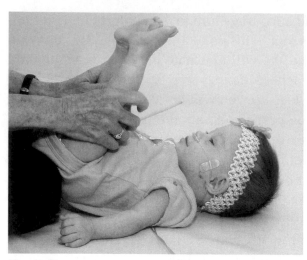

(fig. 2.6)

5. Watch him and see if he is interested in looking at his feet.
6. Hold one foot close to his hand and see if he will reach for his foot. If he does not try to touch his foot, bring his hand to his foot and pat or rub them together. Help him hold onto his foot.
7. Try putting foot jingles or bells on his feet to entice him to reach for the toy on his foot. You can also use colorful socks or foot jingles with faces.
8. Encourage him to reach for one foot while you hold it. You can move his right foot to his left hand (or the reverse).
9. When he consistently reaches for his feet with your support at his buttocks and legs, lower his buttocks slightly and see if he can still reach for his feet.
10. Continue to encourage him to reach for his feet as you lessen your support and gradually lower his buttocks to the floor.
11. Continue to practice until he can engage in hand-to-foot play often by himself.

## Guidelines

*When using toys in this position, you need to pick the right toy for the activity you are doing.*

1. For **reaching** activities, use colorful, movable lightweight rattles, squeeze/squeak toys, and stuffed animals. The toys need to be big enough to touch and grab. You can suspend them from a mobile or play gym or hold them at the proper level.
2. When he is **holding and shaking** toys, use lightweight toys with the proper size handle to grasp. Babies love holding and shaking links. Make sure the toys are safe and won't hurt him if he hits himself with them. Never use a heavy rattle because it is too hard to move and he will tire too quickly trying to play with it.
3. For **hand-to-foot play,** put foot jingles or lightweight rattles on his feet to motivate him to reach for his feet. When he wants to play with his feet, make sure he is barefoot so he can grab his feet more easily.

*When he is not kicking his legs up, watch his legs to see what movements he uses.* When you are not supporting him, watch to see the variety of leg positions that he uses. Observe if his knees are generally in line with his hips or wide apart. During this stage, you want him to learn to move his legs with his knees in line with his hips. Until he is able to move his legs together (neutral hip rotation), support them together when possible.

*When practicing bridging, you want your child to learn to do it actively rather than using equipment to hold his legs together.* There are products such as lycra pants or hip helpers (www.hiphelpers.com) available that hold your child's legs together. These supports can be used if you feel they are helpful, but they are not necessary. What is most important is for your child to strengthen the muscles needed to move his hips to neutral rotation so his knees are together and pointing upward. This can be achieved through stretching exercises and by supporting the legs together to teach him to actively move his knees together (as described in the home programs).

*It is easier for your baby to engage in hand-to-foot play without his diaper or clothes on.* You can let him practice during diaper changes.

# Stomach-lying

Stomach-lying is an important position for building strength, particularly in the neck and arm muscles. Your baby is ready to use this position now that his neck and arm muscles are stronger. He will need to gain the strength to lift his head and prop on his arms for several minutes while watching or playing with toys. He needs to be set up to be successful, by providing the necessary arm, leg, and pelvic support discussed in Stage 1. When his strength improves, this may become his preferred position. If his arms are weak, he can practice supported kneeling as an alternative position.

## Motor Skills

When your baby is on his stomach, the motor skills to focus on are:

1. lifting his head so it is in the center and looking forward towards the toy.
2. propping on elbows, with his elbows forward of his shoulders, and maintaining this position using arm strength for long periods of time
3. propping on hands, with his elbows unlocked and forward of his shoulders, easily shifting weight from side to side, and maintaining this position over time

4. reaching by lifting one hand while weight shifting over the other elbow
5. hips straight, knees in line with hips and pointing down into the surface, with knees either straight or bent
6. pelvis flat on the surface

## Tendencies

The tendencies are:

1. to arch his neck and lift his head back onto his neck and shoulders
2. to arch his back, pinch his shoulder blades together, positioning his elbows behind his shoulders, and not taking much weight on his elbows (like a Superman pose)
3. to lock his elbows straight to maintain the position of propping on hands
4. to position his legs in the "frog leg" posture with the soles of his feet together to stabilize himself
5. to move his legs, lifting his pelvis, so he will not be able to focus on head and arm movements
6. to resist weight shifting and reach with one or both hands, arching his back and head

# Propping on Elbows

Your baby will first learn to prop on his elbows in stomach lying or supported kneeling. When propping on his elbows, his elbows need to be placed forward of his shoulders (side view) and shoulder width apart. With his arms properly positioned, he can push up on his arms better and lift his head more easily. His arms will become stronger with practice, and he will learn to maintain the position for longer periods of time. If he moves his legs and lifts his pelvis, his legs will need to be supported to help him focus on neck and arm strength.

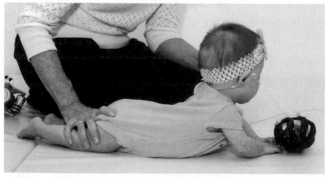

If he stabilizes in the frog leg posture, his legs will need to be supported to teach him to position his legs straight (neutral hip rotation) and together (fig. 2.7). If the frog leg posture becomes a habit, it will inhibit weight shifting for reaching and rolling.

(fig. 2.7)

When your baby is able to prop on his elbows, he will choose between two options. He will either learn to reach while propping on his elbows or he will learn to prop on his hands. You can assist him with both and see what he is interested in doing. To reach, he will need to be motivated to touch toys; to prop on his hands, he will need to have adequate arm strength to push up. He will eventually learn to do both skills.

## Components

The components to focus on are:

1. proper head, arm, and leg posture
2. having the strength to maintain head lift and propping over time

## Tendencies

The tendencies are:

1. to arch the neck
2. to place elbows behind the shoulders (side view) and wider than shoulders, so there is minimal weight bearing
3. to bend his hips so his pelvis is lifted
4. to position his legs in the "frog leg" posture

## ACTIVITY #6: Propping on Elbows and Lifting Head in Stomach-lying

1. Place your baby on his stomach and place his elbows shoulder width apart, with his elbows forward of his shoulders (side view). Support his elbows if needed.
2. Watch the position of his legs and support them if needed. (See Activity #13, step 2, in Chapter 1.) If he uses the frog leg posture or if he bends his hips and raises his pelvis off the floor, support them.
3. Encourage him to lift his head by talking to him or using toys. Place the toys at eye level or slightly lower; do not place them above his head.
4. Encourage him to maintain head lift and propping on elbows as long as tolerated.

# Reaching

After he can maintain propping on his elbows easily, your baby will be ready to practice reaching. If he wants to play with toys, he will be motivated to develop reaching skills. His first method of reaching will be to slide his hand

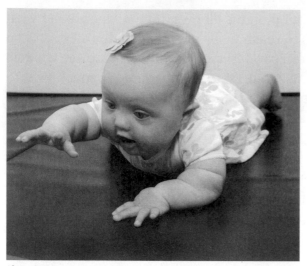

(fig. 2.8)

forward to touch a toy, keeping his hand on the surface. He will want the toy, reach forward for it, and then will grab it and pull it closer to him.

The second method of reaching will be to lift his hand and arm up off the surface to reach and play with a toy. In order to lift his hand off the surface, he needs to learn to lean over his other elbow and weight shift, balancing himself in this position while playing with the toy (fig. 2.8). He will need help to learn this weight shifting movement and to be comfortable with feeling off balance.

## Components

The components to focus on are:
1. weight shifting over his elbow and staying in this position for a few seconds
2. lifting his other arm up off the surface and reaching for the toy, then holding and playing with the toy
3. positioning the leg straight so he weight shifts over his pelvis and leg

## Tendencies

The tendencies are:
1. to reach without weight shifting by arching his neck and back and lifting his arm
2. to position his legs in the frog leg posture so he does not weight shift over his pelvis and leg. This position will also block weight shifting through his pelvis and leg.
3. to be uncomfortable with weight shifting in this partial range and become fussy when feeling off balance
4. to roll over to his back

## Set Up for Learning

To familiarize your child with the weight shift, you can kneel beside him and then weight shift him against your leg. You will support the elbow he is leaning over to make sure it is in the right position (under his shoulder) as he

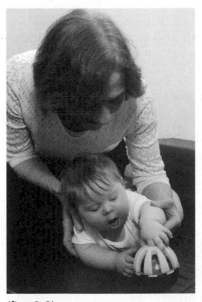

(fig. 2.9)

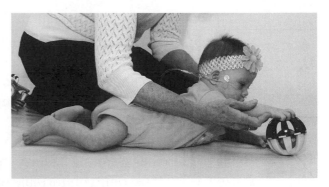

(fig. 2.10)

weight shifts over it (fig. 2.9). You will lift his other hand onto a toy (small ball toy or cube) so he feels how high to lift his arm (fig. 2.10). With his hand on the ball or cube, you can roll it (sideways) so he weight shifts and moves and learns to feel comfortable in the position. You will test each side to see if he prefers reaching with one hand more than the other. If he has a preference, you can practice with this arm until he can do it by himself, and then practice with his other arm.

Your baby will first learn to reach forward and later will learn to reach to the side. Through reaching, he learns how to lean (shift) his weight from one side to the other and balance on one side. This is essential for the development of future motor skills such as moving in and out of positions, creeping, and walking.

## ACTIVITY #7: Stomach-lying and Reaching with Hand on a Ball Toy (fig. 2.11)

1. Sit on your heels (kneeling with your buttocks on your heels) and place your baby beside you (next to your right leg), facing forward.
2. Place his left elbow under his shoulder and stabilize it.
3. Place your right hand under his right arm (near his elbow) and place a 3-4 inch (7.5-10 cm) diameter ball or cube in front of his shoulder.

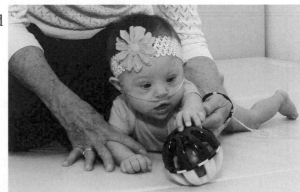

(fig. 2.11)

4. Weight shift him over his left elbow and lift his right arm (with your right hand). Put his hand on the ball and gently rock his body (weight shifting it sideways) while rolling the ball sideways. Do this for about 5-10 seconds (or as tolerated).

5. Repeat these steps with weight shifting over the right elbow and lifting the left hand.

6. Your child will tolerate practicing this activity since he will feel stable because he is leaning against your leg when his weight is shifted. He will become comfortable with being off balance since he can lean against you.

## ACTIVITY #8: Stomach-lying and Reaching

1. Kneel on the floor. Place your baby on his stomach on your bed (raised surface), so you are facing each other.

2. Position him propping on his elbows, with his elbows under his shoulders.

3. Lift his right hand toward your face and weight shift him over his left elbow (and stabilize the elbow if needed). Pat your face with his hand, talk to him, and entertain him while practicing reaching.

4. When he is comfortable with lifting his arm and weight shifting, then place him on the floor and place a toy in front of him and see if he will reach for it. You can use lightweight toys such as tissue paper, or a lightweight rattle. You can also use a 2-4 inch (5-10 cm) diameter ball or weighted toys (with faces) like the Fisher-Price Sparkling Elephant.

5. See if he will stretch his hand forward to touch the toy and place the toy in front of his shoulder to facilitate a weight shift. Then see if he will lift his hand off the surface to touch the toy. Provide the necessary support to be successful. If he just reaches without weight shifting, then assist the weight shift. If he can weight shift but not lift his hand, then assist the lift. If he weight shifts too far, and rolls over, then limit the range of the weight shift with either your hand or body.

6. When he is holding the toy—for example, tissue paper—you can increase the weight shifting and lifting experience by playing tug of war.

7. With practice, your baby will learn to weight shift and reach for toys with each hand. If at first he has a preference for reaching with one hand, let him learn the skill through reaching with that hand, and once established, then practice with his other hand.

# Propping on Hands

Your baby may prefer propping on his hands to reaching if he enjoys watching toys or people and he has the strength needed to push up on his hands (fig. 2.12). With a mirror in front of him he may push up to look at himself or look at a toy. He will be motivated to see something, but not to touch it. He may practice propping on hands first in supported kneeling, since it will be easier to do in this position.

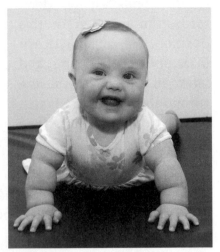

(fig. 2.12)

## Components

The components to focus on are:
1. straightening his elbows and propping on his hands, with his hands slightly wider than his shoulders
2. positioning the legs straight, together, and in neutral rotation
3. holding the head in the mid position, balanced between extending it and using chin tuck

## Tendencies

The tendencies are:
1. to lock the elbows with the hands wider than the shoulders
2. to use the frog leg posture for stability
3. to rest the head back on the neck and shoulders
4. to arch his head and trunk and not bear weight on his hands

## Set Up for Learning

Your baby will first initiate propping on hands with his hands forward of his shoulders (side view). He will be propping on his elbows and from that position, straighten his elbows (fig. 2.13). (If he does not initiate this, you can help him by lifting his chest.) If he does not straighten his elbows, he may not understand how to straighten his elbows and may need support at his elbows so he feels the new position. Once he feels it, he can then imitate it. Once he begins propping on hands (hands forward of his shoulders) and knows the skill, he will practice it on his own and over time will improve arm strength to position his hands under his shoulders. Then he will have fun doing baby push-ups.

Your baby may not want to prop on his hands because he cannot play while propping in this difficult position. He also may resist propping on his hands if his arms are weak. If he shows no interest in propping on his hands when stomach-lying, don't force him to do it in this position. He can practice it in supported kneeling and later in supported sitting (propping hands on a bench but not on the floor). (See Chapter 3.)

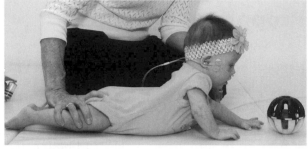

(fig. 2.13)

 **ACTIVITY #9: Stomach-lying and Propping on Hands with Maximal Support** (fig. 2.14)

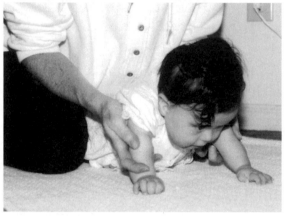

(fig. 2.14)

1. Place your baby on his stomach, facing away from you. Use a firm surface like the carpeted floor.
2. Place his legs together with his hips straight and in neutral rotation and his knees straight. With his legs in this position, his pelvis will be flat on the floor. Sit on your heels over him with your legs supporting his pelvis and legs.
3. Lean your trunk forward and hold his arms with his elbows straight.
4. While maximally supporting his arms, pat his hands against the floor and gently bounce him on his hands until his hands are at a 45 degree angle from the shoulders and the width between his hands is slightly wider than his shoulders. (If his hands are placed under his shoulders, it will be too hard for him to push up.)
5. Try to decrease the support at his elbows as tolerated and see if he will keep his elbows straight for a second or two.
6. When propping on hands, if his elbows bend immediately, use your fingertips to support or tap his elbows and see if this cueing is adequate to guide him to straighten them. Keep decreasing your support or providing intermittent support until he has the strength to straighten his elbows for a few seconds. If he bends his elbows slightly and keeps them up off the surface, he is beginning to learn to do push ups.
7. Encourage him to prop on his hands as long as tolerated, working toward 10 seconds.

## ACTIVITY #10: Stomach-lying and Propping on Hands with Chest Support

(This can be practiced after he has the idea of straightening his elbows with support.)

1. Follow steps 1 and 2 above.
2. Lean your trunk forward and support his chest with your hands holding his trunk (under his arms). Lift his chest and see if he will prop on his hands with his elbows straight (or partially straight), with his hands forward of his shoulders (side view). Make sure his hands are slightly wider than his shoulders to make it easier to prop. (If his hands are close together, it is too hard to maintain the propping position and he will fall.)
3. Have him prop for a few seconds with your support so he learns the game. When he is showing more strength and familiarity with the position, decrease your support and see if he can maintain the position.
4. Continue to practice until he can prop on his own.

## ACTIVITY #11: Stomach-lying and Propping on Hands with Arm Support

1. Kneel on the floor and place your baby on his stomach on a raised (firm) surface above you, like a coffee table or bed. Make sure you are facing each other.
2. Hold his elbows so they are straight and place his hands forward of his shoulders, and slightly wider than his shoulders. You can gently bounce him on his hands while moving him to this position.
3. Gradually let go of his elbows and see if he can keep them straight for a few seconds. If not, tap his elbows intermittently and see if this is adequate support.
4. Use your fingertips to support his elbows as needed until he is able to keep them straight.
5. When he is able to push up and prop on his hands in this position, move his hands so they are closer to his shoulders (at an approximately 60 degree angle).
6. Make sure he bends and straightens his elbows and does not hold them locked. Watch his arm position and now position his hands shoulder width apart. Then when he weight shifts to either side, he will bend his elbows. If he holds his elbows stiff and resists bending them, it is usually because his hands are placed too wide. This can be fixed by repositioning his arms with his hands shoulder width

apart. If he learns to lock (stiffen) his elbows, he will not develop arm strength properly.

7. As his arms get stronger, he will be able to push up and prop on his hands by himself.

### Guidelines

*When practicing propping on elbows and hands, it is best if you place your baby's arms properly and have him prop as long as he can while entertaining him.* I do not recommend using a roll or wedge for propping because your baby will lean and rest on it rather than actively pushing up and propping. He will develop more arm strength by actively propping on his arms rather than by leaning over a roll or wedge.

*If he resists propping and puts his arms along the sides of his body and arches his back, support his arms to help him prop.* As he gains strength, he will be able to prop by himself.

*Use toys that will encourage the skill you are practicing.* For beginning propping, use toys or people your baby is motivated to watch. Place the motivator at eye level or lower. If you place it above his head, he will learn to lean his head back on his neck, which could become a bad habit. When he is reaching forward to touch a toy on the surface, use lightweight rattles that are easy to hold. When he is reaching and lifting his hand off the surface and touching toys, use toys that rock (like a small ball), make sounds, and have bright colors. Examples include: Fisher-Price Sparkling Elephant (wobble toy), Sassy ball toy, squeak toys, and toys with faces. If he can reach for the toy, grip it, and lift it off the surface, then use lightweight toys like tissue paper, and small links or rattles. When propping on hands, use toys or play games that he can watch. Examples are: music boxes, spinning toys, playing peek-a-boo, talking or singing to him, or using a mirror so he can watch himself.

*Watch his leg position and support his legs together if they are predominantly wide apart.* If he has the habit of using the frog-leg posture with his feet together for stability, this will block weight shifting for reaching and rolling. We need to support his legs to teach him to use neutral hip rotation and position his hips straight and legs together. Then he will be successful with learning to weight shift.

## Supported Sitting with Upper and Middle Trunk Support

Your baby will love to look around when you hold him in supported sitting. Since he is motivated to look, he will lift his head up. During this stage he will be able to hold his head up when supported in sitting and he will learn to sit with upper and middle trunk support.

This will be the critical time for your baby to learn how to lift his head to the center and hold it there. In Stage One, he needed support behind his head and he lifted his head up to the sup-

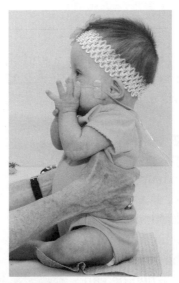

(fig. 2.15)

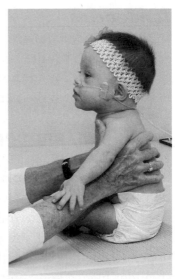

(fig. 2.16)

port. Now the support is no longer needed behind his head and he will need to learn how far to lift his head up so that it does not fall back. He also needs to develop the strength and control to lift his head slowly so he can stop lifting it when it is in the right position. If he lifts it quickly, it will probably fall back.

Your baby will need to have his trunk and pelvis supported up straight so he can learn to lift and hold his head in the proper position (fig. 2.15). If he is held with his back rounded, he will learn to lean his head back on his neck and rest it there (fig. 2.16). This is a bad habit to develop because he will not learn how to lift his head properly and, later, he will sit with his trunk rounded forward and his head tilted back.

## *Components*

When your child is supported in sitting, the components to focus on are:
1. Head lifted and erect, balanced between head lift and chin tuck, and maintaining the position over time
2. Trunk supported up straight and lifted into a little arch in the low back area
3. Pelvis supported up straight and top of the pelvis leaning/tilting a little forward
4. Improved trunk strength, with upper trunk held erect with support below this area; later, middle trunk up straight with lower trunk and pelvic support
5. The ideal sitting posture, learned by practicing with the right support

### Tendencies

The tendencies are:
1. To tilt the head back on the neck and shoulders
2. To round the trunk and slouch (fig. 2.17)
3. To tilt the pelvis back (fig. 2.17)

### Set Up for Learning

To learn to sit properly during Stages 2 and 3, four levels of support will be provided and practiced. During this stage, two levels of trunk support will be practiced. Your baby will start with upper trunk support at the level of his shoulder blades and chest. When he can lift and straighten this part of his trunk while holding his head erect, then middle trunk support will be provided (between his shoulder blades and waist) (fig. 2.18). As neck and trunk strength improves and he can maintain the posture over time (endurance), then the support is placed

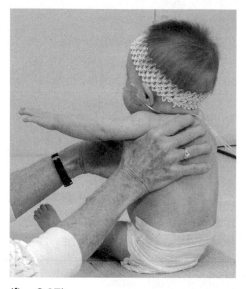

(fig. 2.17)

at a lower level. While practicing at these levels of support, the lower trunk and pelvis are maximally supported in the optimal position.

When practicing supported sitting, **strategic support** is needed to make sure you do it properly for your child to learn the optimal sitting posture and for your child's safety. It is best to take your baby's shirt off when you practice. This way you can see his posture and use the warmth and direct contact of your hands to mold his trunk and pelvis into this new position. As he is developing the neck and upper/middle trunk strength for the optimal sitting posture, this is also the critical time to familiarize him with having his lower trunk being lifted up straight and into an arch, and his pelvis being up straight with the top of his pelvis tilted forward.

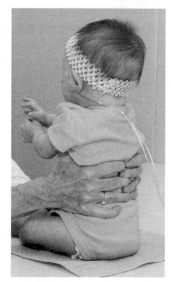

(fig. 2.18)

As your baby is developing head and trunk control in supported sitting, he may want to play with toys. This additional motor skill (reaching, holding, shaking a toy) will challenge his head and trunk control. When he reaches, it will be difficult to keep his head and upper trunk up straight because he will be doing three hard skills at once. You will need to support him more when he is using his arms to play until he develops the strength to do all three activities at once. While practicing sitting, you may need to alternate the goals of practicing the perfect posture and playing with toys.

## Guidelines

· *Place toys or motivators at the level of your baby's eyes or between his mouth and eyes.* When he is working on lifting his head and it is hard for him, have him watch people or toys. You can talk or sing to him or have someone entertain him with toys. When he is able to hold up his head and upper trunk, he will probably enjoy touching toys on a mobile or holding lightweight rattles and shaking them. When he plays with toys, see if his posture changes and give him extra support if he needs it. If he needs a lot of extra support, try to alternate "watching" entertainment and playing with toys.

*When practicing the supported sitting position, take your baby's shirt off to see what his head and trunk really look like.* With clothes on, you cannot see if his back and pelvis are rounded or up straight. With his shirt off, you can hold his trunk more securely with your hands with the skin-to-skin contact and he will be more responsive to this direct touch.

*If he resists the firm upper trunk support, add movement and this may help him tolerate it better.* He will like it if you lean him a little side to side and rock him gently. He may also like it if you playfully rotate his trunk (jiggle him) or add a little bouncing.

*If he resists having his trunk fully straight and wants to bend his trunk (when middle trunk support is provided), he may do better if you use a different method of supporting his trunk.* If he is placed sideways in front of you, and you support the rounded part of his back with one hand and then lift his chest with your other hand, he may straighten his trunk better.

*His trunk will look really long when supported up straight.* He will need to develop the strength to lift his entire trunk up straight and maintain this position. So, if he is very tall, it will take him extra time to gain the strength to learn to sit with this optimal posture by himself.

## ACTIVITY #12: Supported Sitting, Facing You, on a Raised Surface

(Use upper or middle trunk support depending on the level of support needed.)

1. Take your baby's shirt off.
2. Place a piece of nonslip shelf liner (grip liner) on a firm, raised surface like the kitchen table or coffee table. The grip liner will sta-

bilize the pelvis and prevent it from sliding forward on the surface when he is supported in sitting.

3. Place him in supported sitting on the grip liner, facing you, with his legs fully supported on the surface (either "frog leg" or knees bent).

4. Place your hands on his trunk (back, sides, and front, depending on the level of support needed).

   a. Hold the back of his trunk at the level of his shoulder blades to provide upper trunk support.

   b. When he has accomplished sitting with upper trunk support, then lower your support to middle trunk support (between shoulder blades and waist).

   c. Tip: you will support the level of his trunk where it bends (where he has not learned or developed the strength to straighten it).

5. Provide the *strategic support* needed by following these steps:

   a. First overlap your fingertips horizontally on your child's back (fig. 2.19). Your fingers need to support the vertebrae (bones down the center of the back) (fig. 2.20). If your fingers are to the sides of the vertebrae, you will be pressing on the area where the

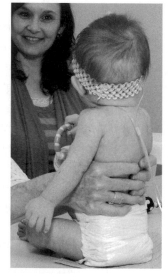

(fig. 2.19)

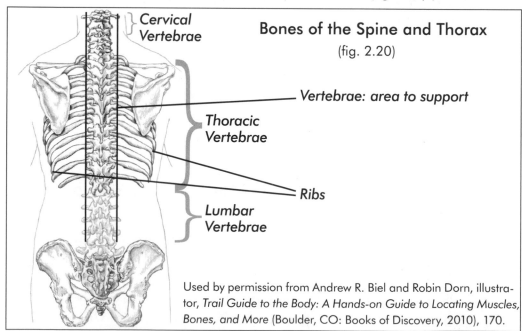

**Bones of the Spine and Thorax**
(fig. 2.20)

Cervical Vertebrae

Vertebrae: area to support

Thoracic Vertebrae

Ribs

Lumbar Vertebrae

Used by permission from Andrew R. Biel and Robin Dorn, illustrator, *Trail Guide to the Body: A Hands-on Guide to Locating Muscles, Bones, and More* (Boulder, CO: Books of Discovery, 2010), 170.

ribs attach to the vertebrae, and these are not stable joints to put pressure on. (See fig. 2.20.)

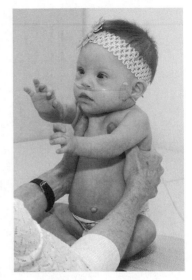

(fig. 2.21)

b. Then place your palms on the sides of your child's trunk.
c. Your thumbs will be vertical and placed on his chest (fig. 2.21).
d. Now that your hands are in the right places, you need to:
   - press inward with your fingers (on his back) to straighten his trunk and lift his pelvis up straight
   - then pivot your wrists as you move his trunk slightly forward, then downward (so he is grounded on the surface), and then upward.
e. Then look at his side view and check his posture to make sure his pelvis and trunk are up straight.

6. Talk to him and have him watch you and engage with you while you talk to him. Make sure you are both at eye level and encourage him to lift his head and maintain the lift for as long as tolerated.
7. Periodically look at him from the side to double-check that he is supported in the ideal position.

## ACTIVITY #13: Supported Sitting, Sideways in Front of You, on a Raised Surface

1. Take your baby's shirt off.
2. Place a piece of grip liner on a firm, raised surface such as the kitchen table or coffee table.
3. Place him sitting on the grip liner, sideways to you, with his legs in the "frog leg" position fully supported on the surface.
4. Place your hands on the front and back of his trunk, providing the level of support needed (upper or middle trunk support).
   a. Place one hand horizontally on his back (where it bends) and press forward and upward to lift and straighten his trunk and move his pelvis upright and tilted a little forward (fig. 2.22).
   b. Place your other hand horizontally on his chest with your thumb and index finger stretched apart and supporting under

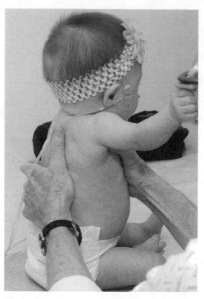

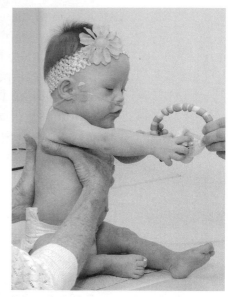

(fig. 2.22)                          (fig. 2.23)

each arm (armpit area). Lift his chest up by pressing in with your palm so he is sitting with the optimal posture (fig. 2.23).

   c. Make sure the hand on the back is lower than the hand on the chest. Use the hand on the back to lead the support (primary action) and the hand on the chest to take up the slack (secondary action). You support his trunk and pelvis in the optimal position by the interplay of pressure between your hands.

5. Encourage him to lift his head to watch a toy or look at people in the environment. Have him hold his head up as long as tolerated.

6. When he can hold his head and upper trunk erect, then you can lower your hands (on his back and front). Place your hand on his back where his trunk bends forward. Place your other hand on his chest with your fingers together and use your palm to press in and lift his chest. Your hand will be just below nipple level. Then follow step 4c above.

7. When your baby can hold his head and middle trunk up with this support, you can introduce toys, having him play by reaching and batting at rattles suspended from a play gym or having him hold and shake lightweight toys (like links). He may need more support since he is activating his arms.

8. This sitting position can also be practiced with your child sitting sideways across your lap. However, it will be more difficult to stabilize his pelvis to keep it from sliding.

# ACTIVITY #14: Supported Sitting on the Floor

1. Take off your baby's shirt and place a piece of grip liner on the floor.
2. Sit on the floor and place him sitting on the grip liner, sideways to you, with his legs fully supported on the surface in the "frog leg" position.
3. Hold his trunk and lift his pelvis up straight. Place one of your legs behind his pelvis and roll your knee against his pelvis to stabilize it and maintain it in the proper position. Place your other leg over his legs ("frog leg" position) to stabilize them.
4. Once his pelvis is supported with your legs, then use your hands on the front and back of his trunk to provide the level of support needed (fig. 2.24).

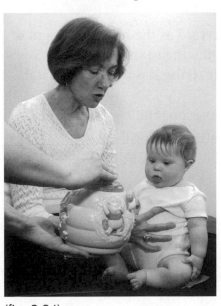

(fig. 2.24)

   a. Place one hand horizontally on his back (where it bends) and press forward and upward to lift and straighten his trunk.
   b. Place your other hand horizontally on his chest (just below nipple level) with your fingers together, and use your palm to press in and lift his chest.
   c. Make sure the hand on the back is lower than the hand on the chest. Use the hand on the back to lead the support (primary action), and the hand on the chest to take up the slack (secondary action). You support his trunk and pelvis in the optimal position by the interplay of pressure between your hands.
5. When he is comfortable with the position, place a 6- to 7-inch (15- to 18-cm) bench over his legs and against his abdomen. (You will need to hold the front of his pelvis (below his navel) or block his legs to stabilize his pelvis, since you won't be able to use your leg.) Then he can prop on the bench while watching toys, and when he is strong enough, he can prop on one hand while playing with toys with the other. (If you don't have a bench, you can use a small plastic stepstool or a sturdy box with two sides cut out to accommodate his legs.)

# Pulling to Sit

Throughout the day, you will be frequently moving your child up to sitting from lying on his back—for example, when he wakes up from a nap or when you are finished changing his diaper. Having your child assist you in moving him to a sitting position is a great game to play with your child. He will learn that when you say "up" and put your hands in front of him, he will get ready to play the game of pulling up to sit. He will enjoy having this game to play with you, and he will be excited. This skill will help your child develop strength in the muscles on the front side of his body in his neck, shoulders, elbows, hands, and abdomen.

## Components

The components to focus on are:

1. Chin tuck and lifting the head forward as the first movement to initiate and then maintain while moving to sit
2. Activation of the shoulder muscles so the shoulder joint is stabilized
3. When held in the semi-reclined position, ability to bend the elbows to pull himself to the midline sitting position
4. Ability to grip an adult's thumbs and hold on while pulled to sit

## Tendencies

The tendencies are:

1. for the child to be pulled to sit with the head leaning back or the head in line with the body
2. for the adult to hold the child's wrists so he does not learn to grip, hold on, and pull
3. for the adult to pull him to sit with his shoulders and arms limp (which is dangerous for his shoulder joints)

## Setup for Learning

In the beginning, your child will need maximum support to learn the first component of tucking his chin and holding the position. The best setup is to place him on a raised surface, and you kneel on the floor. He will do best if semi-reclined on pillows, folded towel(s), or in an infant carrier. You will need to be positioned in the right place so that when he looks at you, he tucks his chin. Then you can provide shoulder girdle support so he only needs to focus on tucking his chin and lifting his head (fig. 2.25). You can initiate the move up to sit (by rolling his shoulders forward) and then wait for him to lift his head and tuck his chin before you move him up to sit. When he knows the game

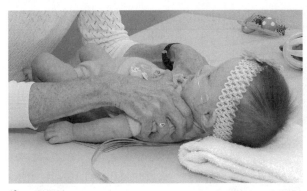

(fig. 2.25)

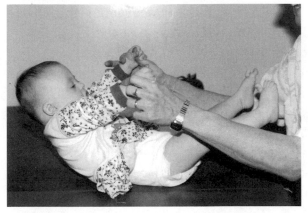

(fig. 2.26)

and consistently lifts his head and tucks his chin from the semi-reclined position, then you can decrease the support under his head and trunk, and eventually move him to sit from lying on his back.

After he has learned the head control needed for moving to sit, you will need to test when he is ready to pull to sit with two-hand support. You can start with your baby in the semi-reclined position to introduce the skill. You will place your thumbs in his palms and use your fingers to hold his wrists (and forearms if needed). You will hold his arms in the diagonal direction with a little traction to cue him that you want him to move up to sit. Give him the verbal cue "up" and wait for him to tuck his chin. Then move him to sit and praise him. When he tucks his chin, you will feel that he activates his upper body and shoulders and then it is safe to move him to sit. If his upper body and shoulders are limp and if he does not tuck his chin, he is not ready to be moved to sit. If this skill is practiced properly each time, then he will learn the right way to do it.

When your baby is familiar with pulling to sit from the semi-reclined position, decrease the support under his head and trunk until he is able to pull to sit from lying on his back (fig. 2.26). Some children do best if allowed to have a folded towel under the head to start the head with a little chin tuck. Continue to provide this minimal support if it helps your child be more successful.

By this time, pulling to sit will be a very familiar game and your baby will be proud to practice it with you. If he consistently tucks his chin and activates his shoulders, then he is ready for the next challenge. When you pull him to sit, stop in the semi-reclined position (approximately 30 degrees from the vertical), then pause and wait for him to bend his elbows to actually pull himself to the midline sitting position. By doing this, he is developing the skill of pulling himself to sit and is gaining elbow strength.

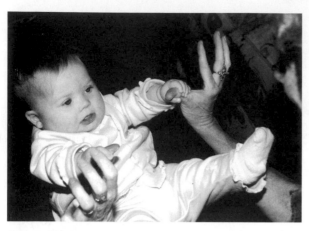

(fig. 2.27)

The last challenge is to develop your baby's grip strength. The goal will be for him to grip your thumbs and maintain the grip while pulled to sit (fig. 2.27). Teaching him to hold your thumbs is best because they are larger than your other fingers and that makes them easier to grasp. In earlier stages, you have placed your thumbs in his palms to stimulate his grasp, but you have always assisted his grasp by supporting his wrists with your other fingers.

After he has mastered the chin tuck and elbow bending, then you can reduce the wrist support you are providing when you pull him to sit. If you do not gradually decrease your support, he will become dependent on it and expect you to support his wrists. To lessen your support, you can place your index fingers over the tops of his wrists. He will feel less support and then learn to use a stronger grip on your thumbs. With practice, he will develop the strength to grip, hold on, and pull to sit.

## Guidelines

*If he is not motivated to pull to sit, does not tuck his chin, and his arms are limp, do not pull him up.* Only practice pulling to sit if he tucks his chin and actively holds on with his hands and pulls with his arms.

*Pulling to sit needs to be done correctly or your child is at risk for shoulder joint damage and too much stress on his neck.* Practice when he actively participates and practice with the level of support that he needs.

*Practice pulling to sit when he will naturally be motivated to do it.* Do it after diaper changes, when he wants to be picked up, or when he wants to sit up.

*Practice when it is functional for him.* He will not like practicing it for several consecutive repetitions. It is best to practice it when it is functional, like every time you move him to sitting.

*If he arches his head and trunk when you hold his hands to practice pulling to sit,* do not practice at that time. Give him a break and tickle his chest and then try again. If he continues to arch, then it is not a good time to practice. If he has a habit of arching when lying on his back, then give him more support with a couple of pillows under his head and trunk to position him in the semi-reclined position to see if this helps.

## ACTIVITY #15: Chin Tuck with Shoulder Support

1. Place your child on a raised surface such as the bed or coffee table (with grip liner under his pelvis to prevent sliding). Position him semi-reclined with one or two pillows under his head and trunk. Add a folded towel under his head to tilt his head forward.
2. Kneel on the floor and have him tuck his chin to look at you.
3. Place the palms of your hands on the tops of his shoulders with your fingers on his back and your thumbs horizontal on his upper chest (to the sides of his breastbone).
4. Talk to him and encourage him to tuck his chin to look at you. Roll his shoulders forward, and, if his chin is tucked, lift him to sitting.
5. As tolerated, decrease the support under his head and trunk and work toward consistent chin tuck when pulled to sit, lying on the surface with a folded towel under his head.

 ## ACTIVITY #16: Pulling to Sit with Two-Hand Support

1. Place your child on a raised surface such as a bed or sofa with grip liner under his pelvis to prevent sliding. Position him semi-reclined with one or two pillows under his head and trunk. Add a folded towel under his head to tilt his head forward.
2. Kneel on the floor and have him tuck his chin to look at you.
3. Place your thumbs horizontally above his chest and say "up" and encourage him to reach for them and hold them. If needed, place your thumbs in his palms. To assist his grasp, use your fingers to hold his wrists (hands and forearms).
4. Position his arms in the diagonal direction with his elbows straight and give a gentle pull (traction). Wait for him to tuck his chin, lift lift his head, and activate his shoulders, and then pull him to sit.
5. As tolerated, decrease the support under his head and trunk and work toward consistent chin tuck and head lift when pulled to sit, lying on the surface with a folded towel under his head (fig. 2.28).

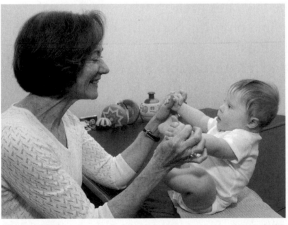

(fig. 2.28)

6. When Step 5 is mastered, pull him to sit and stop at 30 degrees from the vertical position. Wait for him to bend his elbows to pull himself to the vertical sitting position.

7. When Step 6 is mastered, work on his grasp strength and challenge him to hold your thumbs when pulled to sit.

# Supported Kneeling

In Stage 1 you used supported kneeling at a 7-inch (18-cm) cushion to help your child learn to prop on his elbows and lift his head. During this stage, an 8- to 9-inch (20- to 23-cm) high cushion is used to teach him to straighten his trunk in preparation for sitting, while continuing to develop propping on arms and reaching.

## Components

When your child is supported in kneeling, the components to focus on are:

1. Maintaining head lift, balanced between lift and chin tuck
2. Arm strength through propping on elbows (or hands) and reaching
3. Trunk up straight and arched in the low back area
4. Legs supported together with hips and knees bent, and knees together (neutral hip rotation), which will stretch the hips if there is tightness due to the frog leg posture
5. Weight bearing on the legs (preparation for the hands-and-knees position in the future)

## Tendencies

The tendencies are:

1. To arch the head and trunk excessively
2. To bend the trunk in the low back area
3. To keep his knees apart and pointing outward so his toes touch (outward rotation of the hips)
4. To straighten his hips and fall/thrust forward when he arches, if his legs are not properly supported with his hips bent (and if the cushion is not stabilized)

## Set Up for Learning

Supported kneeling will be an easy position for play while your child is developing head, arm, trunk, and leg strength. This position plays a crucial role in this stage because it reinforces the trunk position needed for the ideal sitting posture. It will provide a period of time to practice this posture in a relaxed way while your child is playing. If his arms are weak, this position gives him an easy way to prop and reach.

## Guidelines

*Use a variety of toys to entertain him and encourage him to stay in the position.* Let him prop on his elbows or hands, lean his trunk against the surface, or reach for toys, and you provide trunk or arm support to help him stay in the position.

*Support his legs with his hips and knees bent* to help him be stable in the position with a stable base and to inhibit arching and thrusting forward out of the position.

*Use a soft surface to lean his trunk against* so he is comfortable. Sofa cushions or firm foam cushions are ideal. Also have a soft, padded surface such as carpeting or a blanket under his knees.

*If he resists the position, try to figure out why.* This should be an easy position with your support, so experiment to help him tolerate it.

 ## ACTIVITY #17: Supported Kneeling in front of 8- to 9-inch Cushion

1. Sit on your heels on the floor and hold him sideways across your lap, facing away from you, and position his hips and knees bent and his knees together.
2. Place a soft, firm 8- to 9-inch (20- to 23-cm) cushion in front of you and stabilize it against furniture so it does not slide. Place him in kneeling with his knees together in between your knees and with his elbows (or hands) propping on the surface (fig. 2.29).
3. His knees will be close to the cushion and his pelvis will be slightly lifted, resting on your thighs (not on his heels). His hips and knees

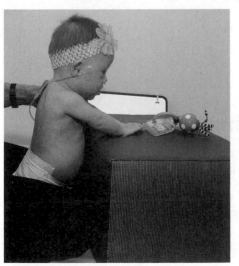

(fig. 2.29)

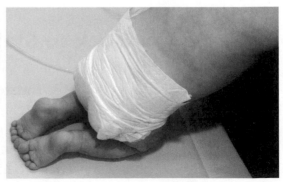

(fig. 2.30)

will be bent and you need to support his trunk so it is straight and arched in the low back area (fig. 2.30).

4. Provide support to the sides of his trunk or his low back to maintain it in the right position. If his trunk is in the right position, then assist in playing with the toys (propping or reaching).

# Rolling

Rolling gives your baby the freedom to move from one position to another or move from one place to another. He can choose when he wants to be on his back or on his stomach, and he can change the position when he wants to. He can also choose to roll across the floor to get a toy. During this stage, he will learn to roll from his stomach to his back and from his back to his stomach. Generally, rolling from stomach to back is easier and develops first. Rolling is a whole body exercise so he will need to activate his head, arms, abdominals, and legs, and he will practice weight shifting.

## Motor skills

The motor skills to focus on are:

1. rolling from back to side, side to stomach, and then back to stomach, and
2. rolling from stomach to back

## Tendencies

The tendencies are:

1. to roll in either direction by arching the whole body
2. to roll better over one side
3. for the arm position to block the roll
4. for the leg position to block the roll

# Rolling from Back to Stomach

Rolling from back to stomach is harder than rolling from stomach to back because it requires two steps. The steps are:

1. rolling from back to side-lying; and
2. rolling from side-lying to stomach.

Your baby will generally learn to roll from his side to his stomach first. Then when he learns to roll from his back to his side, he will be ready to practice putting both steps together.

## Components

The components to focus on are:

1. activating his abdominal muscles and kicking his legs up 90 degrees or more and engaging in hand-to-foot play to help him roll from his back to his side
2. placing his lowermost arm and leg straight so he can roll from his side to his stomach
3. putting 1 & 2 together and moving with momentum to roll from his back to his stomach

## Tendencies

The tendencies are:

1. to roll from back to stomach by excessively arching the head, trunk, and legs
2. to place the lowermost arm with the elbow below the shoulder, which blocks the roll from side lying to his stomach
3. to position both legs or the lowermost leg bent 90 degrees at the hip, which blocks the roll from side-lying to his stomach

## Set Up for Learning

Your baby will generally learn to roll from his back to his side when he can kick his legs up vertically or engage in hand-to-foot play (fig. 2.31). With his legs in this position, he may turn his head to look at something, or his legs may get off balance and then his body will fall or roll to the side. With practice, he will learn to use his legs to initiate rolling to side-lying.

Some children use the total body arching pattern to roll, but this method should be discouraged. It is better for your child to learn to use his stomach muscles to raise his legs to initiate rolling than to use head and trunk arching movements. At this stage, he needs to counterbalance the strength on his backside by developing strength on the front side of his body.

You will need to wait for your baby to develop the strength needed to kick his legs up so he can roll from his back to the side. While you are waiting, you can help him learn to roll from his side to his stomach by providing the proper support, as described in Activity #18.

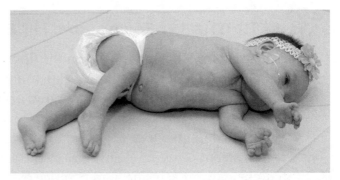

(fig. 2.31)

When he is able to roll from his back to his side and from his side to his stomach, he will be ready to practice rolling from his back to his stomach. You can help him especially after he moves to his side by giving him trunk/pelvic support to block him from rolling to his back. When he is on his side, see if his lowermost arm or leg blocks the roll and provide the support needed. If his elbow is below his shoulder, raise his arm so his elbow is in line with or above his shoulder. If his lowermost hip is bent, straighten it. Removing these "blocks" will help him experience success with rolling. He will need to learn to move his body in a coordinated way to roll from his back to his stomach. It will be easier for him if he moves quickly because the momentum will carry him over to his stomach.

Your baby will roll when he is motivated to do it. If he does not roll right away, it could be that he loves being on his back and has no desire to be on his stomach. When he likes being on his stomach, he will be motivated to roll to that position.

## ACTIVITY #18: Rolling from Side to Stomach

1. Place your baby on his back on the floor.
2. Roll him to side-lying.
3. Place your hand behind his trunk/pelvis to stabilize him in side-lying and to prevent him from rolling back.
4. Place his underneath arm with his elbow above his shoulder and hold it there.
5. Wait and see if he will try to roll to his stomach. If not, see if his legs are blocking the roll because the hips are bent. In particular, straighten the lowermost hip and see if he can roll over with this support.
6. Repeat over his other side. See if it is easier to roll over a particular side and practice over that side first.
7. Continue to practice until he easily rolls from his side to his stomach consistently.

## ACTIVITY #19: Rolling from His Back to His Side

1. Place your baby on his back on the floor.
2. Encourage him to kick his legs up or engage in hand-to-foot play.
3. Place a toy to the side of his face and arm, out of his reach.
4. He will be interested in the toy and turn his head, and he will move to his side. If he does not move to his side, assist him with the gross movement of swinging his legs to the side playfully.
5. Repeat over each side, and practice over his preferred side to help him be successful.

## ACTIVITY #20: Rolling from His Back to His Stomach
(fig. 2.32, 2.33, 2.34, 2.35)

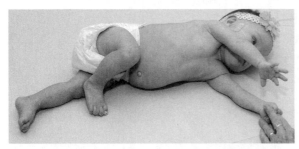

(fig. 2.32)

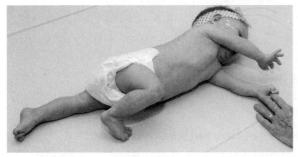

(fig. 2.33)

1. Place your baby on his back on the floor.
2. Place a toy to the side of his face, and slightly above his head. Experiment with toys to find one that highly motivates him.
3. Wait for him to roll to his side. Then provide intermittent support if needed when side-lying to help him continue moving to his stomach.
4. If he is blocked by his lowermost arm or leg in side-lying, provide timely support to help him continue moving to his stomach.

5. Help him practice moving with momentum so it is easier to complete the roll to his stomach. For fun, you can hold his uppermost arm and playfully give him a gentle pull and rock him to assist rolling from his side to his stomach.
6. Repeat over each side, and practice over his preferred side to help him be successful.

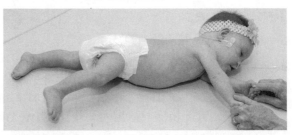

(fig. 2.34)

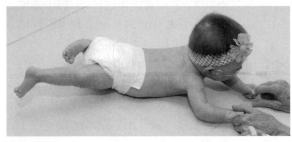

(fig. 2.35)

# Rolling from Stomach to Back

Babies with Down syndrome may accidentally roll from stomach to back very early. If a baby's elbows are under his shoulders and if he shifts his weight to one side by leaning or turning his head, then he will "fall over" and roll to his back. Later, when he is able to prop well on his arms and uses a variety of arm positions, it may be harder for him to roll because his elbows are too wide apart. To learn to roll from his stomach to back, he will need to learn to tuck his elbow in or move it under his shoulder, and then weight shift over it (fig. 2.36).

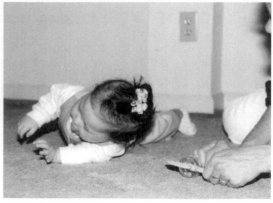

(fig. 2.36)

## Components

The components to focus on are:
1. the elbow or hand he is moving over is positioned under the shoulder
2. the leg he is moving over is in line with his hip
3. he is comfortable with weight shifting and falling to the side

## Tendencies

The tendencies are:
1. to position the elbow or hand he is moving over wider than his shoulder when propping
2. to position his arm along the side of his trunk
3. to place the leg he is moving over in the "frog leg" position
4. to be fearful of weight shifting and falling to the side
5. to try to push off with his leg and foot and rest his opposite arm on the surface beside his trunk so his arm blocks the roll

## Set Up for Learning

It is best to practice rolling from stomach to back when your child wants to move out of the position. You will notice that he is tired or becoming fussy and then you can tuck his elbow under his chest and guide him to roll to his back. He will also become familiar with the weight shift when you practice reaching in stomach-lying. With practice, he will learn the movements for rolling over and will do it with control. Don't worry if it takes him longer to learn to roll from stomach to back at a later time because he will stay on his stomach for longer periods and become stronger in this position.

# ACTIVITY #21: Rolling from Stomach to Back

1. Place your baby on his stomach, propping on his elbows with his elbows under his shoulders.
2. Sit on your heels with your knees at his feet. (Or, place him on a raised surface such as a bed and kneel in front of him at eye level to him.)
3. Make sure the leg he is moving over is straight, in line with his trunk.
4. Hold one elbow and tuck it under his chest and then he will roll over that side and onto his back.
5. If he rolls over quickly, assist him so he does not become scared.
6. Repeat over the other side.

## Guidelines

*Rolling is easier on a soft surface like a bed because it gives.* Your baby will do it there before he does it on the floor. He also will be more comfortable with the ease of weight shifting.

*He may roll better over one side and then learn to roll over the other side later.* Practice over his preferred side so he is successful in achieving the skill. Once he masters rolling over the preferred side, then you can practice over his other side.

*The key in using toys to encourage rolling is to pick toys your child really wants and put them in the right place.* When he is rolling from his stomach to his back, place the toy to his side and upward to see if he will watch it and roll over. You could also position yourself to his side and above him and see if he will roll over to see you.

*When encouraging him to roll from his back to his side, place the toy or yourself to his side and just out of reach.* Place the motivator at head or shoulder level. When he is rolling from his side to his stomach, place the toy above his head and diagonally from his shoulder.

*How he uses rolling will give you information about whether he is an "observer" or "motor driven."* Observers tend to roll to a person or a toy and stop after one or two rolls. Children who are motor driven frequently keep rolling around the room. (See Introduction for more about these two types of children.)

*Practice rolling when it is functional.* When you are moving your baby between his back and stomach or if he shows the interest in changing positions, give the necessary support to have him participate with rolling rather than doing it for him.

## 🏃 MOTOR MILESTONE CHECKLIST

### *Back-lying*

- ❑ He holds onto his clothes on his chest
- ❑ He reaches 2-3 inches (5-7.5 cm) above his chest or shoulder to touch a toy
- ❑ He reaches with elbows straight and holds the position 10 seconds while playing with toy
- ❑ He holds and shakes a lightweight toy
- ❑ He moves his legs to the bridge position and rubs the inside borders of his feet together
- ❑ He kicks his legs up with his feet above his hips
- ❑ With his feet supported above his chest, he holds onto his feet
- ❑ He touches his hands to his knees without support
- ❑ He engages in hand-to-foot play with his pelvis lifted off the surface

### *Stomach-lying*

- ❑ He lifts his head up and props on his elbows for 60 seconds
- ❑ He lifts his head up and props on his elbows for 5-10 minutes with legs straight and together
- ❑ He props on his hands 10 seconds
- ❑ He props on his hands for 1 minute with legs straight and together
- ❑ He reaches forward for a toy with his hand on the surface
- ❑ He weight shifts over one elbow and lifts his other hand up off the surface to reach for a toy

### *Supported Sitting*

With upper trunk support, he holds his head up for:
- ❑ 20-30 seconds
- ❑ 1-2 minutes
- ❑ 5 minutes

With mid trunk support, he holds his head and upper trunk up for:
- ❑ 1-2 minutes
- ❑ 5 minutes

*(continued on next page)*

### Pull to Sit

- ❏ With the tops of his shoulders supported, he tucks his chin when moved to sit
- ❏ With two-hand support, he tucks his chin when pulled to sit
- ❏ With two-hand support, he tucks his chin, and when semi-reclined, he bends his elbows to pull up to sitting
- ❏ With two-hand support, he tucks his chin and has grip strength to hold an adult's thumbs when pulled to sit

### Supported Kneeling at 8- to 9-inch (20- to 23-cm) Cushion

With legs maximally supported,

- ❏ He will straighten his trunk and arch his low back
- ❏ He will prop on his elbows or hands, maintaining the optimal trunk posture
- ❏ He will reach and play, maintaining the optimal trunk posture

### Rolling

- ❏ While on stomach, he leans his head to the side and "accidentally" rolls over
- ❏ He rolls from stomach to back consistently and often
- ❏ In side-lying with underneath arm and /or leg supported, he rolls to his stomach
- ❏ If supported in side-lying, he rolls from his side to his stomach
- ❏ He rolls from his back to his side
- ❏ He rolls from back to stomach

# 3

# Stage 3: Pivoting, Sitting, and Beginning Supported Standing

## Introduction

During this period, your baby will give you lots of surprises. Just as she surprised you with her first roll, she will show you her first pivot to move to toys in her vicinity, as well as how she can sit tall by herself and stand with your support. You will set her up to learn each skill, help her practice the parts, and then she will put them together. You need to wait for the magical moment when she does it by herself. Many of the new positions are off the floor, and your baby will have to practice to develop the increased strength and balance necessary to use them.

### Motor Skills

The motor skills to focus on in this third stage of development are:
1. pivoting after toys in stomach-lying
2. sitting independently on the floor
3. moving to sit with support
4. moving out of sitting with support
5. supported kneeling and moving from kneeling to sitting
6. sitting on a bench
7. supported standing

### Components

The components to focus on are:
1. weight-shifting by practicing pivoting, moving in and out of sitting by moving to the side, and sitting balance

2. sitting (with an optimal posture) with head, trunk, and pelvis fully erect, and using trunk strength to maintain the position (not the arms). With this posture, your child will learn to rotate her trunk to look all around and to move in and out of the position
3. standing (with an optimal posture) with a narrow base, feet pointing straight, mild knee bending (unlocked knees), trunk straight, and hands holding onto an edge or to your fingers

## Tendencies

The tendencies are:
1. to use rolling as the method of mobility and never learn to pivot
2. to sit with a slouched posture and prop hands on the floor to maintain the position
3. to avoid weight shifting and moving off balance to the side
4. to move in and out of sitting through the center moving her legs into a split
5. to kneel with a wide base and with hips and knees turned outward (hip external rotation), which will prevent weight shifting to move to sit
6. to stand with a wide base, feet and knees turned out, inside borders of the feet collapsed into the surface, knees locked, back arched, and abdomen leaning against the surface

This is a crucial time in your child's development because it is during this period that children typically develop "bad habits" or abnormal compensatory movement patterns. (See the Introduction for an explanation of these movement patterns.) In this chapter you will learn the compensatory movement patterns to avoid (the tendencies listed above) and the movement patterns/components to encourage in their place.

## Guidelines

*Your child will show you which skills she likes best.* Practice the skills she is ready to learn even if she briefly uses the less preferred ones. The key is to be sensitive to her preferences and continue to help her with the harder positions until they become easier and she likes them. Do not impose the skills she does not like or she will become more resistant to them.

*Your child's temperament will become more obvious and you will notice whether she is an observer or motor driven child.* Observing and understanding her temperament will give you insight into what she likes to do and why, and it will help you plan strategies to practice the skills she does not like. For example, Samantha was motor driven and loved to pivot, pull to sit, move out of sitting, and move up onto her hands and knees. However, she did not like to sit and would scoot to move out of sitting. Therefore, sitting was practiced for short periods, during her "best" times, and with her favorite motivators. She tolerated sitting under these conditions and learned to sit.

*There is a sequence of steps for each skill.* See what your child is able to do and proceed from there.

*The pace and rhythm will change depending on the skills you are practicing.* When pivoting, pulling to sit, and moving out of sitting, the pace is faster; when using sitting, supported kneeling, and supported standing, the pace is slower. Sequence how you practice the skills to match your child's learning style.

*Vary the way you practice the skills to see what works best for your child.* Some children are able to play and practice for 30-45 minute periods if the skills are changed often. Other children do best practicing for short periods (5 minutes), using a different skill for each practice period. Begin with skills your baby likes and briefly intersperse the skills she does not like. Use the best motivators, particularly with the harder activities. If practice time is limited on certain days, focus on what she wants to do and needs your help to do.

*These skills require a new level of strength, so your child will fatigue faster until she builds up the strength needed for each skill.*

# Pivoting in Stomach-lying

To pivot, your child will need to learn to use her arms to pull her body sideways to move to a toy (fig. 3.1, 3.2). She will be ready to practice pivoting when she has mastered reaching forward when lying on her stomach. The goal will be to pivot in a full circle, in each direction. Learning to pivot will prepare her for the next skill, crawling on her belly, using her arms to pull her body forward on the floor.

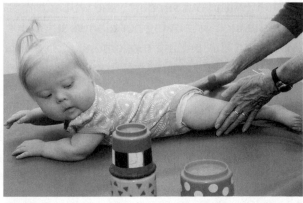
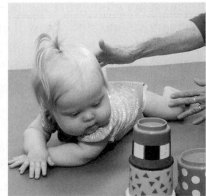

(fig. 3.1)                                          (fig. 3.2)

## Components

The components to focus on are:

1. turning the head to look to the side and side-bending the trunk to move toward the motivator
2. weight-shifting, moving the elbows sideways, and pulling with the leading elbow to pull the trunk sideways to move to the toy, one pivot at a time
3. deliberate, fast, and efficient arm movements to move quickly in a circle
4. coordinated leg movements that develop after your child masters moving her arms

## Tendencies

The tendencies are:

1. to see the toy and want it, but to give up trying to reach it because she does not know how to move there
2. to lie on her stomach with her head on the floor and reach her arm to touch the toy to the side of her shoulder
3. to need help to learn a motor plan because she will not know how to move her arms
4. to position her leg 90 degrees to the side of her trunk (due to her flexibility), which will block moving to the side

## Setup for Learning

It will be difficult for your baby to figure out how to pivot because she has not used her arms for pulling prior to this skill. She will have to grapple with the problem of how to move her arms to move her body to get to the toy. To give her a hint of what to do, wait for her to show an interest in moving to the toy (for example, turning her head and trunk to the right), and then move her left elbow very close to the right, and then she will move her right elbow to the side. Because her elbows are so close together (with your support), she will automatically move one, and this will give her the idea of moving her elbows sideways. Once she has this movement, she will add the pulling movement. Be patient and keep encouraging her while she experiments to discover how to do it.

To teach your child to pivot, her starting position will be propping on her elbows. You will place a toy to the side of her shoulder and encourage her to move to it. She will turn her head to look at the toy and will bend her trunk to turn toward the toy (fig. 3.3). She will then need to shift her weight between her arms, alternating pulling with one elbow and then placing the other elbow closer to the pulling elbow. From this position, she will move her pulling elbow sideways and then reach the toy (fig. 3.4).

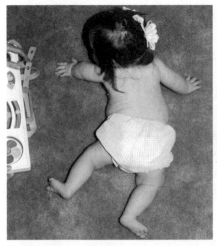
(fig. 3.3)

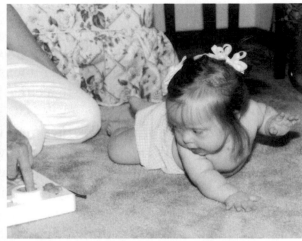
(fig. 3.4)

Once she has learned how to do one pivot to the toy, then you can place the toy at her waist, and she will need to do 2 pivots to move to the toy. She will continue to practice until she can follow the toy and pivot in a full circle. Once she knows how to do it, then practice will make her arms efficient and fast.

When your child first learns to pivot, she will primarily use arm and trunk movements. She may move her legs, but they will not assist her in pivoting. When she can pivot well, she will coordinate her leg movements with the arm movements to move quickly.

## Guidelines

***The Setup is important when teaching your child to pivot.*** You need to position yourself at her feet and make sure no toys or other stimuli are in front of her. Make sure that you or special toys are the only interesting stimuli for her to watch or engage with. With this set-up, she will turn to look at you and try to move to you.

***You will need to be creative to motivate her to keep pivoting.*** You need to use great motivators, such as crinkled tissue paper, a magazine, the TV remote, your cell phone, or a brother or sister calling her. You need to generate hoopla and excitement, and wiggle the toy to keep the momentum going so she moves at a fast pace. The key is to move the toy and yourself quickly so she keeps chasing you and the toy.

When she can pivot more easily, watch to see if she will pivot spontaneously to move to someone sitting on the floor with her or to something she wants. Some children pivot best when they are alone. She may pivot to see where you are if you walk to another room. For example, Joshua loved to be on his stomach and would pivot a couple times to move to a toy. However, he would do his best pivoting when his mother walked from the family room to the kitchen. When his mother moved out of sight, he would pivot to find out where his mother went.

*Encourage her to move toward the right and left sides to see if one direction is easier.* If one side is easier, focus on having her move in that direction. When she is able to move in a circle in that direction, begin moving in the other direction.

*Your child may try to roll rather than work on pivoting, since rolling is easier and established.* If she tries to roll, wiggle or rock her hips playfully to see if she will stay in the stomach-lying position. Or, roll her over a couple times and stop in stomach-lying. Try to get her interested in a toy and see if she will pivot again.

*The longer she uses rolling for mobility, the harder it will be for her to tolerate learning to use pivoting for mobility.* It is important to help her learn to pivot and to introduce it earlier rather than later. Pivoting is a necessary skill to teach pulling with her arms, which she will need to learn for combat crawling.

*Pivoting is a strenuous activity, especially when your child is just learning it.* It is best to practice this skill when your child feels fresh, alert, and active, and to do it for brief periods with the best motivator and setup. When she is tired or no longer interested, it is best to stop.

## Temperament

Children who are **motor driven** love pivoting and practice it more easily than children who are observers. The "motor driven" child keeps going and moves in a circle when she is strong enough to do the skill. The **observer** learns to pivot but prefers to do one or two pivots, play for awhile, and then do a couple more pivots. When encouraged to pivot in a circle, she may do it if the motivator is superb or if she has brief breaks to play with the motivator.

## ACTIVITY #1: Pivoting

1. Use a slippery, firm surface such as a slippery mat or hardwood floor. Dress your child in a short sleeve onesie so her arms and legs are bare. Place your child on her stomach, propping on her elbows.
2. Position yourself at your child's feet and remove all toys and stimuli that are in front of her. (If convenient, have her face a wall and then she will want to move sideways to you and the toys.)
3. Place a toy (best possible motivator) to the side of her shoulder or between her shoulder and waist. See if she turns her head to look at it and bends her trunk to that side.
4. See if she tries to reach for it or use her arms to move toward it.

5. If she is unable to move, then assist her so she learns the game. If the toy is placed to the side of her right shoulder, then move her left elbow close to the right and hold it there. After a pause, she will move her right elbow sideways. Then she can play with the toy. Practice this method until she can initiate moving one pivot by herself.

6. If you need an alternative to step 5, then move her elbows sideways playfully using the movements she would use to pivot (with exaggeration) for 3 pivots to a toy. Use this method to have her feel the movements until she will participate with practicing step 5.

7. Practice in each direction to see if one direction is easier. Continue to practice that direction until your child learns the skill and then have her learn the skill in the other direction.

8. With further practice, she will learn to pivot 2 times to move to the toy. Let her play with the toy and then move it again.

9. Work toward pivoting in a full circle. As your child pivots better, you can place the toy at her waist level and later at her feet, and she will move to it. Move yourself to stay positioned at her feet.

## SITTING ON THE FLOOR

In this stage, your baby will learn to sit on her own (fig. 3.5). She will be familiar with being supported in sitting and playing with toys, and she will initiate trying to move to sit. You may notice that she wants to sit up when you are holding her in your lap or when she is lying on the floor. She will lift her head up and try to move upward to sitting. Or, when she is in an infant seat, she may lean forward and try to sit up.

This is the time to help her learn to sit up tall and play by providing support at the two final levels, at the waist and pelvis. First your child needs to develop the strength (and endurance) in her back muscles to hold her trunk and

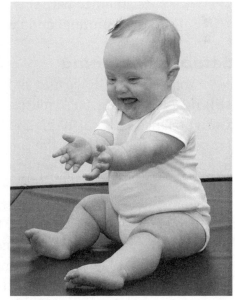

(fig. 3.5)

pelvis up straight, and then she can learn to use her abdominal muscles to maintain her balance.

## Components

The components to focus on are:

1. head maintained lifted and erect, balanced between head lift and chin tuck
2. trunk lifted up straight with an arch in the low back, maintained over time
3. pelvis up straight and the top of the pelvis tilting a little forward
4. legs in the ring sit (frog leg) position (hips and knees bent, knees turned out)
5. balance in sitting when she weight shifts forward, sideways, and backwards
6. trunk rotation with her trunk and pelvis up straight

## Tendencies

The tendencies are:

1. to lean the head forward or rest the head back on the neck
2. to bend the entire trunk and slouch forward; with this posture she will not be able to rotate her trunk
3. to prop hands on the floor for balance
4. to tilt the top of the pelvis back with the lower buttocks tucked under
5. to keep her knees straight and stiff with a wide base
6. to stabilize with this posture (described above) to balance with minimal or no weight shifting tolerated

## Setup for Learning

Your child will learn to sit using trunk strength and control. First she will develop strong back muscles to lift and hold the head and trunk up straight. Once she can do this and has the endurance to maintain the position for several minutes, then she can develop her abdominal muscles to control her balance when moving her trunk forward and back. When she can activate her back and stomach muscles effectively, they will work together to control her balance when she leans side to side. The final goal in trunk control is to rotate her trunk and maintain her balance.

A child with Down syndrome develops sitting differently than a typical child. This is because her arms are shorter relative to the length of her trunk. Because her arms are shorter, she will not be able to use the strategy of propping her hands on the floor to help her learn to sit. To observe the length of your child's arms relative to her trunk, hold her trunk up straight with her arms at her sides and see where her fingertips are. Her fingertips may not even touch the floor. With this short arm length, if she is placed with her hands propping on the floor in front of her, her trunk will be excessively bent forward. If this is how she practices sitting, she will not learn to sit with the optimal sitting posture.

Another consequence of the short arm length is that it will be difficult for your child to effectively use protective reactions when she falls sideways or backwards, especially if she falls fast. (*Protective reactions* refers to a child's automatic response to quickly straighten the arm and prop on the surface in an attempt to catch her balance and prevent a fall.) By the time your child's hand props, she will have fallen halfway to her side, and it will be hard to stop or control the fall so that she can recover her sitting balance. Therefore, she will need to learn to maintain her balance by primarily using her trunk. If she falls slowly, she can use her trunk and arms to stop the fall, and then she can move back up to sitting. It will be useful for her to use her arms to push up to sit and to prop when moving out of sitting and this will be practiced as she learns those skills.

Your child can practice propping her hands forward if they are placed on a raised surface, such as a 6- to 7-inch (15- to 18-cm) high bench, placed over her legs. As long as her trunk and pelvis are erect when she is propping, this setup will work. For a new sitter, it is best to have a large, firm, stable surface to prop on. Later, when she is working on sitting balance, she can prop her hands on her thighs and still maintain the optimal sitting posture.

When she is learning to sit on the floor, she will need her legs in the ring sit (frog leg) position as a stable base to balance over. It is important that her knees are bent so she does not learn to stabilize with stiff knees. After she learns to sit on the floor, then sitting on a bench will be practiced. Through this skill, she will learn to balance with a narrow base with her legs together and her hips in neutral rotation.

Your child will learn to sit following this progression:

1. straightening the middle trunk with support at her waist and pelvis
2. straightening the whole trunk and lifting the low trunk into an arch with support at her pelvis
3. using abdominal muscles to recover sitting balance when she weight shifts in all directions with support at pelvis or upper thighs
4. sitting without support

## Sitting with Waist Level Support

Your child learned to sit up tall with her middle trunk (and pelvis) supported in Stage 2. During this stage, the first goal is for her to learn to lift and hold her trunk up straight with support at her waist level (with her pelvis supported up straight). She will want to bend her trunk at the waist level because this is how her body tends to posture itself and later, after she sits independently, she will try to use this posture because she will feel like she can balance herself better with it. It is critical to be proactive and prevent this "bad habit" as early as possible or else she will not achieve the optimal sitting posture.

### Setup for Learning

When first practicing this skill, your child will do best if placed sideways in front of you, with your hands on the back and front of her trunk. To help her learn to hold her middle trunk up straight, you will hold her pelvis upright and support the back of her trunk just below the ribs and on the top of the pelvic bone. First she will need to feel the specific movement of her low back moving into an arch. This movement will assist her in lifting her trunk vertically. Your hand on the front of her trunk will also guide her trunk up straight.

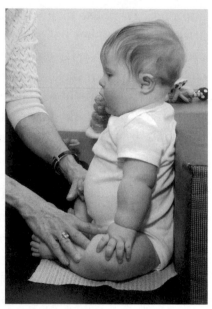

(fig. 3.6)

Once your child is able to straighten the middle trunk area, she will need to develop the strength to maintain the position over time. To do this, you can either seat her in a highchair or place her on the floor in front of the couch or another piece of furniture with firm, soft support down to the floor (fig. 3.6) (Activities 3 & 4). With this support behind her back, it is easier for her to lift her trunk up straight and hold it against the support. Practice using a variety of supported sitting positions. With practice, she will be able to hold her back up straight for 10 to 15 minutes. When she is able to hold her back straight consistently, then lower support can be provided.

### ACTIVITY #2: Supported Sitting with Front and Back Support

1. Take off your child's shirt and place her sitting on grip liner, sideways in front of you. She can be on a raised surface (such as the kitchen table) or on the floor. Position her legs in the ring sit position, feet touching or ankles crossed.

2. Spread your thumb and index finger apart and place them horizontally on your child's back, in the low trunk area, on the top edge of the pelvic bone. Press in and upward with your fingers and palm to

move (scoop) the lower trunk into an arch (fig. 3.7). Place your other hand horizontally on her chest or abdomen at the level needed to support the front of her trunk up straight.

3. If she tries to scoot her lower pelvis forward and under, or if her legs straighten, place your leg over her legs to stabilize her legs and prevent her pelvis from sliding forward. If additional pelvic support is needed, place your other leg behind her pelvis.

4. Entertain her by talking to her, singing, or having her siblings

(fig. 3.7)

play in the area so she watches them. If you want to entertain her with toys, place them on a raised surface such as a 6- to 7-inch (15- to 18-cm) high stepstool or bench. If she cannot hold her trunk up, then she can prop on the bench with one hand and play with the other hand or prop on both hands while you entertain her with toys. If she wants to hold and shake lightweight rattles, make sure she is able to lift her trunk while playing.

5. Encourage her to hold her head and trunk up tall for as long as tolerated.

## ACTIVITY #3: Supported Sitting with Back Supported against Couch or Cushion

1. Take off your child's shirt and place grip liner on the floor in front of a couch or a firm 9-inch (23-cm) high cushion. Place your child sitting on the grip liner with her pelvis up straight and supported against the cushion. Stabilize her pelvis so it does not slide forward.

2. Place her legs in the ring sit position with her knees bent. Place a 6- to 7-inch (15- to 18-cm) high cushion or bench in front of her with toys on it. If you use a cushion, place it against her legs and feet to stabilize them, and then the cushion will be close enough to prop on. If you use a bench, you need to support the front of her pelvis or her legs to stabilize them and prevent sliding or scooting forward.

3. When your child is supported in this position, she needs to learn to lift her trunk up against the cushion (behind her), and maintain it

there as long as possible. Provide intermittent support to cue her to lean back against the support if she moves her trunk forward.

4. Prop her hands on the cushion or bench to help her hold her trunk up straight. Watch how she props and plays and provide the necessary support or the right type of toys to help her maintain her trunk up straight. As she props on the bench and plays with toys, her trunk will move up and down. When her trunk is rounded, see if she straightens it in a few seconds by pushing up on her hands. If she leans forward for longer than 5 seconds, reposition her hands so she can prop and hold her trunk up straight. With practice, she will learn to hold her middle trunk up straight and maintain it while propping and playing with toys on this raised surface.

5. If she slowly leans slightly to one side, see if she will try to move back to the center. When she is in this position, you want her to be calm and stable while playing. If she is stable, she may have the control to recover her balance if she does a mild and slow weight shift. If she is unstable in the position, figure out the support or type of play needed to help her be stable and use organized movements.

## ACTIVITY #4: Supported Sitting in a Highchair or Reclining Chair

1. Put grip liner on the seat of a highchair, feeding chair, or feeding seat.
2. Place your child's pelvis up straight against the back of the seat and stabilize it there. Buckle the hip strap and tighten it.
3. Hold her trunk up straight against the back of the chair and see if she can maintain it. If needed, place a rolled-up towel on each side of her trunk to fill up the space.
4. Put on the tray and adjust it close to her chest/abdomen. If there is space between her trunk and the tray, use a small rolled-up towel to fill the space.
5. Place toys on the tray and play with her.
6. Use this sitting position for play if she can hold her trunk erect. Practice as long as tolerated.

## Sitting with Pelvic Support

When your child can sit and maintain her trunk up straight with support at her waist, you can lower your support by placing one hand on the back of her pelvis and your other hand on her lower abdomen, below her navel (fig. 3.8).

Your hand on the back of her pelvis will hold her pelvis up straight and lift it so the top of the pelvis tilts forward. Your hand on her abdomen will anchor her pelvis from sliding and will help her begin to activate her abdominal muscles for balance if she weight shifts in the small (mild) range.

When your child is familiar with this lower support, you can use your leg or a 5-inch (12.5 cm) cushion behind her pelvis to provide the support (rather than your hand) and continue to use your hand across the front of her lower abdomen to anchor her. With practice, she will develop the strength to hold her trunk up straight for several minutes. It will be helpful to place

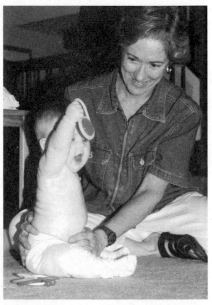

(fig. 3.8)

toys on a bench in front of her so they are raised and it is easy for her to play with them while maintaining her trunk erect. If toys are on the floor, they will be too low and she will lean her trunk forward to play with them.

When providing low trunk support, your child's pelvis needs to be positioned up straight rather than allowed to slouch back. If her pelvis leans back, her trunk will be rounded and she will not be able to sit tall.

## ACTIVITY #5: Supported Sitting with Pelvic Support

1. Take off your child's shirt and place her sitting on grip liner, sideways in front of you. Sit on the floor with your legs apart in front of you.
2. Place her legs in the ring sit posture and support them if needed.
3. Support the front and back of her pelvis. Place one hand horizontally on the back of her pelvis (middle of the pelvis) and press forward and upward with your palm to hold it up straight. Place your other hand horizontally on her lower abdomen under her navel, with your little finger at the crease of her thighs, pressing inward and down. The hand on the back of the pelvis leads the movement and the hand on the front stabilizes the pelvis. You will help her sit erect by the interplay of pressure between your hands.
4. Place a bench in front of her with toys on it. Use toys that encourage her to sit tall.
5. Practice as long as she is able to sit up straight and play with the toys.
6. If she leans back or to the side slowly, see if she will move back to the center.

7. When she is familiar with this position, provide less support by using your leg or a sofa cushion behind her to support the back of her pelvis. Place the grip liner under her pelvis and support the back of her pelvis up straight against your leg or the cushion. Place your hand on her lower abdomen as described above (step #3). Then follow steps 4-6.

## Sitting with Support to Balance Herself

By this time your child knows the sitting position, how to play in it, and how to hold her trunk and pelvis up straight with support. She knows the centered or balanced position. She is now ready to work on balancing herself when she leans to the side or backward. She needs to be given strategic and intermittent support so she can work on moving back to the center when she weight shifts. She also will learn that she needs to move herself back to the center to recover her balance rather than depending on you to catch her and move her.

The support you provide will depend on how far she leans and how quickly she falls. If she leans slowly and just a little bit, you can firmly support her opposite side at her pelvis or upper thigh and see if she will move back to the center. If she falls fast, you need to catch her to stop the fall and then hold her in the leaning position. From here, wait to see if she can move herself back to the center to regain her balance. As your child learns how to recover her balance, she will need less support to help her move back to the center.

Since your child has shorter arms, using her hands to catch herself when she falls will be less effective. She will need to learn to use her trunk control to balance herself effectively and maintain the centered position. When sitting on a firm surface and playing with toys, she will lose her balance frequently, and this is the best time to work on how she can move to recover her balance.

 **ACTIVITY #6: Supported Sitting with a Sofa Cushion for Support** (fig. 3.9)

1. Place your child sitting on the floor on grip liner with a sofa cushion behind her pelvis. Make sure her pelvis is up straight and firmly supported against the cushion. Stabilize the cushion against furniture or the wall to prevent sliding. Place her legs in the ring sit position.
2. Position yourself in front of her or sitting at her side.
3. Entertain her by talking to her or singing songs with gestures. Play pat-a-cake or so-big, clap her hands, and see if she can maintain her balance. Also test her balance using toys placed on a bench, having

her prop if needed. If she can maintain her balance, then test her further and let her hold and shake toys.

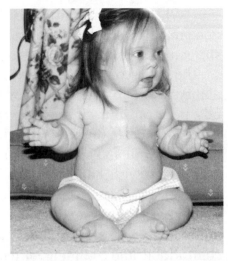

4. When your child weight shifts, provide intermittent and strategic support and see if she can move back to the center. If she leans back slowly, place your hand below her navel or on her upper thigh and see if she will move back to the center. If she leans to the side slowly, hold the opposite hip (pelvis or up-

(fig. 3.9)

per thigh/crease) and see if she will move back to the center. If she leans back quickly, catch her with the palm of one hand and place your other hand below her navel and see if she will move back to the center. If she leans to the side quickly, use the fingertips of one hand to catch her at her shoulder or trunk and use your other hand to firmly support the opposite pelvis or upper thigh to see if she will move back to the center.

5. Practice this position until she can maintain her balance consistently and controls the range and speed of weight shifting. When she masters her balance in this position, she will be ready to practice balance without support behind her pelvis.

## Sitting without Support

After your child has practiced these supported sitting positions, you will notice she has learned to sit tall and to balance herself with less support, and sometimes briefly without any support. She may continue to sit when you slide the sofa cushion away from behind her pelvis. Or, she may prop her hands on her thighs and sit while you entertain her (fig. 3.10). You will need to watch her cues because she will show you when she is ready to learn to sit without support.

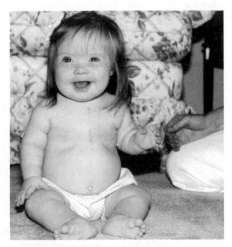

(fig. 3.10)

When she starts sitting by herself, you need to help her gradually increase the time she can maintain sitting. The longer she can sit, the more confidence she will have in her ability to sit. To help her sit for longer periods, position yourself at eye level to her and entertain her. If you are above her, she will look up at you and lose her balance. You can sing songs with hand motions ("Itsy Bitsy Spider"), play pat-a-cake or peek-a-boo, or talk to her. Try to keep the play calm, quiet, and centered in the midline. When she is comfortable and confident with maintaining her balance in sitting, she can play with toys or hold rings or lightweight rattles.

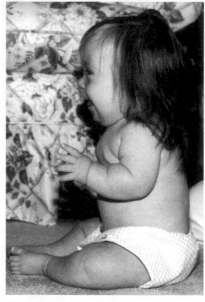

(fig. 3.11)

When she practices sitting by herself, she will be figuring out how to be stable and balance herself. She will experiment to see how far she can lift her trunk before she falls backwards and how much she can play with her hands before she falls over. She probably will learn that if she leans her trunk forward a little, she will not fall backwards. You can use pillows around her so she is safe while practicing on her own. This is the time to let her discover what she needs to do with her body to sit by herself.

All of a sudden, your child will consistently sit when you place her in sitting (fig. 3.11). She will still need supervision, though, until she develops effective balance when leaning in all directions, particularly backwards. For all children, learning to regain balance when they lean backwards is the hardest.

## ACTIVITY #7: Sitting Independently

1. Place your child sitting on the floor (or firm surface) on grip liner, facing you, with her legs in the ring sit position. (Alternative position: she sits sideways in front of you and you place your leg behind her pelvis, if she needs help to maintain her balance.)
2. Prop her hands on her upper thighs and see if she can hold the position and maintain her balance.
3. Entertain her by talking or singing, or with toys at eye level. If you have her look up above eye level, she will lose her balance and fall back.
4. Encourage her to balance in this position as long as tolerated. Begin with 10 seconds and work toward 2 to 3 minutes.

5. If she leans back or to the side, provide intermittent support at her upper thighs, and see if she can recover her balance and move back to the center.
6. When she can maintain her balance in the position for 2 to 3 minutes, see if she can let go with one hand to touch or hold a lightweight toy or bubbles.
7. With practice, she will learn to sit for 5 minutes or longer and will not need to prop her hands on her legs to maintain the position.

## Guidelines

*You need to use the supported sitting positions while she is playing.* Then she will become used to sitting, learn what the position is, how to use it, and how to hold it. She will learn the value of the sitting position for playing and will become motivated to sit.

*When your child is practicing sitting, take her shirt off to check her back.* By looking at her trunk from the side, you can see which section she holds up straight and which sections are rounded. This will help you determine the support needed so she sits with her trunk and pelvis erect.

*Use a firm surface for sitting—the floor, a table, or highchair.* With a firm base, your child will learn to sit up straight and she will know when she is off balance and try to move back to the center. On a soft surface, such as a bed or sofa cushion, she will easily lean and fall to the side because the surface will give as she leans into it. She will have difficulty balancing herself, as the surface will not allow her to move back to the center when she is off balance.

*Move at your child's pace and challenge her when she is ready to learn the next step.* Sitting takes time to develop properly, and you need to complete each step before moving on to the next step. This will help your child avoid common "bad habits," including leaning the trunk forward, tilting the pelvis back, holding the legs wide apart with the knees stiff and straight, and propping hands forward on the floor.

*Use toys appropriate to the level of sitting you are working on.* When your child is using her hands to prop or hold on, use toys or entertainment she can watch. If she is reaching for toys, suspend them on a play gym so she can touch and watch them rather than hold them. When she is watching toys, keep them at eye level or shoulder level. When she is working on holding her trunk up and balancing herself, it is best to do simple, calm hand activities. For example, a good activity is propping and playing with an activity center placed on a bench or stabilized over her thighs because it supports her in the centered position and keeps her attention focused in the center. If she plays with a rattle, waving her arm and shaking the toy will make it harder for her to hold her trunk up straight and maintain her balance.

### Temperament

Your child's temperament will influence her desire to sit. If your child is an **observer,** she will love to sit and will sit as long as she can physically tolerate it. Since she is motivated to sit, she will work to maintain her balance in sitting. She will enjoy playing and watching what's going on around her in sitting.

If your child is **motor driven,** she will not like to sit for long. She will prefer to move out of the position. She will need the best motivators to entertain her so she uses the position as long as possible. For example, Trey was motor driven and sitting had no value to him at first. He felt stuck and confined in the position. He preferred to roll, pivot, or move on his belly. When he did not want to sit, he would arch his back or scoot his buttocks forward to move out of sitting. Later, he worked on balancing himself in sitting when he was motivated to use the position.

## Moving to Sit with Support

After your child has learned to pull to sit from back-lying with two-hand support using chin tuck and grip strength, she will be ready to learn a more advanced way to move to sit that will prepare her for moving to sit on her own. In order to move to sit on her own, she will need to learn to push up with her arms and weight shift through her pelvis. In the next stage, she will learn to move to sit from her stomach or hands and knees. In this stage, she will learn how to push up to sit from lying on her side and to initiate the pelvic weight shift when moving from supported kneeling to sitting. By teaching her this new method, she will learn to move to sit by moving to the side, which is the goal. This will prepare her to move to sit by herself the proper way.

### Components

The components to focus on are:
1. moving from lying on her side up to sitting
2. propping on arms and pushing up to sit
3. weight shifting the trunk over the pelvis to move from side-lying up to sitting
4. weight shifting through the pelvis and pushing the pelvis into the ground (from the vertical position to the horizontal position)

### Tendencies

The tendencies are:
1. to resist this new movement pattern of moving to sit because she knows the old game of pulling to sit, and she wants to do this

2. to be uncomfortable with weight shifting and to dislike the transition of moving from side-lying to sitting
3. to resist weight bearing on one arm
4. to resist weight shifting over and through the pelvis
5. to move to sit without weight shifting, using her excessive hip flexibility and moving through the center with legs in a split

## Setup for Learning

To introduce this new skill, your child will need maximum support. You will place her on her side, in the "L" position, and then you will support the front and back of her trunk and move her up to sit (fig. 3.12, 3.13) This will be a new sequence for her to become familiar with, so she will need extra support to learn this new game. Once she is used to this movement and tolerates it, you

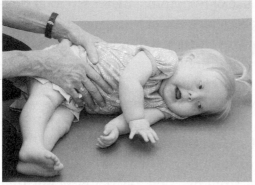 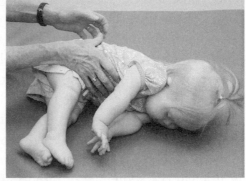

(fig. 3.12)                    (fig. 3.13)

can support her middle to lower trunk and weight shift her through her pelvis, and this will elicit lifting her head and propping on her elbow (fig. 3.14). From propping on her elbow, she will press her hand into the surface and then prop on her hand (fig. 3.15). From this position, you will move her to sitting in the midline (fig. 3.16). With practice, she will learn the sequence of steps to move to sit with the beginning (lying on her side in the "L" position), the middle (halfway between side-lying and sitting and propping on her arm), and end

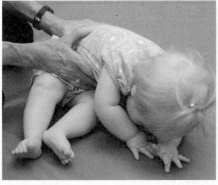 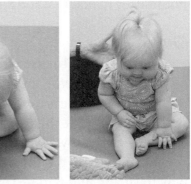

(fig. 3.14)                    (fig. 3.15)                    (fig. 3.16)

(playing in sitting). With your handling and support, she will learn how to participate and become comfortable with weight shifting.

In the beginning, you will move her quickly from her side to sitting so she participates but is not stressed, and ends in the desired sitting position. When she knows what to do and is comfortable with the transition, then you can move her slower and provide lower trunk or pelvic support, and she will need to use more control with her arms and trunk to move to sit.

Your child will only learn this method of moving to sit if you introduce it and practice it. She will not discover it on her own. If she does not learn this method, she may develop her own method of moving to sit by spreading her legs far apart and doing a wide split to move from her stomach up to sitting through the center. When she does this, she will also hold her knees stiff and straight. Children with Down syndrome figure out this method of moving to sit because it is easy for them to do because of hypotonia, increased joint flexibility in the hips (ligamentous laxity), and shortness of the arms. If they only use this method of moving to sitting, however, they will not learn to weight shift, which is critical for future skills, including moving out of sitting, moving in and out of kneeling, pulling to stand, standing balance, and walking. Instead, they will continue to use the wide leg position and stiff knees when standing and walking. This is the time to teach your child the preferred way to move to sitting before she figures out the split method.

Your child will not learn to move to sit by herself during this stage. She will learn the sequence of moving to sit from her side, particularly pushing up with her arms. She will also practice weight shifting through the pelvis with your support when she moves to sit from her side and when moving from supported kneeling to sitting (page 100, Activity 10). In the next stage, when she moves to sit from her stomach or hands and knees, she will move through side-lying and will know how to move from side-lying to sitting from her practice during this stage. Each child learns to sit using her own preferred method (from stomach or hands and knees). As long as she learns to move to sitting by moving to the side with weight shifting through the pelvis, it does not matter which method she chooses.

## Guidelines

*When using toys to encourage moving to sitting, place the toy in front of your child's feet.* When she is in side-lying, she will see the toy and move toward it. Once she is in sitting, the toy will be in the right place for her to play with it. If you place the toy at the level of her trunk, then she will stop halfway to play with the toy. If you move the toy when she reaches it, she will be upset. You want to place the toy at the endpoint. Then she will learn to move all the way to sitting and will be rewarded with the toy.

*Practice moving to sitting often during the day when it is functional for your child and she wants to do it.* If you practice moving to sitting after changing her diaper, when picking her up, and every time you move her to sit, she is naturally motivated and you will make the transition a habit for her. Just like she learned to pull to sit, she will learn to push up to sit. By practicing it when it is functional for her within her daily routine, she will practice it often and will give you her best performance since she is doing it for one repetition when it is meaningful to her.

*Practice moving over each side to see if one side is easier.* If it is easier over one side, practice over that side while your child is learning the skill so she is successful. When she has mastered moving to sitting over the easier side, then she can practice over the other side.

## Temperament

If your child is **motor driven,** she will like the movement of going from one position to another. Although she may not want to stay in sitting, she will like pushing up, weight shifting and moving over her side, and then moving up to sitting. She will not be fearful and will go with the flow of movement. If your child is an **observer,** she may resist the new movement sequence initially and will need practice to become familiar with it. She may be fearful with the weight shifting as she moves from side-lying up to sitting, but once she is sitting, she will be happy.

### ACTIVITY #8: Moving from the "L" Side-lying Position up to Sitting

1. Sit on your heels on the floor.
2. Place your child on the floor on her back, facing you. Roll her to her side with her hips bent 90 degrees and her knees straight (L position). Place a motivating toy at her feet and have her look at it so she is interested in moving to it. If she resists moving from her back to side-lying, then start her on her stomach and then roll her to her side (to the L position).
3. Maintain her in the L position on her side and use your knees (temporarily) to maintain her knees straight if she tends to bend them. (Once you start moving her to sit you will need to move your knees or else you will block her.) Her knees have to be straight when you are weight shifting her through her pelvis, or they will block her from moving completely to sitting.
4. Place your hands vertically (lengthwise) on the front and back of her trunk and then move her to sit so she becomes familiar with the movement.

5. When she is comfortable with the movement in step 4, place your hands on the front and back of her trunk, horizontally at her waist level. Begin the transition by weight shifting through her pelvis and moving her pelvis from the vertical position toward the horizontal position. (You will press her pelvis into the ground as you weight shift her.) After she has become familiar, when she feels you begin to weight shift her pelvis, she will lift her head and prop on her elbow. After you weight shift her pelvis halfway, and she props on her elbow, pause and then she will press her hand into the surface and push up onto her hand. After she props on her hand, then move her to the midline sitting position.

6. When she is comfortable with the support provided in step 5, and she knows how to push up with her hand, then provide less support and place your hand on the top of her pelvic bone. Use the web space between your thumb and index finger (and stretch your thumb and finger wide apart). Place your hand on top of her pelvic bone and weight shift her pelvis with this support. Wait for her to prop on her elbow and hand, then continue to provide the pelvic support and wait for her to move her trunk to the midline sitting position.

7. Practice moving over her right or left sides to see if one is easier and then practice over the easier side until she learns the skill. Then practice over the other side.

## Moving Out of Sitting

When your child can sit by herself, she needs to be taught how to move out of sitting. The goal will be to learn to move out of sitting by moving to the side. To do this, she will need to be comfortable with falling to the side, propping on her hands with both hands to one side, rotating her trunk, moving down to the floor, and landing on her stomach. You will begin with having her tolerate the gross movements with support and become familiar with the beginning (weight shifting to the side or initiating the fall), middle (propping her hands to one side with trunk rotation), and end (landing on her stomach) (figs. 3.17, 3.18, 3.19). With practice, she will learn to do the transition with balance and control.

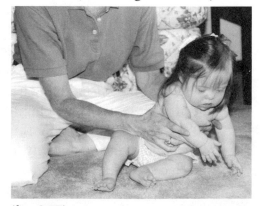

(fig. 3.17)

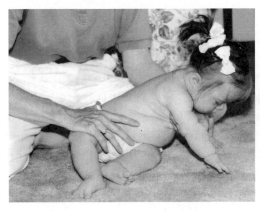 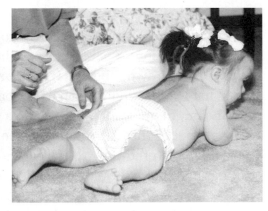

(fig. 3.18)                                  (fig. 3.19)

She will need to be taught this method with your support because she would feel too unstable to initiate it on her own.

## Components

The components to focus on are:
1. weight-shifting her trunk a little forward and mostly to the side
2. bending the knee she is moving over and tucking that leg under her so she can weight shift over it when she is ready to move down to her stomach
3. propping her hands to one side
4. bending her elbows to lower herself with control to her stomach
5. rolling her lower body over to her stomach

## Tendencies

The tendencies are:
1. to avoid the weight shift to the side and instead lean the trunk forward to move down to the floor with her legs in a split
2. to fall backwards and have you catch her, especially if you are sitting behind her
3. to stiffen her knees and hold them straight to feel stable in sitting and resist having the knee bent (that she is moving over) and be fearful of weight shifting
4. to resist moving out of sitting because she loves the position and wants to stay in it
5. to move back up to sit after you place her propping with her hands to the side
6. to avoid the fall to the side and down to her stomach
7. to move to her side and then roll onto her back

## Setup for Learning

Your child needs to have a way to move out of sitting when she chooses to change positions. If she is not taught to move to the side, she will not discover it on her own, and she will figure out her own way, which could lead to bad habits. She might learn to fall backwards, especially if you are behind her. She might move forward and do a wide split with her legs to move down to her stomach. She will prefer to use forward or backward movements rather than moving to the side. Children with Down syndrome tend to prefer the split method, but it should be avoided for the reasons already discussed.

At first, your child will need full support, and it is best to practice on the bed, since it is a soft, comfortable, and safe surface to fall into. You will place a toy to the side of your child. Once she shows an interest in it, you will bend the knee she is moving over and place both hands far to one side and prop them on the bed. Then you will support her at the trunk/armpit area on the side she is moving over and wait for her to bend her elbow to move her chest down to her stomach.

When she is supported with her hands propped on the bed, see what her reaction is and wait to see what she will do. She may bend her elbow and fall down and roll over to her stomach easily, or she may stay in the propped position for a few seconds. She may feel stuck and not know what to do, and she might be scared because she feels off balance. When she does bend her elbow, you will guide her to land on her stomach, not on her back. By supporting her in this way, she will participate with each step of the transition rather than being passively moved through it. You will need to be sensitive to her reaction when practicing this skill and proceed at the speed that she feels most comfortable with. Some children want a slower pace and other children like to move fast.

When you place both of your child's hands to the side, you will weight shift her and rotate her trunk. Both of these movements will be a challenge for her. It will be a challenge to weight shift in this vertical sitting position relative to the prior weight shifting performed on the floor lying on her stomach or back. This is the first skill that has used trunk rotation, so she will not be familiar with it and may be stiff. It is also important to understand that your child's trunk needs to be straight in order to rotate it. (If the trunk is bent and rounded, your child will have limited range of motion when she tries to rotate her trunk.) After a few practices, she will become familiar with these new movements and then tolerate them.

When your child is familiar with moving out of sitting with support on the bed, then you can set her up with the toy to her side and see what she will do. Most likely her first strategy will be to fall to the side and roll to her stomach quickly. If she is not willing to weight shift to the side on her own, place her arms to the side and she will move out of sitting. When she is familiar with moving down, wait for her to initiate moving down rather than helping her. She will learn to lift her head and lower her arms as she is moving down to her stomach on the bed. When she moves slower and with control, she can practice moving out of sitting on the carpet. Always practice on a padded surface so she is safe.

Your child will learn to move out of sitting by herself with control during the next stage. In this stage, the focus is teaching the components of moving out of sitting by moving to the side and having her feel comfortable with weight shifting, falling, and moving to her stomach. When she learns to do it on her own, she does not need to do it the perfect way you practiced it. As long as she moves partially to the side and can move over her legs with her knees bent, she has learned an acceptable method of moving out of sitting.

## Guidelines

*To help motivate your child to move out of sitting, use her favorite toys.* Watch where you put the toy, because she will move to the toy. If you put it in front of her, she will move forward; if you put it to the side, she will move to the side. Place the toy just out of reach. If it is too far away, she will not even try. If it is just out of reach, she will keep reaching for it and will move to get it if she thinks it is worth it. If she quits, try again or get a better toy.

Try to use soft toys so she will not get hurt if she falls on them. If the toy is hard, be ready to move it as she moves out of sitting. She will move farther than you think.

*Practice moving out of sitting when she becomes fussy in sitting and wants to change positions.* You can also encourage her to move out of sitting if you place a favorite toy to the side of her knee.

*Try moving out of sitting over both sides and see if one side is easier.* If one arm is stronger, it is usually better to move over that side first because her stronger arm can lower her weight more gradually.

*See if your child moves back up to sitting after you prop both hands to one side.* She might use her hands to push herself back up to sitting. If she does, congratulate her for using her arms so well! However, to help her learn to move down to her stomach, you will need to place her hands further to the side to make it harder to push up to sitting and easier to go down to her stomach.

*Some children will be motivated to move out of sitting on their own after they learn to move to sit.* Your child may love being in sitting so she will not want to initiate moving out of sitting. Once she is able to easily move to sit, then she will be willing to move out of sitting.

## Temperament

If your child is an **observer,** she will not like the feeling of being off balance or falling when you first introduce moving out of sitting. She also may not want to move out of sitting because she likes to sit. When you help her move out of sitting, she might get fussy or scared. She might feel stuck when you place both hands to the side of her leg. You will need to support her until she is familiar with the position. She will do better if you are in front of her face and arms so she can move to you. For example, Katie was scared when moving out of sitting for the first time. She was able to sit with stability and was scared to be positioned off balance. With practice and with her mother in front of her face, she learned to tolerate moving out of sitting.

If your child is **motor driven,** she will like falling out of sitting and will enjoy the ride. You will need to clear the area to make sure she is safe when she moves quickly out of sitting.

### ACTIVITY #9: Moving from Sitting to Stomach-lying

1. Place your child sitting on the bed with a toy to the side of her right thigh, out of her reach.
2. Position yourself behind your child. Hold her trunk and lift it straight, then rotate it and prop both of her arms to the side of her thigh, so her trunk is leaning far to the side.
3. Place your right hand under her upper trunk (near her armpit), and let her lean against you until she decides to bend her elbow to lower herself down to prop on her elbow. As she is moving to her elbow, guide her to roll to her stomach.
4. If she is scared or does not want to move downward to the toy, position yourself on her right side in front of her arms and face. She will feel better seeing you and moving toward you. Gently hold her elbows and rock them to help her move down to her stomach.
5. With practice, she will move down by herself after you place her hands. Later, she will move down all by herself.
6. When she is able to move out of sitting on the bed, you can use a padded surface like the carpet or a mat.
7. Practice moving over her right and left sides to see if one is easier and then practice over the easier side until she learns the skill. Then practice over the other side.

## Supported Kneeling, Preparation for Quadruped, Moving from Kneeling to Sitting

Supported kneeling was used in Stage 1 to help your child develop head control and propping on arms. It was used in Stage 2 to develop trunk strength for sitting. In this stage, it will be used to develop leg strength for the hands and knees position (quadruped) and supported standing and to practice the pelvic weight shift for moving to sit. Your child will like using this position for play (fig. 3.20) and when she wants to move out of the position, she can move to sit.

(fig. 3.20)

## Components

The components to focus on are:
1. having the mobility and strength to move her hips to neutral rotation, hold her knees together, and take weight on her knees
2. using her abdominals to maintain the position and to move from kneeling to sitting
3. using her buttock muscles to bounce up and down and lift her pelvis off your thighs
4. being comfortable with weight shifting to move to sit, and learning to initiate the transition when she chooses to change positions
5. using hands to prop and hold onto the surface, maintaining the position, playing with toys, and helping to control moving to sitting
6. maintaining the position with control with the hips bent and the trunk up straight

## Tendencies

The tendencies are:
1. to hold the knees wide apart and turned outward and the feet together ("frog leg" position)
2. to arch the trunk and straighten the hips, thrusting forward out of the position or sliding the legs backwards to move out of the position
3. to resist weight shifting through the pelvis to move to sit or to be blocked from moving to sit due to the frog leg or wide knee position
4. to overuse the back muscles to arch the back and be unable to use the abdominals to develop an interplay between the muscles of the front and back
5. to fuss when she wants to move out of the position because she does not know how to do it

## Setup for Learning

Supported kneeling is the best way to teach the components needed for quadruped, and when your child is strong enough to move to quadruped, she will do it. It will be difficult for your child to learn to use the quadruped position on her own. She will learn to prop on her hands first, but then it will be hard for her to move her legs into the position since her tendency will be to position her legs in the frog leg posture. She will not have the leg strength or know how to move her legs into the quadruped position. She will need to learn to bend her hips and knees, move her knees together, and hold this position. Once she develops the arm and leg strength for quadruped, then the last component to develop is abdominal strength, which will help her get into the position, maintain it, and playfully rock forward and backward in it.

The best way to practice supported kneeling is to put a sofa cushion on the floor and put your child's hands on the cushion and her knees on the floor. With her hands on the cushion, her shoulders are positioned higher than her buttocks. This puts more weight on the legs and helps to keep the hips and knees bent. There is also less weight on the arms so she can more easily use her hands to play. The height of the surface will be 5-9 inches (12.5-23 cm) high, and you will choose the height depending on her trunk length and what you are practicing.

When you first use the position, you need to use your legs to hold your child's knees together, with hips and knees bent, while kneeling behind her. When she is comfortable with this position, you can lessen your support by holding her knees together with your hand (using your thumb/index finger web space) (fig. 3.21). With this hand support, it will be easier for her to practice moving from kneeling to sitting. If she needs help to initiate the pelvic weight shift, you can guide this by tilting your hand to one side. Without support, her knees will be apart and will block the weight shift and moving to sit.

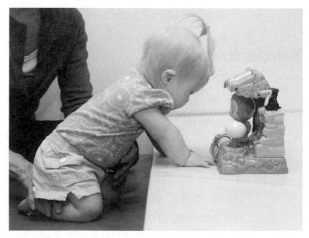

(fig. 3.21)

While your child is practicing supported kneeling, she will experiment with moving her pelvis up and down. The up and down movements will strengthen her abdominals, buttocks, and hip muscles, which will develop strength for supported standing. When she is tired of supported kneeling, you can help her move to sitting by moving to the side (fig. 3.22, 3.23). She will learn to weight shift her pelvis and move to sit by herself during this stage as long as you help her be comfortable with this movement transition. In the next stage, she will use the pelvic weight shift to move to sit from her stomach or hands and knees.

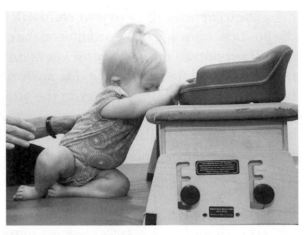

(fig. 3.22)

## Guidelines

*Use the supported kneeling position as an alternative position for play.* When your child is supported in kneeling with her hands on the cushion, you can use any entertaining toy, such as a pop-up box or busy box/activity center, musical toy, xylophone, stacking cups, ring stack toy, or spinning toy. She will easily use her hands to prop and play.

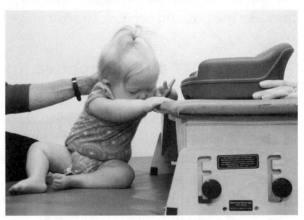

(fig. 3.23)

*Encourage your child to use the position as long as tolerated.* She will play as long as she wants and when she wants to move out of the position, help her move to sitting. Place the toy down on the floor and teach her to weight shift her pelvis to the side to move down to sitting on the floor. For example, when Junior first started using supported kneeling, he would only tolerate the position for brief periods. He would arch his back and keep looking at me when he wanted to get out of the position. He did not care what motivator I used at that point. He was ready to change positions, and he was persistent with giving me the sign.

*Take steps to prevent your child from stiffening and straightening her hips and knees, causing her to thrust forward or fall out of the position.* To avoid these leg movements, support her with her hips and knees bent and her pelvis weight shifted back toward her heels (but not resting on her heels). These movements tend to occur in combination with arching the head and trunk, so minimize these movements too.

*Use a carpeted floor so your child will be more comfortable.* If she resists the position, try using extra padding on the carpet, like a blanket or comforter.

*If supported on hands and knees on the floor, she frequently will be frustrated and fuss, resisting this position.* She will not be able to use her hands to play and will feel stuck in the position. She will be more tolerant if you playfully practice rocking forward and back (with support) and only ask her to stay in the position briefly. She will like the supported kneeling position because she can play. That is why it is the preferred position to use to prepare her to use hands and knees.

### Temperament

If your child is an **observer,** she will like supported kneeling because she can stay in one place and play with toys. If your child is **motor driven,** she may like the position because she can move up and down and move to sitting.

### ACTIVITY #10: Supported Kneeling on a Cushion, and Moving to Sitting

1. Sit on your heels on the floor. Place a 5- to 9-inch (12.5- to 23-cm) cushion on the carpet and stabilize it against furniture.
2. Position your child kneeling in between your legs with her elbows or hands propping on the cushion. Support her knees together with hips and knees bent, and her pelvis lifted a little and resting on your thighs (not on her heels).
3. Place a toy on top of the cushion and entertain her while she maintains the position.
4. While playing, she may bounce up and down and lift her pelvis. Support her at her pelvis to help control her movements and prevent falling out of the position. Watch her to make sure she does not arch her trunk and straighten her hips and knees because then she will thrust herself forward.

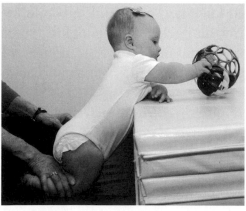

5. When she is comfortable with the position, sit to the side of her and use your hand to hold her knees together. Stretch your thumb and index finger apart and then place them on the outsides of her knees (fig. 3.24). (With this support, you can hold her knees together and assist her in moving from kneeling to sitting.)

(fig. 3.24)

6. When she is tired of supported kneeling and wants to move out of the position, move her to sitting by weight shifting her pelvis a little to the side and then lowering it down to the floor. Make sure her knees are together. You will guide her to help her land safely in sitting. When she is familiar with this movement, provide less support and have her learn to do it by herself. In the beginning, she will lower herself with a plop (without control) but will learn control with practice.

# Sitting on a Bench

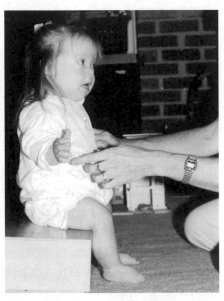

When your child is able to sit well on the floor, the next challenge is for her to sit on a bench with her hips and knees bent 90 degrees (fig. 3.25). This is called *90/90 sitting.* By practicing this skill, your child will refine her sitting posture and balance. She will learn to sit with her trunk up straight, hips in neutral rotation, balance with a narrow and short base, and take weight on her legs and feet. Her feet will be flat on the floor and she will need to actively use her feet and legs to help her maintain her balance when she leans forward. Once she is comfortable in 90/90 sitting, she will learn to stand from this position.

(fig. 3.25)

## Components

The components to focus on are:
1. head, trunk, and pelvis fully erect
2. hips in neutral rotation and knees in line with the hips with the full length of her thighs fully supported on the bench
3. balance in sitting when she weight shifts forward, sideways, and backwards
4. weight bearing on her feet and legs to maintain the position
5. trunk rotation with balance to look in all directions and reach for lightweight toys

## Tendencies

The tendencies are:
1. to sit in the slouched position (head, trunk, and pelvis)

2. to sit with knees apart and hips externally rotated, with the thighs only partially supported
3. to stiffen and straighten the knees for balance
4. to avoid taking weight on the feet
5. to be fearful of the position

### Setup for Learning

Your child will feel challenged in 90/90 sitting and when first placed in the position may need support to become comfortable. If you sit in front of her on the floor and place your legs on the sides of her pelvis, this may be all that she needs to help her feel stable. If she needs additional support, she can hold your fingers, or you can hold her hands and sing gesture songs. When she is familiar with the position, you can lessen your support so she does not become dependent on it. If it helps, you can prop her hands on her thighs.

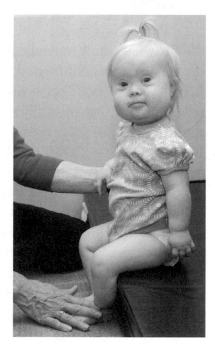

Once your child is familiar with the new position, and she is sitting without your support, she will realize that she needs to balance herself. She will respond to this challenge once she figures out how to do it. She will feel the new leg position, shorter and narrower base, and weight bearing on her feet. She will also notice that if she weight shifts to the side, forward or back, that she will fall more easily. With her heightened responsiveness, she will learn to quickly balance with her trunk or by weight bearing on her feet. You can give in-

(fig. 3.26)

termittent support while she is figuring out how to balance herself (fig. 3.26).

In 90/90 sitting, your child will learn to hold her trunk up straight because if she leans her trunk forward, she will fall forward off the bench. When sitting on the floor, it is easy to lean forward, and she may do it to feel more secure and balanced. By practicing sitting tall in 90/90 sitting, she will strengthen her back muscles and learn to maintain her trunk up straight. This will carry over to sitting on the floor.

When you begin using 90/90 sitting, supervise your child closely. She will easily fall forward or backward until she learns how to lift her trunk to the balanced position and maintain it there. You need to keep your eyes on her at all times because she could fall in a split second and become scared. If you help her learn to use the position properly and safely, she will be comfortable with using it and learn what she needs to do to maintain it.

The setup for 90/90 sitting is crucial. The surface that she sits on needs to be at the right height, so her knees are bent at a 90 degree angle to the floor. It also needs to be firm (e.g., a wooden bench or folded mat). The correct height of the bench is determined by your child's leg measurement from the back of her knee to the bottom of her foot. Her feet need to be flat on the floor so she can work on her balance using a stable position. If the bench is too low, her pelvis will tilt back and her trunk will be rounded. If it is too high, she will need to weight bear on her tiptoes and will feel off balance and insecure. She will also need grip liner on the surface to prevent her pelvis from sliding. She will have a short base and her thighs need to be stabilized on the surface to learn to balance in the position. Place her thighs on the bench with her knees at the front edge to give her the longest base possible on which to balance. Place the bench on a firm surface. If you place it on the rug, make sure it does not rock. If it rocks, your child will not feel secure enough to try this activity.

You can build a bench the appropriate height (usually between 5 and 6 inches) (12.5 and 15 cm) or you can improvise and find something around the house that is the right height. The sitting surface of the bench should be at least 15 inches (38 cm) from side to side and 10-12 inches (25-30.5 cm) from front to back. Your child will feel less stable if the surface is smaller. Do not use a chair with back and side supports, because she will lean against the supports rather than sit tall and learn to balance.

## Guidelines

*Make sure her knees are bent and her feet stay flat on the floor.* It is best if she is barefoot so she feels the surface, presses her feet into the surface, and balances with her feet. If her knees are straight or she cannot keep her heels under her knees, then you support her feet (with your feet or leg) and stabilize them until she can do it.

*When first balancing in the position, use lightweight rattles for play.* She will want to play and if the toys are lightweight it will be easier for her to maintain her balance. If she does not have the balance to play with toys, then sing gesture songs or talk to her to entertain her.

*Place the bench on the floor in front of the sofa (or other soft surface) for safety.* With the bench placed here, if she falls backwards, she will be safe. She will not lean back against the sofa for support if the bench is 10-12 inches (25-30.5 cm), measured from front to back.

## ACTIVITY #11: 90/90 Sitting on a Bench with Her Feet Flat on the Floor

1. Use a bench that is the right height (measure from the back of her knee to the bottom of her foot). Place grip liner on the bench. Place the bench on a firm surface in front of the sofa. Test the stability of the bench and make sure it does not rock or tip.
2. Place your child on the bench (with her back to the sofa) with the full length of her thighs supported. Then bend her knees 90 degrees and place her feet flat on the floor with her heels under her knees. Stabilize her feet if needed.
3. Sit on the floor in front of her and entertain her with a toy held at her eye level.
4. If she needs extra support, place your legs on the sides of her pelvis to help her feel stable. Take away this support when she is comfortable so she does not become dependent on it.
5. If needed, she can prop her hands on her thighs (fig. 3.27). Entertain her by talking to her or singing gesture songs so she enjoys the position. Blow bubbles and catch one bubble with the wand and place it in front of her hand to pop it. When she feels stable, let her hold and shake lightweight rattles.

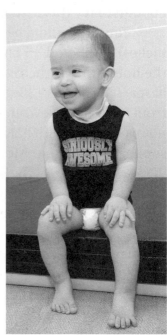

6. When she weight shifts while playing, watch her to see if she is safe maintaining her own balance. If not, provide intermittent support when needed.
7. Closely supervise her so she is safe and does not fall off the bench. Help her gain confidence in her ability to maintain the erect sitting posture and her balance.
8. As she gains confidence in the position, encourage her to reach forward and maintain her balance.

(fig. 3.27)

9. Next, encourage her to rotate her trunk to turn to each side to pop a bubble, or reach for tissue paper or a lightweight toy that is easy to grasp. When rotating her trunk and reaching, she will shift her weight and will need to work on maintaining her balance. When she can manage turning to the side, move the toy further back and see if she can reach and maintain her balance.

# Supported Standing

When your child is able to sit by herself on the floor and in 90/90 sitting, she is ready to practice supported standing (fig. 3.28). This is the critical time to teach her the perfect standing posture, because at this point she will only be able to stand when you place her in the position and support her. Therefore, you have the opportunity to control how she stands and you can make sure she learns the right way to stand with your support. Later, when she can move to stand by herself, you will not be able to control how she stands and she will stand the way she has learned to stand. If you know the best posture to teach her to use, you can give her the support needed to establish this method of standing. The goal is to ensure she learns to stand properly and to maintain the position with hand support. By teaching her this skill now, you will set her up to be successful when she pulls to stand in the next stage.

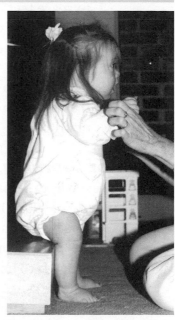

(fig. 3.28)

## Components

The components to focus on are:

1. hips in neutral rotation with knees pointing straight ahead
2. knees unlocked and slightly bent
3. feet 2 to 3 inches (5 to 7.5 cm) apart (narrow base) and pointing straight ahead
4. trunk straight with balance between front and back muscles
5. hands holding onto your thumbs or a surface with an edge

## Tendencies

The tendencies are:

1. to rotate the hips so the knees and feet turn outward
2. to lock and stiffen the knees, and maybe to use the *back-knee position* (to move the knee past the vertical position of the thigh and lower leg due to excessive mobility; see fig. 3.29)

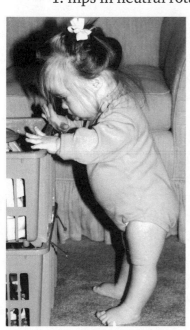

(fig. 3.29)

3. to space feet wide apart (wide base) and turned outward with collapsing of the inside borders of the feet (flat feet)
4. to arch the trunk and lean it against the surface, with the pelvis leaning back behind the heels (side view)
5. to try to keep the hands free to play with toys by leaning the trunk against the surface instead of using hands for holding on or propping

## Setup for Learning

The best way to begin practicing supported standing is to help your child move to stand from 90/90 sitting. The set-up is critical for your child's success:

- The bench must be the perfect height to provide support behind her knees (at the crease behind the knee).
- It needs to be solid from seat to floor, with no empty space under the seat.
- You must stabilize the bench against furniture so it does not slide.
- Your child's feet need to be placed 2-3 inches (5-7.5 cm) apart, pointing straight, with her heels against the bench. You can maintain them by placing your toes on her feet gently.
- Then support her under her arms (at her trunk) and assist her with taking weight on her legs and moving to stand.

The goal now is to practice standing up and sitting down. The focus is on straightening her knees to move to stand and then bending her knees to lower to sitting. It will be easier for her to move to stand and harder for her to lower herself to sitting.

When your child is comfortable with the up-and-down movements, taking weight on her legs, and straightening and bending her knees, then you can have her practice maintaining standing for a few seconds with support (fig. 3.30). The focus now will be her foot and knee position. Her feet will need to be supported with a narrow base, pointing straight, with her heels against the bench. Then the next focus will be standing with her knees unlocked and slightly bent. With her feet in the right position and the proper height bench, if you move her pelvis gently backwards so it is over the bench (side view), you can unlock her knees. This needs to be done gently and slowly because if it is done too fast, it will cause your child to sit down.

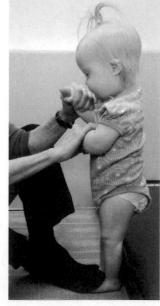

(fig. 3.30)

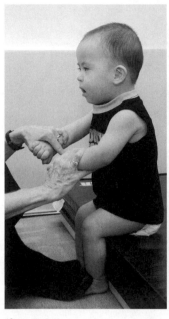 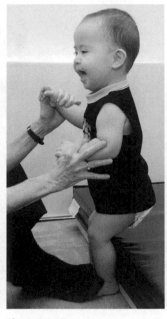 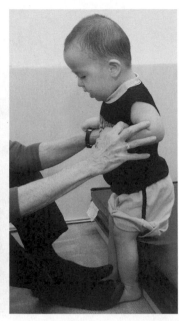

(fig. 3.31)　　　　　　(fig. 3.32)　　　　　　(fig. 3.33)

When your child is familiar with and participates in the desired knee and foot posture for standing, then you can test whether she can hold your thumbs and pull to stand (fig. 3.31). At this point, the focus is on her trunk posture and on having her hold on to pull to stand (fig. 3.32) and maintain standing (fig. 3.33). After she stands, she will arch her trunk and will need to learn to activate her abdominal muscles to hold her trunk straight with balanced control between the front and back muscles. As she holds your thumbs, you can move her hands toward her abdomen (and even place them on her abdomen) and cue her to activate her abdominals. With your hands at her abdomen, you can also provide gentle support to move her pelvis backwards slightly. This will help her bend her knees and activate her abdominals.

Since your child's tendency will be to arch her trunk and lock her knees, you will guide her to develop the opposite (and desired) pattern of activating her abdominals and bending her knees (fig. 3.34, 3.35).

The next component to focus on is holding onto a surface to maintain the standing position. You will need to teach her to hold on since her preference will be to lean her trunk against the support so her hands are free to play. She will need to learn to hold on with both hands to maintain her balance. She will be most stable if she holds a surface with an edge or holds your thumbs. When she holds your thumbs, her hands need to be in front of her chest, and no higher than her shoulders. With this hand support, she will be responsible for moving herself back to the center if she leans sideways or backwards. When she is able to hold your thumbs, then you can teach her to hold a surface with an edge. Gripping the edge helps her maintain standing

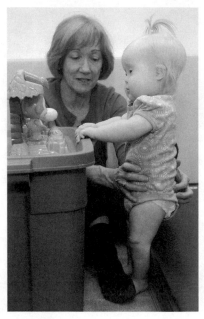 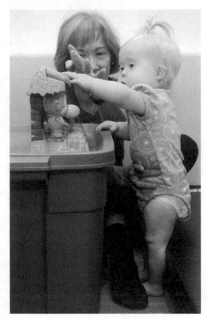

(fig. 3.34)                          (fig. 3.35)

and balance herself. Examples of surfaces with an edge include: a weighted laundry basket, an open drawer, a crate, a toy box, or a plastic storage box. She will need to be entertained since she will not be able to let go with one hand to play. You can sing gesture songs, dance to music, or watch videos.

When your child can use the ideal standing position (feet, knees, trunk, and arms), then she can increase time in the position with support. If a child begins standing too early before her legs are strong enough or does not learn to stand properly, she will develop bad habits that will persist and later affect walking skills.

## Guidelines

*Be prepared to be the primary motivator, since your child will be standing holding your thumbs or a surface with an edge.* You can entertain her by singing, talking, saying "up" and "down," or listening to music and dancing. You can also help her touch your nose, hair, and parts of your face. You can kiss her hands or belly and play peek-a-boo.

*When your child is learning to stand, do not allow her to stand and lean her belly against the surface.* If you teach her to hold on, this will be the method she learns to use and will become her habit. If you let her lean her trunk in the beginning and only later try to teach her to hold on, she will prefer to lean her trunk.

*You can use an Activity Jumper/Jumperoo or Exersaucer/Entertainer as an alternative play position.* Think about what your goal is. The Activity Jumper/Jumperoo allows your child to bounce playfully in supported standing with her knees bending. The Exersaucer/Entertainer allows your child to play between sitting and standing positions and she can spin to turn in a circle to look at people in her environment. If this equipment is used for brief periods and you monitor your child's leg posture and adjust the equipment for the best posture, your child will benefit from using these alternative positions. When using these pieces of equipment, adjust the seat so that your child's hips and knees are bent about 90 degrees. Avoid a seat height that encourages her to stand with knees locked and feet wide apart.

*When she is learning to stand with support, have your child go barefoot.* Then you can observe her feet and see how they are positioned. She will also be able to move them more easily and begin to develop strength and to feel weight shifting movements. If it is cold, she can wear socks with nonskid bottoms or slippers such as Bobux or Robeez. Do not use regular socks because they are slippery. Shoes are not recommended because: 1) you cannot see how your child's feet are positioned inside the shoes, 2) the firmness of shoes around her ankles will prevent her from moving her ankles, and 3) she will tend to stiffen her knees and feet.

## Temperament

If your child is **motor driven,** she will like moving to stand, rocking in standing, and bouncing. She probably will be bored with stationary standing and will only use it for brief periods. If your child is an **observer,** she will like to stand and will stand for longer periods. She will stand up and sit down if you are playing something fun. She may initiate bouncing if you put music on and dance together.

 ## ACTIVITY #12: Moving from 90/90 Sitting to Standing and from Standing to Sitting

1. Sit on the floor with your child sitting in front of you, facing you.
2. Place her in 90/90 sitting. Use a bench that is the right height (measure from the back of her knee to the bottom of her foot). Place grip liner on the bench. Place the bench on a firm surface in front of the sofa. Test the stability of the bench and make sure it does not rock or tip.
3. Place your child's feet flat on the floor with her feet 2 to 3 inches (5 to 7.5 cm) apart, pointing straight, and her heels against the bench. Place your toes over her feet to stabilize them in this position.
4. Hold her under her arms at her trunk and begin lifting her to stand. See if she will take weight on her legs and activate her legs to move to stand. Once she takes weight on her legs, have her use her leg

strength to maintain the position, and you balance her in standing (fig. 3.36).

5. In the beginning, encourage standing up and sitting down so she is familiar with straightening her knees and then bending them. If she resists bending her knees, it is usually because she is arching her back and locking her knees. You will need to assist her with bending her head and trunk to help her bend her knees. Encourage her to look down; this will help her bend her knees. If she continues to resist bending her knees, first make sure the backs of her knees are resting against the bench (fig. 3.37). Then place one hand across her lower abdomen and press gently backwards, waiting for her to bend her knees (fig. 3.38, 3.39). She may be fearful until she learns how to move to sitting, so help her be comfortable with this transition.

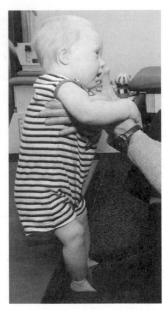

(fig. 3.36)

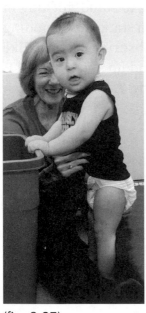

(fig. 3.37)

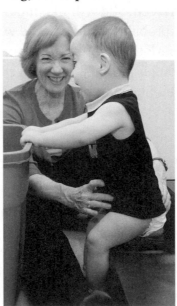

(fig. 3.38)

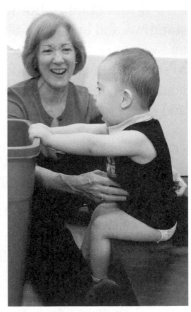

(fig. 3.39)

6. When she is comfortable in supported standing and will stand for a few seconds, observe her posture. Place your toes over her feet to help her keep her feet pointed straight ahead, spaced 2 to 3 inches (5 to 7.5 cm) apart, and heels against the bench. Help her bend her knees slightly by leaning her pelvis back over the bench (with

her heels against the bench and the bench height at the crease of her knees). When she is standing with mild knee bending (knees unlocked), observe her trunk and guide her to activate her abdominals rather than arch her back. You can support her hands at her abdomen and tickle or tap her belly to focus her attention there.

7. When your child uses an optimal leg posture in standing, see if she can hold your thumbs (when sitting on the bench) and pull to stand. Use your fingers to support the tops of her hands if she needs help holding on or maintaining her grasp. Have her continue to hold on while standing and support her hands in front of her chest below shoulder level. Have her practice holding on while lowering herself to sitting with control.

8. When she stands with an optimal posture holding your thumbs, then you can encourage her to maintain standing while you entertain her with singing, playing pat-a-cake, peek-a-boo, and so-big, listening to music, or bouncing, dancing or rocking.

9. When your child is ready to sit down, encourage her to hold onto your thumbs, bend her knees, and lower herself to sitting on the bench.

10. When she can easily hold your thumbs for steps 7–9, encourage her to repeat those steps holding onto a surface with an edge (fig. 3.40).

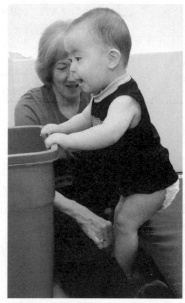

(fig. 3.40)

**MOTOR MILESTONE CHECKLIST**

### Pivoting
- ☐ She pivots one time
- ☐ She pivots 180 degrees
- ☐ She pivots 360 degrees in both directions

### Sitting
- ☐ She sits with waist-level support for 5 minutes
- ☐ She sits with pelvic support (front and back) for 5 minutes
- ☐ She sits with a sofa cushion behind her pelvis and maintains her balance for 5 minutes
- ☐ She maintains sitting without support for 1 minute
- ☐ She sits independently for 5 minutes

### Moving to Sitting
- ☐ She moves to sit from the "L" position with trunk support, pushing up with her hand
- ☐ She moves to sit from the "L" position with her pelvis supported, pushing up with her hand

### Moving out of Sitting
- ☐ After her hands are placed to one side, she moves down to her stomach

### Supported Kneeling
- ☐ She maintains supported kneeling (hands on a cushion) with knees supported together
- ☐ She moves from kneeling to sitting with her knees supported together
- ☐ When supported in kneeling, she moves her pelvis up and down

### 90/90 Sitting
- ☐ She maintains 90/90 sitting for 1 minute
- ☐ She maintains 90/90 sitting with her trunk up straight for 5 minutes without propping
- ☐ She rotates her trunk and maintains her balance in 90/90 sitting

(continued on next page)

### Supported Standing

❑ From 90/90 sitting, with support under her arms, she takes weight on her legs and practices standing up and lowering herself to sitting on the bench

❑ From 90/90 sitting, she stands with support with her knees unlocked and slightly bent

❑ From 90/90 sitting, she stands with support with her trunk erect, not arched

❑ From 90/90 sitting, she holds on (to your thumbs or a surface with a edge) to pull to stand, maintain standing, and lower herself to sitting on the bench

❑ From 90/90 sitting, she stands holding onto a surface with an edge for 5 minutes using the ideal posture with feet 2 to 3 inches (5 to 7.5 cm) apart and pointing straight, knees unlocked and mildly bent, and trunk erect without arching

❑ Bounces (dances) holding your thumbs or a surface with an edge

# 4

# Stage 4: Crawling, Climbing, Quadruped, Moving Into and Out of Sitting, Pulling to Stand, and Standing

## Introduction

During this stage, there will be an explosion of skills that your child can do by himself. These skills will make him independent and capable of exploring on his own. You will have many firsts to celebrate. You will experience the first time he crawls, the first time he sits up by himself, and the first time he pulls to stand. It will be an intense period, with many skills to practice.

What skill your child chooses to do next will be influenced by his temperament, by what he is motivated to do, and by his strength. If he is very motivated to sit, he will find a way to move into sitting. If he is an observer, he will love to sit and play for a long time. If he is motor driven, he may love to crawl. If his arms and legs are strong, he may move into the quadruped position and learn to creep on hands and knees. If he wants to stand, he will learn to pull to stand.

### Motor Skills

The motor skills to focus on in this fourth stage of development are:
1. crawling
2. climbing
3. moving into quadruped

4. creeping
5. moving to sit
6. moving out of sitting
7. pulling to kneel
8. pulling to stand
9. moving from standing to sitting on the floor
10. standing, holding on

## Components

The components to focus on are:
1. arm strength: using forearms to pull his body forward with his belly on the floor (combat crawling); propping on hands to move to hands and knees and creep; holding on and pulling to kneeling and standing; and holding on and maintaining a grip on the surface to maintain standing
2. trunk strength, focusing on abdominal muscles: using core strength to move onto hands and knees, climb, and creep; using abdominals to move between positions; and to stand with the abdominals activated so the trunk is up straight but not arched
3. leg strength and posture: moving hips in neutral rotation and keeping knees and feet in line with hips (for hands and knees, creeping, kneeling, and standing); using controlled knee bending to move from standing to sitting; using leg strength to move from kneeling to standing
4. foot strength: to rise up on tiptoes in standing and push off with toes when climbing; and to weight shift through the feet in standing, especially to the outer borders of the feet
5. feeling comfortable with weight shifting so he moves in and out of positions by moving over his side

## Tendencies

The tendencies are:
1. to skip combat crawling because your child does not learn to use his arms to pull
2. to depend on adults to hold his hands and not learn to grip and hold on to pull to kneel and stand at a surface with an edge
3. to arch his back and overdevelop his back muscles and not gain adequate strength in his abdominals (which is especially needed for moving in and out of positions and for kneeling and standing)
4. to position the legs in the frog leg posture when in kneeling and quadruped, which will also prevent moving to sitting

5. to stand with a wide base, knees and feet turned out, knees stiff, and weight bearing on the inside borders of the feet
6. to be uncomfortable with weight shifting so he will move to sit by moving his legs into a split, move out of sit with a split, and pull to stand from sitting on the floor with legs wide apart
7. to learn to scoot in sitting and not learn crawling, moving into quadruped, and creeping

Your child practiced the foundation needed to learn these skills in the last stage by learning weight shifting and the proper movement patterns for moving in and out of sitting with support, supported kneeling, and supported standing. In this stage, you will practice the skills with your child until he can do them by himself. Since there are many skills to practice, you can be strategic and combine the following skills according to the *themes of sitting, crawling, and standing.*

For **sitting**, you will practice moving to sit, sitting, and moving out of sitting. For **crawling**, you will follow the progression of first learning combat crawling, then climbing. In the meantime, you will practice kneeling and wait to see when your child initiates moving onto hands and knees. After he climbs up the flight of stairs and moves into quadruped, then he will be ready to learn creeping. For **standing**, you will first practice pulling to stand from 90/90 sitting, holding on and maintaining standing, and then lowering to sitting on the bench. When your child is interested in standing and can pull to kneel, then he can learn to pull to stand from sitting on the floor. He will practice pulling to kneel, moving from kneel to stand, standing, and moving from standing to sitting.

## Guidelines

*Do not expect your child to develop the skills of this stage in a particular order.* Your child will show you what he is interested in doing, and he will determine the order. Let him practice what he wants to do, and if he is not interested in doing a skill, practice it briefly just to keep it familiar for when he does become interested in it. Casey made this point very clear. She had learned to sit on the floor so I started practicing belly crawling with her. Every time we practiced, she looked very sleepy and tired. Then, one day, after we had practiced 90/90 sitting, I encouraged her to pull up to stand from sitting on the bench. She was ecstatic! She would pull up to stand, stand holding on to the edge of the toy bin, sit down, and then repeat the sequence again for many repetitions. She was showing me what *she* wanted to do and she was energetic again!

*Try concentrating first on the easier skills to learn, and the ones that are most functional based on what he is able to do.* Since your child is able to sit, practice moving to sit from his stomach and kneeling, and moving out of sitting. Since he is able to pivot, start practicing combat crawling to give him the idea of moving forward on his belly. Since he is familiar with playing in supported kneeling, have him learn to move from kneeling to sitting and then sitting to kneeling. Practicing kneeling will also prepare him for the leg strength needed for assuming hands and knees. Since he has learned to stand with support, practice moving from sitting on a bench to standing, holding on in standing, and lowering to sitting on the bench.

*Moving onto hands and knees (quadruped) tends to develop later, so work on the skills related to quadruped after your child initiates this skill. (While waiting, continue practicing kneeling.)* After he moves into quadruped, then he is ready to learn to move from quadruped to sitting. After he can climb up a flight of stairs, he is ready to practice creeping on hands and knees. When he likes creeping and wants to move to stand, then you can teach him to pull to kneeling from quadruped, and then to stand.

*Practice the skills when your child is strong and giving you his best performance. Use his favorite motivators to generate his interest.* Watch him and practice each skill as long as he is interested. Try to do a minimum of 2-3 repetitions to make the skill more familiar and automatic. Change the position or activity when he is no longer interested, and do it before he becomes fussy.

*Practice skills for 5-10 minute periods and then give your child a break for independent play.* Planning an hour-long practice session is not recommended. At this stage, he has many skills that he can do and likes to do, and he wants to be independent. You may be considered an interruption in his plan of exploration or playtime. So, you need to be subtle and try to weave your agenda into his.

*If he dislikes a position but is ready to learn the skill, try to do it briefly with the best motivator to help him learn to tolerate it and become familiar with it.* If you do it briefly with the best motivator, he will be distracted and tolerate it. With practice, he will learn the value of the position and then his resistance will decrease. If he still does not cooperate with this ideal setup, then stop working on the skill and try again later. You can test when he is ready to do it. Never force a skill. You will make your child grow to hate the skill if you practice it too often while he is resisting it. There are plenty of other skills to work on, so focus on them until he is ready to try the skill he dislikes.

*Be strategic with the order of the skills you practice.* Keep in mind that he will be strongest and most tolerant at the beginning of the practice time. Practice the more challenging skills first and practice the skills in a functional way. If you practice the themes, you will do skills that naturally go together and that combine movement and stationary positions. He will like this pace of moving to a position and then playing in it. For example, if he practices moving to sit every time he wants to sit (or is placed in sitting), it will become a habit and he will learn the skill the best way. When he is done sitting, you can set him up to practice moving out of sitting.

# Crawling

In order to understand this section, you need to know the definitions of crawling and creeping. These terms tend to be used interchangeably, and they do not have standardized definitions. For the purposes of this book, the definitions I will use are:

- *Crawling* refers to your child moving forward with his belly on the floor, pulling with his arms and pushing with his legs (also called combat or army crawling).
- *Creeping* refers to your child moving forward on hands and knees, stomach up off the floor, in quadruped.

Most children with Down syndrome crawl before they creep. Creeping is harder due to the arm and abdominal strength required. Therefore, I teach crawling first so children learn the idea of moving forward to get something, and I wait for them to learn creeping when they are ready. Your child will need to develop arm, leg, and abdominal strength to crawl and creep.

Your child will be ready to learn crawling when he can pivot 360 degrees in both directions. Through pivoting, he will learn to pull with his arms to move his body sideways. What initially limits learning to crawl is a child's lack of arm strength to pull his body forward, so that is the first component that your child needs to learn. **It will not be helpful to hold his foot,** since pushing off with his legs will easily develop after he can pull himself forward with his arms. If your child does not learn how to pull himself forward with his arms, he will learn to use rolling, pivoting, or scooting in sitting to move in his environment rather than crawling and creeping.

The goal will be for your child to crawl approximately 10 feet (across a room). Once he can do that, he will move everywhere.

### Early Crawling Patterns

Your child will not begin crawling using a coordinated crawling pattern. He will begin with one of six basic methods. They will not look like what you might think of as crawling, but over time, they will develop into an efficient crawling pattern. You need to be aware of them so you recognize them as early attempts to crawl and can encourage them. Any method of moving forward is the goal.

The methods commonly seen are:
1. "reach and roll,"
2. pull forward with both elbows at the same time,
3. prop on hands and move forward,
4. "inchworm,"
5. pull forward with one elbow at a time, and do alternating movements,
6. move onto hands and knees and thrust forward.

The **"reach and roll"** method (fig. 4.1, 4.2) is done by reaching with one arm and then when the child does not reach the motivator, rolling or leaning over that elbow, and reaching with the other arm. As he leans over the elbow, he bends it and presses it into the surface, and he pulls his body forward slightly so his reaching arm is then able to touch the toy. When reaching with the first arm, the child's hand is stretched as far forward as it will go; then, when that hand cannot touch the toy, he reaches with his other hand. With these movements, he does one pull with his elbow and moves his body forward enough to touch the toy.

If your child chooses to use the method of **pulling forward on both elbows,** he needs to have his elbows in front of his shoulders (side view) (fig. 4.3, 4.4. 4.5). He will lean his head forward and press his elbows into the surface,

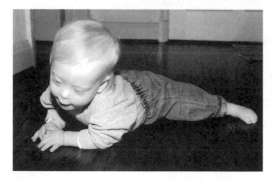

(fig. 4.1)

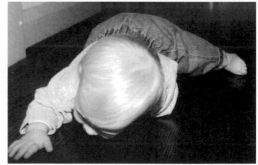

(fig. 4.2)

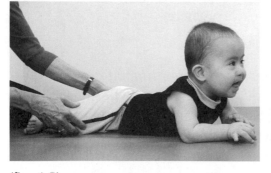

(fig. 4.3)

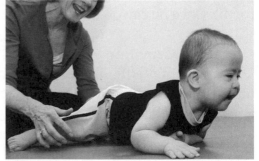

(fig. 4.4)

and this will pull his body forward. When he pulls with both elbows at the same time, he pulls his body forward like a log or as one unit and does not weight shift.

Some children who love to **prop on hands** figure out a method of moving forward from this position (fig. 4.6, 4.7). While propping on hands and keeping their elbows straight, they push up and then lean the head and trunk forward over their hands (side view) and slide the body forward. They tend to keep their legs straight and the primary action is using the arms. This is another method that moves through the center, without side to side weight shifting.

Savannah figured out what her mother called the "**inchworm**" pattern, moving up and down to move herself forward (fig. 4.8, 4.9, 4.10). From prone, she moved onto her elbows and knees (with her knees wide apart), and then pushed up with her hands to move forward.

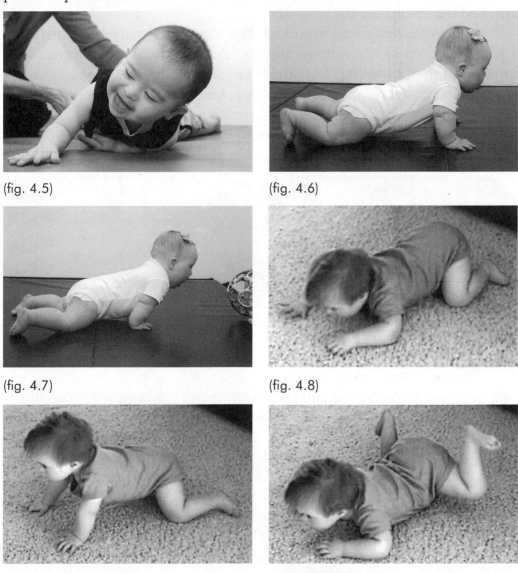

(fig. 4.5)

(fig. 4.6)

(fig. 4.7)

(fig. 4.8)

(fig. 4.9)

(fig. 4.10)

With practice, many children develop the pattern of alternating the arms, **pulling with one elbow** at a time (fig. 4.11). They will lean to one side and pull forward with that elbow and then lean to the other side and pull forward with that elbow. With this method, the child shifts his weight from side

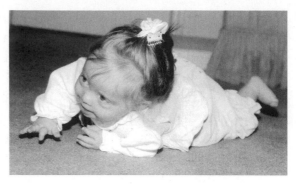

(fig. 4.11)

to side and his legs can participate when they are ready. As he becomes efficient with this pattern, he will use a reciprocal pattern, moving the opposite arm and leg simultaneously.

If your child has strong arms and abdominals, and can move onto hands and knees, then he may choose the method of **moving onto hands and knees and then thrusting forward** to get the toy (fig. 4.12, 4.13). When he is really motivated to move to something, his spontaneous method will be to move onto hands and knees to try to reach it. He will find that he cannot move his arms and legs to move forward, so instead will just thrust himself forward, falling onto his belly.

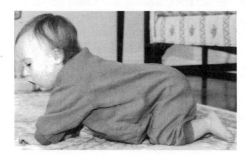

(fig. 4.12)

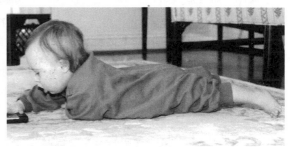

(fig. 4.13)

## Components

The components to focus on are:

1. arm strength to pull the body forward while propping on elbows
2. weight shifting over each forearm, combined with pulling, to move forward
3. the desire to move forward, the determination to figure out a method, and the persistence to keep going to move to the motivator
4. use of the legs to assist the arms with crawling forward, after the arm movements are established
5. use of the abdominal muscles to move with an efficient pattern, working toward the refined pattern of moving the opposite arm and leg simultaneously.

## *Tendencies*

The tendencies are:

1. to just continue using rolling for mobility, and, after your child can move to sit, to scoot in sitting
2. to have weak arms, so he becomes frustrated with trying to move forward and then quits because he is not setup to be successful
3. to have the habit of propping on his hands in prone and since this is his primary position, to slide backwards (and not be able to move forward)

## *Setup for Learning*

Children with Down syndrome often have trouble learning to crawl because their arms are not strong enough to pull their body weight forward across the floor. Their legs may be strong enough to help push, but if the arms are too weak to pull, they cannot move forward. If your child is having a hard time moving forward, it could be because he has weak arms or because he cannot figure out a way to use his arms to pull his body forward.

To learn to crawl, your child will need to figure out his own way to move forward, using his arms. At first, we need to give him the idea to move forward to get a toy, just like we introduced the idea of moving his body sideways to pivot. Then we need to help him learn how to pull with his arms to move forward. We need to set him up to want to move forward by placing a toy in front of him, just out of his reach. If he has the intent to move and if we give him a method of moving forward, then he is setup to be successful to learn this new skill.

The easiest way to support him to move forward is to straighten his elbows in front of him, have him hold your index fingers while you stabilize his hands on the surface, and then wait for him to bend his elbows and pull his body forward (fig. 4.14, 4.15, 4.16). His hands need to be on the surface and then he will also feel his forearms against the surface on which he is lying. By providing this support, you want him to learn to pull himself forward by bending his elbows, pressing his forearms into the surface. Once he can do this well, you can place the palms of his hands on the surface and stabilize them, pressing them into the surface, and he will pull himself forward with this support. When you are using this strategy to teach crawling, your child needs to wear a onesie so his arms and legs are bare. He also needs to be on a slippery surface to help his body slide forward easily.

After you have set him up to want to move forward and have given him a method, your main role in helping him initiate crawling by himself is to place the "ultimate" motivator in front of him, just out of reach. If it is too far, he will just quit. If it is too close, he will be able to stretch out his arm and reach it. You will also be amazed how far he can reach without moving forward!

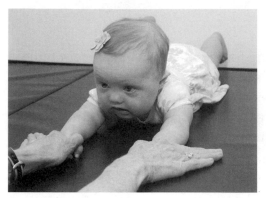

(fig. 4.14)

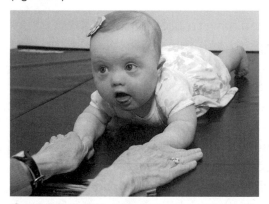

(fig. 4.15)

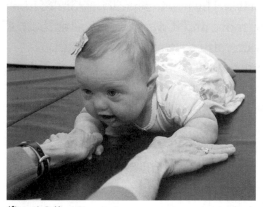

(fig. 4.16)

Wait and see if he tries to move forward. If he does, reward him with the toy and clapping. If he is excited but does not use any arm movements, help him by having him hold your index fingers and pull himself forward to the toy. With practice, he will initiate arm movements to move himself forward.

The hardest part of learning to crawl is doing the first one or two pulls forward, and moving forward the first one or two feet. Once he has the desire to move forward and has a potential method, he will build on it and improve his method with practice. We need to let him figure out the method that works best for him, with his arm strength and body size. (See "Early Crawling Patterns," above.) When you see the method your child uses in the beginning, you will agree it is his method and that it probably is not how you would have taught him. That is why it is so important for your child to figure out how he wants to do it; then, he can do it by himself.

As your child continues to practice moving forward and develops a method of moving his arms, he will begin using his legs to become more efficient, so that he can move faster and for longer distances. In the beginning, his legs may be straight and he may try pushing off on his tiptoes. If he uses the "reach and roll" method or pulling forward with one elbow at a time, he will shift his weight from one side to the other and one leg will bend and the other leg will straighten. With these leg movements, he will learn to push off with the foot of the bent leg.

After he has a crawling method and consistently moves forward 3 to 5 times in a row, you can gradually work on increasing the distance. Place the toy about 18 inches (half a meter) in front of him and see if he will move himself forward to touch the toy. When he does this easily, place the toy 2 feet (.6 meters) in front of him. Continue to increase the distance up to 5 to 10 feet (1.5 to 3 meters). When he can crawl 10 feet, he will be able to crawl around a room and begin crawling around the house.

## Guidelines

*To stimulate beginning crawling, use the "ultimate" motivators.* You may want to save your child's favorite motivator just for when you practice combat crawling. Some examples are: shiny crinkly tissue paper, a tower of stacking cups to knock down, small balls, TV remote, cell phone, Slinky, brother or sister, paper or magazine, a book, "push button" toy or radio, spin toy, toy with music and lights, or veggie sticks. Use the best motivators so your child will work on moving forward to the toy no matter what he has to do with his body. He just thinks about getting the toy and tries whatever movements he can to move forward. By experimenting with different movements, he will develop a method of crawling. For example, ten-month-old Mendy had the "observer" temperament and would only crawl if he was highly motivated. His mother discovered that if she took the parakeet out of the cage and placed it on the floor in front of him, he would do whatever was necessary to pull himself forward to try to get the parakeet.

*Remember that your child's size will affect his ability to crawl.* If he is small, it will be easier for his arms to pull his body across the floor; if he is large, he needs more arm strength to succeed in crawling.

*When he is first figuring out how to crawl, experiment to see which surface works best for the method of crawling he chooses.* Try linoleum, tile, hardwood floors, and different types of carpet. The linoleum, tile, and hardwood floors will provide a slippery surface, which may make it easier to slide forward. If you have a deep pile carpet, your child may grip the carpet to help pull himself forward. If you have a shorter pile or berber carpet, he may prefer this because it is easier to move across than a deep pile carpet.

*Cover areas of your child's body that need to slide across the surface and expose the bare skin on areas of his body that need to pull or push.* For example, a onesie with short sleeves will cover his belly for easy sliding, and his bare arms and legs will make it easier to pull with his elbows and push off with his legs.

*Practice only for brief periods, when he is most alert and active, and with the best motivators.* At the beginning crawling stage, your child may only tolerate practicing for 2 or 3 repetitions and then be tired or lose his motivation. It will take time for him to develop the arm strength required for crawling. If he rolls over, it is probably a sign that he is finished. You can try again later when he is motivated and ready.

*Don't give up; be patient. Your child will succeed at crawling, so make it fun and keep practicing, and he will do it on his own timeline.* If your child has not learned to move to sit by himself, this will be the best time to help him figure out a way to move when he is on his belly. If he has learned to move to sit, he may choose to sit rather than practice crawling. You will need to be creative with motivating him to have him stay on his stomach and try to crawl forward.

*Set him up to practice when you are not there to help him or entertain him.* If you place a toy out of his reach and you are out of the room but nearby (watching him), he may be more persistent on his own with figuring out how to move to the toy. If you are there, he may rely on you to help him or may engage with you socially rather than figure out how to crawl.

## Temperament

If your child is **motor driven,** he will love to crawl and will be motivated to move as far as he can. If your child is an **observer,** he will learn to crawl when he thinks it is useful for him. After he learns to crawl, you may change your mind and think he is motor driven because his activity level will increase. However, you will see some observer characteristics, such as being cautious, return when he is learning to walk.

 ### ACTIVITY #1: Crawling with Belly on the Floor

1. Dress your child in a onesie. Place him on his stomach on a slippery surface (slippery mat or floor). If his habit is to prop on his hands, then place his feet against the wall (to prevent sliding backwards).
2. Place a motivating toy in front of him, just out of his reach. Place the toy close enough so he is motivated to try to get it, but not so close that he can reach it.
3. Watch and see if he wants the toy and if he tries any movement to try to move forward to touch the toy. Watch his arms and his feet.
4. If he tries any of the 6 early crawling methods described above, or just tries to push off with his tiptoes, that is great. Make sure that you praise him and that he reaches his toy so this is a successful experience.

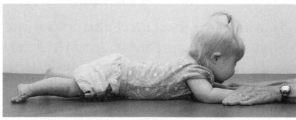

(fig. 4.17)

5. If he wants the toy but has no idea how to move forward, then help him learn to pull with his elbows. The easiest way to support him to move forward is to straighten his elbows in

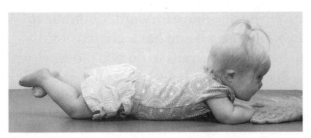

(fig. 4.18)

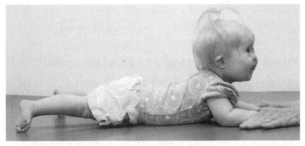

(fig. 4.19)

front of him, having him hold your index fingers. Place his hands on the floor and stabilize them with your thumbs on top of his hands or wrist. With this support, wait for him to bend his elbows and pull his body forward. His hands need to be on the surface and then he will also feel his forearms against the surface. By providing this support, you want him to learn to pull himself forward by bending his elbows, pressing his forearms into the surface.

6. Once he can do the steps in #5 well, you can place the palms of his hands on the surface, pressing them into the surface, and he will pull himself forward with this support (fig. 4.17, 4.18, 4.19).

7. If helpful, you can also practice weight shifting and gently pulling each side forward. You place your index fingers on his shoulder blades/trunk and your other fingers gently hold the outsides of his upper arms. You will lean him over his left elbow and gently pull his right side forward. Then you will alternate and lean him over his right elbow and gently pull his left side forward. You can do this for four moves forward to a motivator. By practicing this method, you will give him the idea of weight shifting and pulling with each forearm.

8. Each time you setup your child to crawl, test the first trial to see if he tries to move forward on his own. If he initiates, then let him use his method. If he is interested but does not have a method, then practice step 5 and/or 6.

9. Constantly test the setup (the types of surfaces, use of clothes, and motivators) to see what works best to help him try to crawl.

10. The next goal is for your child to figure out how to initiate crawling on his own without your support. Test how you can lessen your support. You can try a mild incline and see if he can do one or two pulls, moving down the incline. To make an incline, you can use a mat, a sofa cushion, or a card table and raise one end about 4 inches (10 cm).

11. With practice, he will learn to do one move forward. Continue to practice this until he knows he can do it and has a chosen consistent method. Then move the toy so he needs to do two moves to get it. Gradually increase the distance to three feet, five feet, and ten feet. When he is able to do ten feet, he will move within a room or from one room to another.

# Climbing

Once your child is able to combat crawl, he is ready to practice climbing. If he crawls but does not move into quadruped or creep, climbing will teach him the movements needed to learn to use quadruped and creeping. If he can creep, then he can learn the skill of climbing on furniture and up a couple of stairs. The first goals will be to climb up onto the sofa cushion (placed on the floor) and to climb up the top 2 stairs (of the flight of stairs) onto the landing. When he knows how to climb, he can practice the next goals of climbing up the top three to four stairs and climbing up onto the sofa, with the seat cushion removed.

By practicing climbing, your child will learn to pull to kneel, maintain the quadruped position, prepare for creeping, and pull to stand from kneeling, and he will improve arm, leg, and abdominal strength. In this stage the primary focus is climbing up. You can familiarize him with climbing down (off your lap or off the sofa) when it is functional for him, but he will need your direction and support to do it during this stage. In the next stage, he will learn to climb down by himself.

## *Components*

The components to focus on are:

1. arm strength to pull to kneel from lying on his stomach, from sitting, or from hands and knees; the strength to pull his body forward on the cushion, landing, or sofa; and the ability to prop and advance his arms to move up the stairs
2. abdominal strength to maintain the hands and knees or hands and feet position, and to stabilize the core as he moves each arm and leg
3. leg strength to move each knee and each foot onto each stair, to move from kneeling to standing, and to hold the hips in neutral rotation and knees and feet in line with hips
4. ability to remember the sequence of steps needed to climb
5. developing the habit of always climbing to the top (of the cushion or landing or sofa) and away from the edge for safety

## Tendencies

The tendencies are:

1. to have weak arms or be unable to figure out how to use the arms to climb
2. to have weak abdominals or have the tendency of arching the trunk, so it is difficult to use the abdominals when pulling to kneeling and when moving the hands or knees
3. to have weak legs and to be unfamiliar with how to weight shift and move the legs to climb on the sofa cushion, up the stairs, and onto the sofa
4. to have difficulty weight shifting from side to side when climbing up the stairs
5. to be overwhelmed with the many steps required to climb up one stair (or onto the cushion)

## Setup for Learning

To succeed in climbing up, your child will need to use his whole body. It is best to start practicing climbing by using a low surface, like a sofa cushion (approximately 5 to 6 inches or 12.5 to 15 cm high) placed on the floor. You will place him in front of the surface and he will need to pull to kneel. You can test which position is easier for him to pull to kneel from: lying on his stomach, on hands and knees, or sitting in front of the surface. Once kneeling, he will then need to move forward onto the cushion. He will lean his trunk forward over the cushion and then will need to pull with his arms, and he may push off with his feet, pushing his tiptoes against the floor. After his trunk is on the cushion, he will continue to move forward using his combat crawling pattern.

After your child is able to climb onto the sofa cushion, you can practice *climbing up the top two stairs of the flight* (fig. 4.20, 4.21, 4.22, 4.23), *onto the landing* (fig. 4.24, 4.25). He will need to learn the sequence of moving each knee (fig. 4.20, 4.21), then moving onto one foot (into the half-kneel position; see fig. 4.22), and then moving up to stand and weight bearing on his other foot (fig. 4.23). (The sequence will be knee, knee, foot, foot.) Once he has moved his legs, then he can advance his hands, one at a time. He will need to repeat this sequence to move up each stair. With his short leg length and the standard height of stairs, he will need to use this unique method to be successful. (The typical child climbs up by moving each knee.)

It will be difficult for your child to climb up on the sofa because of his short legs. You can lower the height of the sofa by removing the seat cushion. With the seat cushion removed, check to see if the top of the sofa is even with his hips when he is in the standing position. If it is the right height, then you can assist him with lifting his knee and placing it by providing support behind

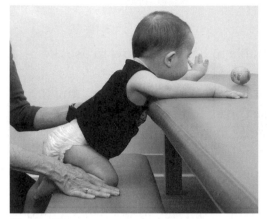

(fig. 4.20)

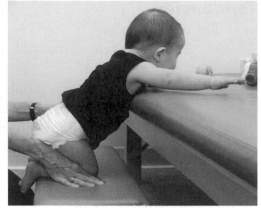

(fig. 4.21)

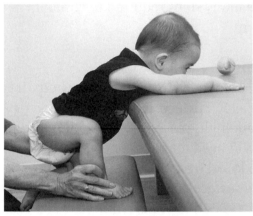
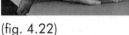

(fig. 4.22)

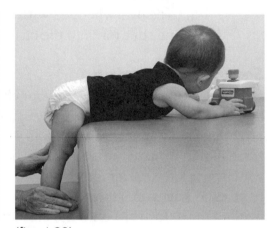

(fig. 4.23)

his knee. If the sofa is still too high, then you can place the sofa cushion on the floor in front of the sofa and have him stand on the cushion, with his trunk leaning over the sofa.

Since your child will want to climb down off the sofa or off your lap, you can familiarize him with the movements. When he shows the desire to climb down, roll him to his stomach, straighten his legs (especially the hips), and then have him push with his arms and slide down and land on his feet in standing (fig. 4.26, 4.27). On his own, he will see what he wants and try to climb down, moving toward it, head first. He will need to be taught the sequence of steps to climb down safely. With practice, he will learn to climb down safely during the next stage.

## Guidelines

*The climbing sequence is difficult, so assist him with each step so he can participate and be successful.* Know the sequence of steps for each climbing activity and anticipate his next step so you are ready to support him

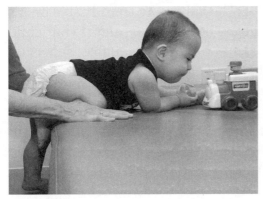

(fig. 4.24)

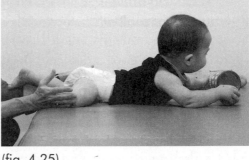

(fig. 4.25)

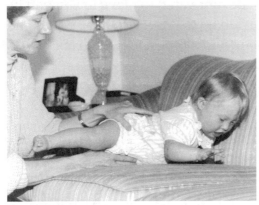

(fig. 4.26)

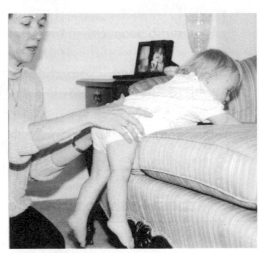

(fig. 4.27)

after he initiates it. By practicing this way, you are building on his attempts, which helps him be successful and allows him to do what is next. If he does not initiate the next step, then assist him.

*When you are helping your child learn to climb up stairs, support behind his knee or foot after he moves it, so it is stable and does not slide.* If his knee or foot slides backwards after he places it, he will fail and not feel the success of his action. Have your hand ready to support his knee or foot so he can continue to progress to the next step of the sequence.

*It is best to teach climbing up stairs beginning at the top of the flight, and always have him climb to the landing so this is his habit, and he is Setup to be safe.* If he is setup to climb to the landing every practice, he will develop safe climbing habits. He can practice climbing one or two stairs and when he masters them, then the number of stairs can be increased, until he can do the flight. If this method is not practiced and he is setup to climb up more stairs than he is ready to do, when he no longer wants to climb or wants to take a break, he will try to sit on the stair and will not know how to do it safely. He will move his pelvis and try to sit and probably will not be able to maneuver in this small space. He could then fall down the stairs if you were not there.

*When possible, use carpeted stairs.* They are more comfortable on his knees and less slippery than wooden stairs. They are also safer if your child accidentally bumps his head. If carpeted stairs are not available, supervise your child closely so he does not bump his head on the edge of the stair above him, when he is first learning to climb up.

*If you do not have stairs, try to use stairs at a relative's or friend's home, or improvise by stacking sofa cushions.* Climbing is a valuable skill to practice to prepare your child for moving into quadruped and creeping, and for developing arm, leg, and abdominal strength. If possible, find an alternative setup if you do not have stairs at home.

*Your child may enjoy the game of climbing over your legs or trunk when you are lying on the floor.* He will be motivated to move to you and he will be able to hold onto your clothes and pull up to kneel. It will be easier and fun to pull to kneel on you by holding onto your clothes, legs, or arms.

### ACTIVITY #2: Climbing onto a Sofa Cushion Placed on the Floor

1. Place a 5-inch (12.5 cm) sofa cushion on the floor. Place your child on the floor in front of it. You sit behind your child, sitting on your heels.
2. Test whether it is easier for your child to pull to kneel from lying on his stomach or from sitting, and then place him in that position in front of the cushion. (If placed in sitting, place him with his side next to the surface, with a 4-5 inch (10-12.5 cm) space between him and the cushion.)
3. If he pulls to kneel from his belly, place his arms and hands on the cushion with his armpits at the edge (and stabilize them if needed). See if he will activate his abdominals and lift his abdomen and then move each knee forward. If he can assume quadruped, he will move from prone to quadruped, and then place his hands on the cushion.
4. If he pulls to kneel from sitting, see if it is easier to move over one side and then practice with that setup. Place him sitting with his side next to the surface, with a space in between him and the cushion. Then he will lean his trunk against the surface and prop on his arms. After he leans, his legs (hips and knees) will bend, and you can support his knees together, and then wait for him to lean his trunk over the surface and lift his pelvis to move to kneeling. Make sure the knee he is moving over is maximally bent, or it will block him from moving to kneeling. (See "Pulling to Kneel" section, Activities 14 and 15.)

5. Once your child is kneeling, place a motivating toy at the far edge of the cushion and lean his trunk forward over the cushion. See if he will try to move forward on the cushion, by pushing off with his legs or pulling with his arms. If he does not initiate moving forward, then support his hands (with his elbows straight, like you did for combat crawling) and wait for him to bend his elbows to pull his body forward. He will learn to use his combat crawling pattern when climbing forward on the cushion. If he can use his arms to move forward, but tends to arch his trunk and straighten his legs so he slides backwards off the cushion, then block his feet so he can figure out how to use his arms to pull forward to bend his knees to climb or kneel. Keep assisting him as needed to move forward to the toy.

6. After he can climb on the cushion successfully, then he can practice climbing off (head first) with support for safety. He will need to lift his head while climbing off with control, using his arms. (Later, when he is on higher surfaces, he will need to learn to climb off feet first.)

## ACTIVITY #3: Climbing Up the Top 2 Stairs to the Landing

1. Place your child on his feet on the second stair from the top, and place his hands on the landing.
2. Place a toy on the landing, out of reach.
3. See if he will try to move his knee onto the #1 stair from the top, to climb after the toy. If not, bend one knee and place it on the #1 stair. Hold his knee (using your thumb in the crease behind his knee) to stabilize it and wait for him to move his other knee onto the #1 stair. If he does not move it, then you assist him and stabilize that knee also. To help him move his other knee, lean his pelvis to the opposite side, and he may be able to move his knee with this support.
4. From this position on the #1 stair, wait to see if he tries to move one leg into the half-kneel position (moving onto one foot). (See photo of half-kneel in fig. 4.22.) Loosen your support behind his knees in anticipation of him moving his foot. If he does not initiate moving into the half-kneel, then assist him. To help him move into the half-kneel position, lean his pelvis over the opposite side and see if he moves his foot onto the stair. Once his foot is placed, then stabilize it behind his heel with one of your hands. Wait and see if he will move onto his other foot, so his legs are standing. (Weight shift him at the pelvis and lean him over the opposite side to help him move his other foot.) Now both feet are on the #1 stair and

hands are on the landing. Stabilize both heels by kneeling behind his feet and see if he will climb onto the landing.

5. To climb onto the landing, your child will either combat crawl or creep on hands and knees. Support him so he learns to climb onto the landing and end the activity (and get his toy). If he does not initiate moving forward, then help him so he completes the skill. If his preference is to combat crawl onto the landing, lean his trunk forward on the landing and then he will combat crawl forward (similar to climbing on the sofa cushion placed on the floor). If his preference is to creep, then place one knee and hold it (step 3 above) until he moves his other knee and creeps forward.

6. Continue to practice this activity until he can climb up by himself with you supporting his knee or foot (after he places it) to prevent it from sliding. The sequence he will need to learn is knee, knee, foot, foot.

7. When he masters climbing up the top two stairs, then place his feet on the #3 stair and his hands on the #1 stair, and have him climb up onto the landing. As tolerated, increase the number of stairs until he can climb up the flight.

8. Supervise your child so he is safe and help him as needed. Position yourself behind him and help him learn the movements required.

## ACTIVITY #4: Climbing on the Sofa without the Cushion

1. Remove the seat cushion of the sofa. The height of the sofa needs to be even with your child's hips when he is standing for him to be successful. If the sofa is still too high, place the sofa cushion (or other surface like a mat) on the floor in front of the sofa and stabilize it so it does not move.

2. Place your child standing, facing the sofa. Put a toy on the seat and encourage him to climb up on the sofa to get it.

3. If he is motivated to move after the toy but cannot figure out how to do it, help him by bending one knee, placing it up on the seat, and stabilizing it with your thumb (in the crease behind his knee). Place and support his knee under his abdomen (hip in neutral rotation) and support his trunk on the opposite side under his armpit. Then lean his trunk over his knee and see if he will move his other knee up on the sofa.

4. An alternative way to help him climb up is to weight shift him (with support on the sides of his lower trunk or pelvis) to one side and see if he can move his knee up on the sofa with this support.

5. After he climbs up, help him move to sit and play with the toy.

## ACTIVITY #5: Climbing Off Your Lap or Off the Sofa with Support

1. Practice this skill when your child is interested in climbing down off your lap or off the sofa (so it is functional for him).
2. When he is ready to climb off, move him to his stomach and straighten his hips, then let him slide down to standing on the floor. He can use his arms to push and you want him to "catch" with his feet when he lands in standing.
3. He will need to practice this many times to learn the sequence of steps to climb down safely. Let him do what he can and you do the rest. The hardest parts for him to learn will be to roll to his stomach and to straighten his hips to slide down safely.

# Moving into Quadruped

Moving into quadruped (hands and knees) is a hard skill for children with Down syndrome to develop due to the tendency to have weak arms, the habit of using the frog leg posture, and weak stomach muscles. This skill occurs at a unique time for each child depending on his interest, and the strength in his arms, legs, and abdominal muscles. Some children like being on their stomachs, develop combat crawling, and wait to use quadruped until later, after they learn to climb. Other children may playfully move into quadruped, and then enjoy rocking forward and back in the position. Some children will move into quadruped briefly as an intermediate (interim) position on the way to moving to sit.

Until your child can assume the quadruped position, you will continue to practice the missing components. The goal is for your child to move into quadruped by himself, and to maintain the position once assumed.

## Components

The components to focus on are:

1. strong arms so that your child can push up on his hands and then maintain propping on hands
2. mobility and strength in the legs to hold the hips in neutral rotation and adduction, so that the knees are together and the feet point straight behind
3. strong abdominals to initiate moving into quadruped by lifting the pelvis and bending the hips, and then maintaining the quadruped position once achieved

4. use of chin tuck in combination with activating the abdominals to assist with initiating moving into quadruped
5. weight shifting the trunk backwards over the legs to move into quadruped
6. the ability to maintain the position and playfully rock forward and back with control

## Tendencies

The tendencies are:
1. to have weak arms and prop on hands with the hands forward of the shoulders (side view)
2. to position the legs in the frog leg posture or weight bearing on the knees with the knees wide apart and the feet together (hip external rotation)
3. to arch the head and trunk when prone propping on hands, so he cannot do the head and trunk bending movements to move into quadruped
4. to have weak abdominals so he cannot lift his pelvis and bend his hips to initiate moving into quadruped, or to be unable to use abdominal strength once in the position to maintain it (while stationary or when rocking)
5. to have difficulty figuring out how to coordinate and sequence the movements to move into quadruped
6. to overuse the back and hip muscles when in quadruped so he tends to thrust forward
7. to have difficulty controlling the range of motion, when rocking forward and backward in quadruped

## Setup for Learning

Your child practiced supported kneeling during the last stage, which prepared him to develop the leg strength (neutral hip rotation and adduction) for quadruped. The next step is to develop the abdominal strength needed to move into quadruped from lying on his stomach. To move into quadruped, he will need to be able to push up on his hands, tuck his chin, activate his abdominals, bend his hips and knees with his knees close together, and weight shift his trunk

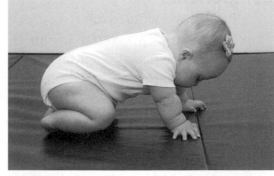

(fig. 4.28)

backwards over his legs (fig. 4.28). He will develop the arm position first. To test to see if he can move his legs into the position, wait for him to prop on his hands and then lift his abdomen, and activate his abdominal muscles (4.29). With this support, see if he will move his legs into position. If he can, he has the arm and leg movements needed to move into quadruped

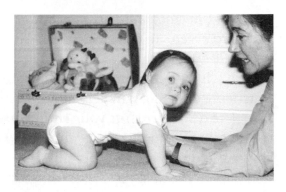

(fig. 4.29)

and just needs to learn to activate his abdominals, and then coordinate and sequence the movements to move into quadruped.

When your child is able to move into quadruped, he will be able to learn many new skills. Quadruped is a key position from which a child learns to move to sit, creep, pull to kneel, and pull to stand. If he does not develop quadruped until later he will need to learn other ways to move into these positions.

Using quadruped gives your child a more efficient way to move from one position to another and from one place to another. When he is able to use quadruped, he will move from sitting to quadruped, creep to the sofa or table, pull to kneel, and then pull to stand. If he is not able to use quadruped, he will move from sitting to stomach-lying, belly crawl to the sofa, move from stomach-lying to sitting, pull to kneel from sitting on the floor, and then pull to stand.

## Guidelines

*To encourage your child to move to quadruped and stay in the position, place a motivating toy on a raised surface (approximately 10 inches or 25 cm high) so his weight is shifted back over his legs.* If the toy is placed there, when he looks up at it, he will weight shift his trunk backwards over his legs and then it will be easier for him to maintain the position. If his weight is shifted forward over his arms (shoulders forward of his hands—side view), he will fall forward out of the position.

*Do not force your child to use quadruped or to maintain it when he is resisting it.* Use supported kneeling (Activity #10, Stage 3) until he is interested in being placed in quadruped and rocking on hands and knees, or he is ready to move into quadruped with your help. If he resists, figure out which component needs to be developed (arm, leg, or abdominal strength) and then work on it using other skills. If he is able to combat crawl and does not use quadruped, continue working on climbing skills (previous section of this chapter) and have him practice the quadruped position that way.

*Just because he assumes quadruped does not mean he is able and ready to creep.* To creep, he will need to balance himself using his abdominals as he weight shifts and moves each arm and leg. Since creeping is so complicated, it will take time for him to figure out how to do it. In the meantime, practicing climbing will help him learn the components.

*Use a surface that your child can sink his knees into.* Then his knees are stabilized and it is easier for him to activate his abdominals and weight shift his trunk back over his legs. It is easier to assume quadruped on soft, non-slippery surfaces like sand, the crib mattress, a bed, or the sofa. It is harder to assume quadruped on hard and slippery surfaces like a hardwood floor.

*To assume quadruped, your child needs his head in line with his trunk, looking down at the surface (side view), with his chin tucked.* If his head is looking up and lifted while in prone, his head and trunk are in the arched position and he cannot activate his abdominals and bend his hips to initiate moving into quadruped.

### Temperament

If your child is **motor driven,** he will like to experiment with pushing up on his arms and legs when on his stomach. Once he finds quadruped, he will like the movement of rocking forward and back. If your child is an **observer,** he will use quadruped when it is helpful. He may learn to use it to move to sit or to position himself close enough to the sofa to pull to kneel and stand.

### ACTIVITY #6: Moving into Quadruped

1. Place him on his stomach on a soft, raised surface like the bed. Sit on the floor in front of him so you are at eye level to him.
2. Wait for him to push up on his hands. Watch his head position and encourage him to look down at the bed, rather than look up at you (or lower your head to help him look downward). Then place your hands in between his arms and press your fingertips into his abdomen while lifting his abdomen. When you press your fingertips into his abdomen, use a tickling motion to activate his abdominals.
3. With this support, watch what his legs do. Wait for him to bend his hips and knees and assume quadruped. (If he keeps his legs straight, then you bend them so he is in quadruped.) If needed, move his knees together if they are too wide apart.
4. Then rock his trunk back over his legs, and play the "rocking game." While rocking him, keep his trunk and pelvis primarily over his legs. When rocking him forward, just move his shoulders over his hands but not forward of his hands (side view).

5. After he is in quadruped, you can encourage him to raise his head and look up at you or a toy and the action of lifting his head will help him maintain the position since it will cause his trunk and pelvis to weight shift back over his legs.

6. As tolerated, lessen your support so he learns to move into quadruped and maintain it by himself.

7. With practice, he will surprise you and you will find him moving into quadruped and rocking in his crib.

# Creeping

Creeping is moving on hands and knees from one place to another (fig. 4.30). The goal will be for your child to creep at least ten feet. Once he can do that distance, he will use it for mobility in his environment. Creeping is

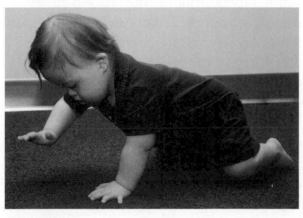

(fig. 4.30)

important because it teaches your child valuable movement patterns. He will strengthen his abdominal muscles, move his legs in an alternating, repetitive pattern with neutral hip rotation and adduction, strengthen his arms, and, when creeping is refined, he will coordinate his arms and legs to move in a reciprocal pattern (opposite arm and leg moving together).

Children with Down syndrome develop creeping at different times, depending on when they are strong enough and motivated to use it. For some children, creeping is easy because they have strong arms, and it is the first and only method of mobility that they use. Most children, however, crawl first and creep later, after they have learned to climb up a flight of stairs. Some children choose to use creeping when they see it is functional for them, like when they want to pull to stand. They may combat crawl across the room fast. Then when they approach the sofa, they move to quadruped and creep to pull to stand more efficiently. Some children choose to use creeping later when they are cruising and stepping with support.

Each child chooses his own time to start creeping, so do not give up. Your child can use combat crawling for mobility, keep practicing climbing up the stairs, and then creep when he is ready.

## Components

The components to focus on are:

1. arm, leg, and abdominal strength to assume and maintain the quadruped position
2. weight shifting with control, side to side and forward and back
3. abdominal strength to maintain balance in quadruped as your child moves his legs and arms
4. ability to coordinate the repetitive arm and leg pattern to move longer distances
5. maturation of the arm and leg pattern into a reciprocal pattern (opposite arm and leg moving simultaneously)
6. ability to move quickly and efficiently over long distances

## Tendencies

The tendencies are:

1. to have weak arms or difficulty positioning the arms to move them forward with control, so your child ends up falling forward
2. to position the legs in the frog leg posture or with a wide base (knees wide apart), which hinders weight shifting and movement of the legs forward
3. to have weak abdominals so it is difficult to move the arms and legs
4. to have difficulty tolerating or controlling weight shifting in all directions (forward, backwards, and sideways)
5. to continue to use combat crawling because it is such a fast and efficient form of mobility

## Setup for Learning

When your child is able to move into quadruped and rock, he is not necessarily ready to move forward and creep. By moving into quadruped and rocking, he is developing the strength and balance needed to hold the position and move forward and backward over a stable base. More complex, coordinated movements are needed for creeping. When he is first learning to creep, he needs to be able to shift his weight and maintain his balance while he moves his arm or leg forward.

The best way to teach your child the components for creeping is by practicing climbing up stairs. Therefore, I generally recommend that you practice creeping after he can climb up the flight of stairs. Usually, I do not advise working on creeping earlier unless you have a child with strong arms who is very interested in the skill. These self-motivated children will assume quadruped, rock forward and back, weight shift to each side (moving into and out of sitting), and may experiment with trying to move forward. If they cannot figure out how to do it, then you can practice creeping with them.

When teaching your child to creep, the leg movements are easier to develop, so start there. He needs to be setup with his trunk weight shifted back over his legs. If his trunk leans forward over his hands (side view: shoulders forward of his hands), he will fall forward onto his face and be upset. It will be harder for him to control his arm movements and trunk posture, so this needs to be totally managed so he can learn to initiate the leg movements. To help him weight shift back onto his legs, set him up to look at a motivator (toy) on a raised surface (9 inches or 23 cm high), placed 1 to 2 feet (30 to 60 cm) away from him.

To help him feel the creeping movements, you can place him in quadruped and kneel over him with your legs on the sides of his legs, supporting his legs with a narrow base. Use your hand to support his chest so his trunk is weight shifted back over his legs and his hands are forward of his shoulders (side view). With this support, you can initiate weight shifting (side to side) with your legs and see if he will move each knee after you weight shift him. After he moves each knee, then you move each hand forward. Continue this sequence until you reach the surface with the toys and he is kneeling at the surface. When he reaches the surface, place his hands on the surface and wait for him to move each knee forward. At this point, your goal is for him to become familiar with moving his knees, one at a time. As needed, support his trunk and arms to provide stability so that he is more comfortable moving his knees.

When your child tries to move forward on hands and knees, his first movements will be slow and uncoordinated. He will experiment with moving each knee and then his arms, using very small steps in order to keep his balance. His first creeping pattern will be with his knees wider than his hips. To help him be successful, set him up so the endpoint is very close, about 2 feet away, with the motivating toy up on a raised surface (about 9 inches or 23 cm high). This setup will help him persist with using quadruped since he is close to the toy and he is at the level of the toy. (If the toy is on the floor, then he will move to the floor and combat crawl to it.) With practice, he will learn to creep longer distances. With the repetition of using creeping for mobility, his speed and efficiency will improve and he will ultimately learn to use a reciprocal pattern (moving opposite arm and leg at the same time).

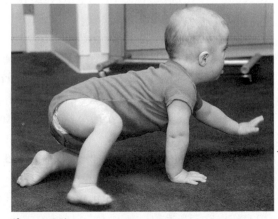

(fig. 4.31)

Some children initially learn to creep on one foot and one knee (fig. 4.31). Using this method makes it easy to move up to stand or to move back to sitting. Frequently, this is a temporary pattern and then the child progresses to creeping on both knees. If your child uses this pattern, you do not need to try to change it because he will be upset and frustrated if you interfere with his method of mobility. If this pattern persists, you and your physical therapist can check his legs in standing to see if his knee and foot are turned outward on the side where he uses his foot. Generally, this is not the case, but if it is, this posture should be addressed when practicing standing skills.

Some children develop even more creative ways to move around their environment. For instance, Sam moved around in sitting by using his arms to scoot himself backwards. Melissa moved around in sitting by using her feet to pull herself forward. Jordan was able to scoot himself along the floor by moving himself from sitting to hands and knees and back to sitting again until he had moved himself sideways across the floor to where he wanted to be. If your child is motivated to move and figures out his own unique method, let him use it. In the meantime, continue to practice climbing up the stairs and your child will learn to creep when he is ready.

## Guidelines

*Place the toy close enough that your child will be motivated to creep to it, and place it on a raised surface at eye level so he needs to be on hands and knees to see it.* Start him in quadruped facing the toy. If the toy is too far away or it is placed on the floor, he will automatically belly crawl to it.

*Do not try to rush your child into creeping.* If he does not creep during this stage, he will do it during the next stage. If he is an excellent belly crawler or if he has created a scooting pattern he likes, he may not want to change his method to creeping yet.

*Binding your child's legs together to create a narrower base is not necessary.* It is best if your child learns to actively hold his legs together rather than passively supporting them together. If support is needed when he is first learning the skill, you can provide intermittent support with handling, and then decrease your support as tolerated. Your child will learn to keep his legs together if you practice supported quadruped, supported kneeling, 90/90 sitting, moving in and out of sitting, and supported standing.

*Try a variety of surfaces to test which surface works best for creeping.* Creeping on a hardwood floor or other slippery surface is very difficult. If you use a slippery surface, your child may prefer to combat crawl. If your child is outside on the sidewalk or grass, he may bear walk. If he is on the carpet, he may creep. Your child will use whatever method is most efficient on each surface.

*Test to see what clothes work best for creeping.* Creeping is difficult in a dress or skirt. Some children prefer to creep with pants on (on a carpeted surface) and others prefer bare knees. Your daughter will move her knee onto the edge of the dress or skirt and then will be frustrated that she is stuck. Make it easy for her by dressing her in a onesie or shorts. Watch to see when creeping is easiest, observing what clothes and surfaces work best.

## Temperament

Whether your child is motor driven or an observer, he will learn to creep. He will develop this skill when he is ready, motivated, and strong enough to do it. All of a sudden, he will begin practicing it and that will be your cue to help him learn to do it. If he does not initiate it and is able to climb up a flight of stairs, then you can introduce creeping to him so he learns this new method of mobility. When he is able to creep, you will begin to see how active he is. Even if you said he was an observer before, you will probably think he is motor driven now. If he is truly an observer, however, you will notice the observer traits (being careful) return when he is learning to walk.

## ACTIVITY #7: Creeping on Hands and Knees

1. Place your child on his stomach on the floor. Place him 2 feet away from the surface you will put the toy on. The surface needs to be 9 to 10 inches (23 to 25 cm) high, at eye level when he is on hands and knees. It is best if it is a soft surface (like a folded mat or two stacked sofa cushions), in case he bumps into it as he is moving toward it.

2. If he can move onto hands and knees, have him do it. If not, place him on hands and knees and kneel over him with your knees around his. With this support, you will provide stability and narrow his base. Then place the palm of your hand on 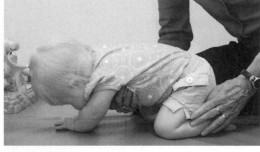 (fig. 4.32) his chest and weight shift him so his pelvis is back over his heels (fig. 4.32). This will keep him from diving or thrusting forward.

3. From this position, encourage him to creep to the toy. Watch his legs because it will be easier to move his knees than his arms. If he does not move his knees, then weight shift him to the side and see if he moves the opposite knee. Repeat the weight shift to the other side and he will move his other knee. Then move each hand forward.

4. Support his chest and move his arms until he can move his knees. Once he is at the surface, place his hands up on the surface and wait for him to move each knee forward to kneel and play.

5. With practice, your child will learn to move his knees and hands over this short distance with this setup.

6. When he can creep a distance of 2 feet to the toy and does it well, gradually increase the distance to 3 feet. Continue to increase the distance as tolerated.

7. If your child resists creeping farther than 2 feet, place the toy 2 feet away and have him creep to it. Let him play with it briefly and then move it 2 feet away again.

8. Work toward creeping within a room and around the house.

# Moving to Sit

During this stage, the goal will be for your child to learn to move to sit by himself by moving over one side (rather than moving through the center). In the last stage, he learned the individual components of pushing up to sit with his arms (from the "L" position) and weight shifting through his pelvis (moving from kneeling to sitting) with your support. Now he will learn how to combine these components in an organized sequence to achieve the skill of moving into sitting by himself. He will learn to move to sit from his stomach or after he assumes quadruped (hands and knees). Until he can do it by himself, you will continue to help him practice moving from kneeling to sitting.

## *Components*

The components to focus on are:

1. arm strength to prop and the ability to move the hands until he has moved to the midline sitting position

2. pelvic control to stabilize the pelvis and then weight shifting through it as he moves up to sit

3. trunk control (side bending and rotation) and use of abdominals to initiate and assist throughout the process of moving into sitting

4. leg strength to hold the knees together (in quadruped), weight shift the pelvis over the legs, assist with balance, and move the legs to the midline sitting position

5. ability to sequence the timing of the arm, trunk, pelvic, and leg movements in a coordinated and organized way to move to sit

6. desire to sit and the persistence and determination to keep going until he achieves the balanced sitting position

## Tendencies

The tendencies are:

1. to have difficulty pushing up with the arms due to weakness, placing the hands too far away from the trunk, or lack of perseverance to keep repositioning the hands for several repetitions while moving to the midline sitting position

2. to have difficulty initiating the weight shift through the pelvis to begin moving to sit

3. to move to sit through the midline (without weight shifting) by moving the legs into a wide split

4. to arch the trunk and hold it straight and centered (for stability) rather than use side bending and rotating movements. (Your child will tend to overuse the back muscles and underuse the abdominal muscles)

5. to hold his knees apart when in quadruped, and then not be able to weight shift the pelvis to move to sit

6. to have difficulty in sequencing and coordinating the timing of the arm, trunk, pelvic, and leg movements to move to sit

7. to choose to stay in the prone position because it is a preferred position

## Setup for Learning

### Methods of Moving to Sitting

**Moving to Sit from Quadruped.** The easiest and most efficient method of moving to sit is from hands and knees (figs. 4.33, 4.34). Once your child can get onto his hands and knees, you can help him move to sit using this method. From quadruped, he will need to hold his knees together and weight shift his pelvis back over his feet and then to the side. After his pelvis moves to the ground, then he will push up to sit with his hands. Until he can do it by *himself,* you can help him with the missing components by holding his

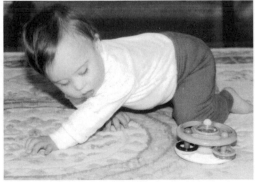

(fig. 4.33)

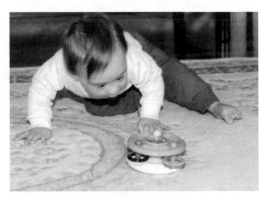

(fig. 4.34)

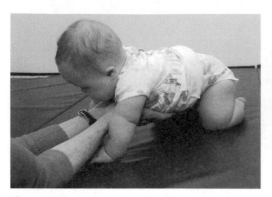

(fig. 4.35)

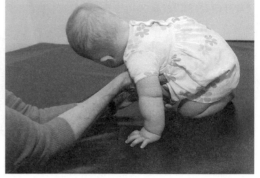

(fig. 4.36)

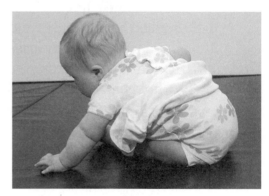

(fig. 4.37)

knees together, helping him with the weight shift (two directions: back over his feet and then over to the side), or supporting his pelvis after it lands on the floor to anchor it until he begins pushing up with his hands (figs. 4.35, 4.36, 4.37). It is best if you provide strategic support, only helping the specific component needing assistance. You want him to be successful and learn to do it by himself and you want to be sure he does not learn to become dependent on you to do the skill.

**Moving to Sit from Prone.** Since many children with Down syndrome do not learn to assume quadruped until later, they need to practice other methods of moving to sit. From observing many children with Down syndrome, I have learned a new method that is a good option for many children. It is easy for them due to hip flexibility, and they are comfortable with the amount of weight shifting through the pelvis. From prone, I support the child's lower leg in the frog leg position (fig. 4.38a) and his opposite armpit, holding under his arm at his trunk (fig. 4.38b, p. 154). Then the timing and coordination of the next

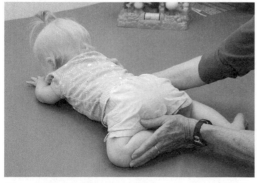

(fig. 4.38a)

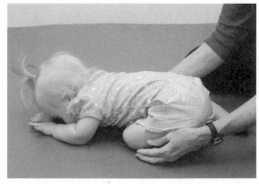

(fig. 4.39)

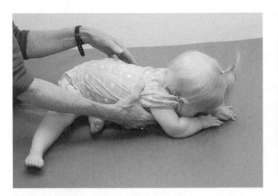

(fig. 4.40)

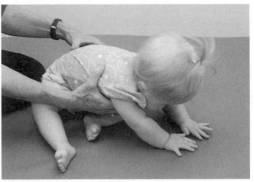

(fig. 4.41)

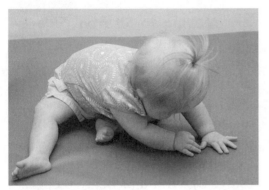

(fig. 4.42)

movements are critical. I begin to scoop or tuck his leg under his trunk and then (after a brief pause) slightly lift his armpit to weight shift his pelvis over his hip (figs. 4.39, 4.40). Once you have done these movements, he is propping on his hands and he can push up to sit (figs. 4.41, 4.42. 4.43). If needed, you can slightly support his pelvis (to gently stabilize it) to make it easier to push up to sit. Sometimes the child's hands are too far from his trunk and you will need to place the hands closer so he is successful with pushing up to sit.

Some children with Down syndrome learn to move from stomach-lying to sitting by spreading their legs wide apart and doing a split, and then they push up to sitting with their hands (fig. 4.44–4.47). Some children figure out this method even though you have practiced the methods of moving over one side using weight shifting. If your child develops this method, let him use it during his free play because it enables him to move to sit independently. When you are on the floor

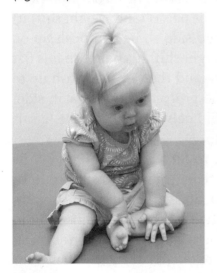

(fig. 4.43)

playing with him, continue to practice the methods of moving to sit by moving to the side, and moving from kneeling to sitting. When he can assume the quadruped position, he will learn to move to sit by moving to the side. The important component to learn is weight shifting since this is needed for many gross motor skills and ultimately for an efficient walking pattern.

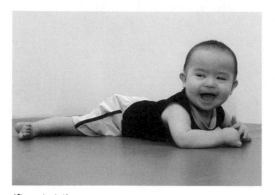

(fig. 4.44)

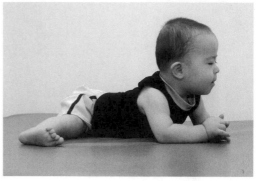

(fig. 4.45)

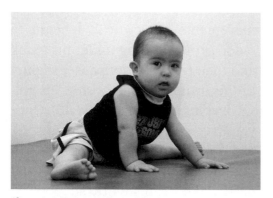

(fig. 4.46)

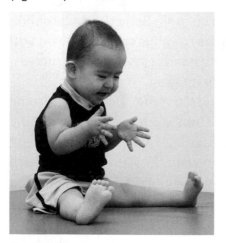

(fig. 4.47)

***Moving to Sit from Side-Lying.*** Sometimes a child with Down syndrome will try to move to sit from the side-lying position (figs. 4.48, 4.49). He will move from his back or stomach to side-lying, propping on his elbow or hand. To be successful, place his legs in the "L" position (Stage 3), with hips bent 90 degrees and knees straight. From this position, support his pelvis (and weight shift it) on the opposite side so he can push up on his hands. Weight shift his pelvis so it is flat on the surface and then he will push up to sit. Later, if he props on his elbow in side-lying, give mild pelvic support so he learns to move to sit.

***Moving to Sit from Kneeling.*** While you are practicing moving from prone or quadruped to sitting, continue to simultaneously practice moving from kneeling to sitting since it is an easier skill and reinforces the components needed. When your child plays in kneeling, have him practice moving from kneeling to sitting (Activity #10) when he wants to move out of kneeling (figs. 4.50, 4.51, 4.52). You will need to make sure his knees are together. Then, when he weight shifts his pelvis to one side, he will move his pelvis to the ground and then use his arms to push up to sitting in the midline. When he first practices this skill, it will be easiest if he is kneeling at a low surface, like a 5-inch (12.5-cm) sofa cushion placed on the floor.

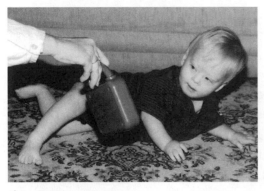

(fig. 4.48)

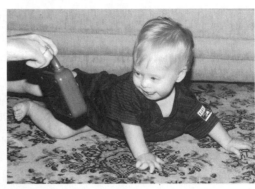

(fig. 4.49)

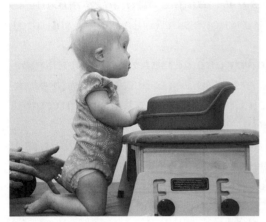

(fig. 4.50)

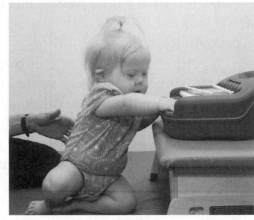

(fig. 4.51)

**The Best Method for Your Child.** Your child will figure out the best method to use (for his body and his learning style/temperament) to move to sit. You will help him learn the components and give him experience with the possible methods, and then you need to wait and see what he initiates. While you are practicing the methods, you may be able to feel

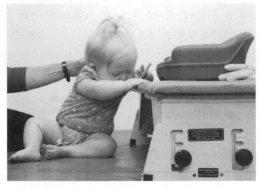

(fig. 4.52)

which method is easier for him. You may feel him moving with ease with one method and resisting another particular method. If you feel this difference, then practice the method that he likes. It is likely that he will learn to use this method first. Watch to see what works for your child and build on it.

## Guidelines

*Practice moving to sit every time you place your child in sitting.* If you are carrying him, place him on the floor and then have him assist with moving to sit. Anytime he is on his stomach and he wants to sit and play, assist him with moving to sit. It is best to practice this skill when it is functional for him rather than doing it in a repetitive way. By practicing it in this way, it will become a habit for him and he will practice it often during his day.

*Place a motivating toy to one side at the level of his feet, so that the toy is in the right place after he moves to sit.* If you place the toy to the side of his trunk, he will want to stop and play with it when he is halfway to sitting. If you do not let him play with it and move it again, he will be upset and frustrated. It is best if the toy is placed at the endpoint to motivate him and to set him up to achieve the goal of moving to sit.

*Do not worry if he figures out his own unique method of moving to sit.* As long as he moves to sit by moving over one side (with weight shifting), his variation is acceptable.

*If your child's hands are too far away and he is struggling with moving to sit, place his hands closer to his trunk so he is successful with pushing up to sit.* You do not want him to quit or fail, so help him be successful. With practice, he will be able to do it by himself.

*Watch his pelvis and help him fully shift his weight through it so it is stable and on the ground.* When moving to sit, he will initially have his weight on one side of his pelvis. As he pushes to midline sitting, he will weight shift to the other side and his pelvis will be horizontal and stable on the floor. As he weight shifts through his pelvis, the legs will follow to move into the circle-sit position when his pelvis is stable on the floor.

*Make sure his knees are together when he is moving from kneeling or quadruped to sitting.* If his knees are even slightly apart or if his hips are in slight external rotation (knees apart and feet together), this will block the weight shift of moving to sit. With his knees totally supported together, the slightest weight shift will initiate moving to sit. You want this transition to be easy and the knee position is critical.

*When your child is moving from prone or quadruped to sitting, remember that he will need to weight shift his pelvis in two directions, backwards over his legs and to the side.* In the beginning, you will need to emphasize and support these two directions. When he is familiar with these movements, he will use the mature pattern of moving in the diagonal groove by combining the two directions to weight shift backwards and over. If he only weight shifts to the side, then his hands will be too far away from his trunk to be able to effectively push himself up to sit.

The weight shifting movements are complicated and difficult to explain but you will understand them if you practice them with your body. If your child is having difficulty, you can imitate his movements and then understand why he is stuck, and adjust the support you are providing.

## *Temperament*

If your child is **motor driven,** he will like to experiment with moving from one position to another. He will try to move to sit as he is moving around. He may not want to sit for long, but he will enjoy moving to sitting. If your child is an **observer,** he will want to sit. Since he loves to sit, he will be motivated to figure out how to move to the sitting position.

## ACTIVITY #8: Moving from Quadruped to Sitting, on Raised Surface

1. Place your child on his stomach on a raised surface (like the bed), with him facing you.
2. You sit on your heels on the floor.
3. Wait for him to push up on his hands.

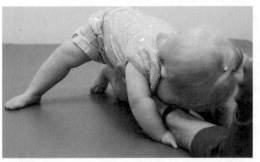

4. Encourage him to look down at the surface so his head is in a neutral position (not looking up).
5. Place your hands on his abdomen and lift it, and use your fingertips to activate his abdominals (tickling movements). Wait for him to bend his hips and knees to move to quadruped.

(fig. 4.53)

6. Once he is on hands and knees (with your hands on his abdomen), weight shift him back onto his legs and then over his side until his pelvis is on the bed (fig. 4.53, 4.54). Then give mild pelvic support (to stabilize it) so he can push up to sit (fig. 4.55). If his knees are wide apart, you will need to move his knee in (so it is under his hip) before you do the weight shift.

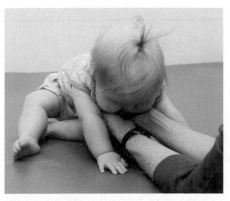

(fig. 4.54)

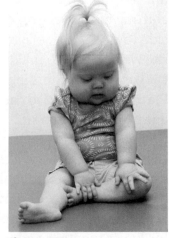

(fig. 4.55)

7. In Step 5, if he does not bend his hips and knees to move into quadruped, then move one knee forward and place it on the bed, and then assist the pelvic weight shift (Step 6). The closer you place his knee to his hands, the easier it will be to push up to sit.

8. With practice, your child may initiate the pelvic weight shift over a preferred side once you do Step 5 and he is on hands and knees. If so, then assist the weight shift to make sure he moves in both directions (back over his legs and then to the side). He probably will know to weight shift to the side and you can assist the backwards direction.

9. Place a motivating toy between his knees and feet to encourage him to move to sit.

10. Continue to practice until he can move to sit by himself, gradually decreasing your support. To make it easier to move to sit from Step 6 and 8, move his hands closer to his knees.

## ACTIVITY #9: Moving from Quadruped to Sitting, on Floor

Sit on your heels on the floor with your knees apart.

1. Place your child lying on his belly in front of you, facing away from you, with his legs together in between your legs.

2. Lift his trunk and move his pelvis back over his legs, so he is on hands and knees, with his knees together (fig. 4.56). Place the palm of one of your hands on his chest to keep his pelvis weight shifted over his feet. Then move your legs away from supporting him and see if he initiates weight shifting his pelvis over one side (fig. 4.57). If so, assist

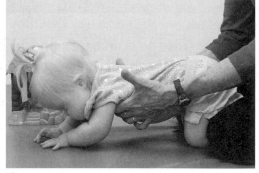

(fig. 4.56)

the weight shift to make sure he moves fully in both directions (pelvis back over his legs and then to the side) (fig. 4.58).

3. Place a motivating toy at the level of his knees and feet to encourage him to move to sit.

4. From this position, he will use his hands to push up to sit (figs. 4.59, 4.60). Provide mild pelvic support (if needed) so he can push up to sit. To make it easier to move to sit, move his hands closer to his knees or move his knee closer to his hands.

5. If he does not initiate the pelvic weight shift in Step 3, then place his knees together and hold them with your hand (between your

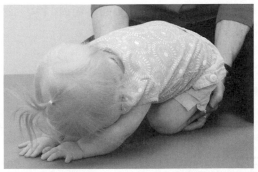

(fig. 4.57)

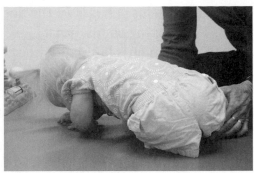

(fig. 4.58)

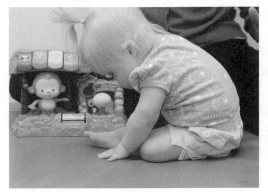

(fig. 4.59)

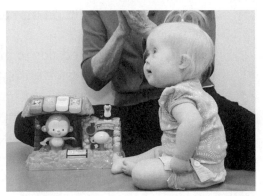

(fig. 4.60)

index finger and thumb), and weight shift his pelvis back over his heels. With this support, see if he will initiate the weight shift. If he still does not weight shift his pelvis, lean his pelvis to the side until it touches the floor. Then follow Steps 4 & 5.

6. See if he has a preferred side to move over and practice moving to sit in that direction.
7. Continue to practice until your child can move to sit by himself, gradually decreasing your support.

## 🏃 ACTIVITY #10: Moving from Kneeling to Sitting

1. Place your child kneeling at a 5-inch (12.5-cm) sofa cushion placed on the floor. Stabilize the cushion against furniture to prevent sliding.
2. Hold his knees together with your thumb and index finger.
3. Weight shift his pelvis so it is back over his heels.
4. Wait for him to weight shift his pelvis to one side to initiate moving to sit. If he does not initiate the weight shift, then guide it with your hand (the one that is holding his knees together).
5. If needed, place a toy on the floor (between his knees and feet) to motivate him to initiate the weight shift.

6. Once his pelvis is on the floor, assist him to move to sit safely by propping on his arms.
7. When he is familiar with these movements, decrease your support until he can move from kneeling to sitting by himself.
8. When your child can move from kneeling to sitting at the 5-inch (12.5-cm) surface, then teach him to do it when kneeling at higher surfaces.

## ACTIVITY #11: Moving from Stomach-lying to Sitting

1. Position yourself on the floor sitting on your heels.
2. Position your child on his stomach in front of you, facing away from you
3. If he has a preferred side to move over, practice over that side. If not, practice over each side until you notice which side is easier for him.
4. To move over his left side:
   a. Place a toy on his right side below hip level.
   b. Place his left leg in the frog leg posture and place your left hand alongside his lower leg.

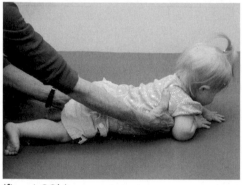
(fig. 4.38b)

   c. Place your right hand under his right armpit, with your hand holding his trunk (fig. 4.38b).
   d. With a scooping motion with your fingers, slide his left leg under his abdomen and then lift his trunk with your right hand and weight shift the left side of his pelvis over his left hip. Remember that the weight shift needs to be in two directions: pelvis back behind foot and to the left side.
   e. When the left side of his pelvis is on the floor, he will be propping on his hands. At this point, he will probably need you to give gentle support to the right side of his pelvis while he pushes up to sit.
5. To move over his right side, practice the above steps with his right leg and left armpit supported, and the toy placed on his left side.
6. The timing and coordination of the movements in Steps 4 and 5 are critical.
7. Continue to practice until he can move to sit by himself, gradually decreasing your support. To make it easier to move to sit from Step 4e, move your child's hands closer to his knees so he is successful with pushing up to sit.

# Moving Out of Sitting

During this stage, your child will learn to move out of sitting by himself with control, by moving over one side. In the last stage, he practiced the components needed for this skill: tolerating falling to the side, propping on his arms, and moving down onto his belly. He needed your supervision and guidance for safety. It was important to familiarize your child with this weight shifting method of moving out of sitting as soon as possible since he would not have chosen this method on his own. Now that he has had this preparation, during this stage, he will choose to use this method consistently and spontaneously, whenever he wants to move out of sitting. The ultimate goal will be to move out of sitting by moving over one side with weight shifting. As long as he moves to the side and moves over his leg with his knee bent, he will have accomplished the goal.

## Components

The components to focus on are:

1. propping hands to the side, then bending his elbow to lower himself down to the floor with control
2. trunk mobility and control (side bending and rotation) to prop his hands to the side and weight shift, to begin the transition of moving out of sitting
3. bending the knee that he is moving over, and moving easily over the leg so it does not block moving down to his stomach
4. ability to tolerate weight shifting over one side, as well as the risk of falling down, and choosing to initiate these movements
5. ability to sequence the parts of the skill, and ultimately land on his stomach rather than his back
6. having the desire to move out of sitting and deliberately choosing to do it with control

## Tendencies

The tendencies are:

1. to move from sitting to his stomach by spreading his legs into a wide split and moving through the center (see the box below).
2. to resist placing his hands to the side to prop (because of his short arms) and to stiffen his elbows for stability when propping (because he is afraid of letting go and falling down)
3. to resist trunk rotation and prefer to hold his trunk erect and centered
4. to straighten and stiffen his knees in sitting so he feels stable and balanced in the center, which prevents weight shifting

5. to stabilize himself by positioning his legs in a wide base with the frog leg posture, which blocks moving out of sitting
6. to resist weight shifting and moving down out of sitting because it feels too risky, or he is fearful of feeling off balance
7. to choose to stay in sitting if it is his preferred position for play. If he reaches for a toy but it is out of his reach, he will choose to stay in sitting and move back to the centered position. When setup and assisted to move out of sitting, he will push back up to sitting.

## Setup for Learning
### Methods of Moving Out of Sitting

There are three methods of moving out of sitting. The first method your child will learn will be to move from sitting down to his stomach. Later, when he likes to creep, he will learn to move from sitting over to quadruped. The third method is moving upward from sitting to kneeling. All three methods involve weight shifting over one side and will be taught when he is ready to use them, depending on what gross motor skills he is ready to learn.

**Moving from Sitting to His Stomach.** To practice moving from sitting down to his stomach, you need to test what your child is willing to do on his own. You will place a motivating toy to the side of his knee (in front of his knee and to the side of it), just out of his reach, and then wait for his reaction. If he reaches for it and props his hands to one side, then he is willing to start the weight shift. If he does not, you will need to do this for him. By placing his hands to the side, you will set him up to be in a predicament that will provoke him to move. (He will not like feeling off balance so will either move back to the centered sitting position or down to his stomach.) Then you will wait to see if he will bend his elbow and weight shift more, to begin moving down to his stomach. You will assist as needed to help him land safely on his stomach.

When your child first moves out of sitting, he will do it fast and without control. As he practices moving down to his stomach, he will learn to lift his head so he does not bump it on the floor, and he will learn to lower himself down slowly, using his arms. He will learn to slowly bend his elbows to lower himself with control rather than falling fast (figs. 4.61–4.63). By choosing the most motivating toy and placing it in the right location, you will set him up to move out of sitting with weight shifting. With practice, he will sequence the movements to move out of sitting by himself with control.

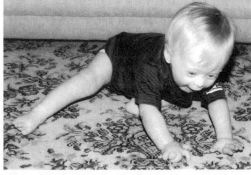

(fig. 4.61)

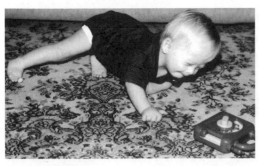

(fig. 4.62)

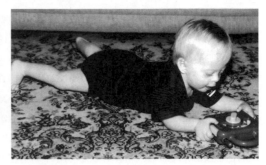

(fig. 4.63)

***Moving from Sitting to Quadruped.*** When your child can use the quadruped position and is able to creep on hands and knees, he will be motivated to learn to move from sitting to quadruped. From sitting, he will prop both hands to one side and then lift his buttocks up to move onto hands and knees. You can help him practice this using Activity #13.

***Moving from Sitting to Kneeling.*** When your child is able to kneel to play (even if he needs your support to hold his knees together) and can move from kneeling to sitting, you can practice moving from sitting to kneeling (figs. 4.64–4.66). By practicing this skill, you are beginning to teach him to pull to stand from sitting on the floor (which will be discussed in the next section). Another way to think of it is that moving from sitting to kneeling is having your child move out of sitting and moving upward. So, it is a way to reinforce weight shifting and moving over one side. If your child is not initiating moving down to his stomach or if he needs more practice with weight shifting, he can be setup

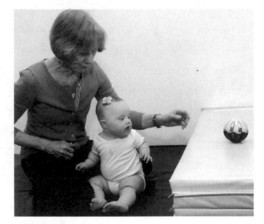

(fig. 4.64)

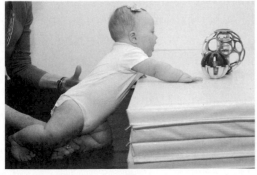

(fig. 4.65)

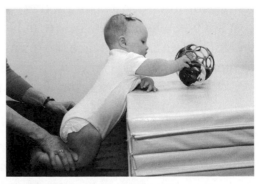

(fig. 4.66)

to assist with moving from sitting to kneeling when it is functional for him. Rather than just placing him in kneeling, he can learn to do specific parts of the skill of moving to kneeling with your support.

Keep practicing the methods of moving out of sitting with weight shifting over one side until your child chooses to do it on his own. Your child will choose to do it at his own unique time, when it is functional for him and he feels comfortable doing it. He may not want to move out of sitting because it is his preferred position for play. When he is setup with the toy placed just out of his reach, he may lean and initiate moving toward the toy but when he sees that he cannot reach it, he will choose to move back to the centered sitting position. He may wait to move out of sitting and choose to do it later after he can move to sit by himself.

---

### Doing the "Splits"

Even though you have practiced weight shifting over one side, your child may learn to move from sitting to his stomach by spreading his legs with his knees straight and doing a wide split. If your child chooses this method, be happy that he figured out a way to move from one position to another and has the desire to change positions. When you are playing with him on the floor, continue to practice weight shifting over one side (to move down to his stomach or up to kneeling). After he can assume quadruped and creep, he will learn to move in and out of sitting by moving to the side. In the meantime, he will use this "split" method until he feels comfortable using another method. Just remember, the real goal is for him to learn how to weight shift to move in and out of sitting.

---

## Guidelines

*He will go where the motivating toy is, so place it in the right location to guide him to move out of sitting with weight shifting, moving over one side.* To motivate your child to move from sitting to his stomach, place the toy to the side and forward of his knee (forward lateral diagonal), just out of his reach. Then when he reaches for it, he will be setup to move out of sitting with weight shifting. If you place the toy in front of him, you will be setting him up to move through the center without weight shifting.

- To encourage moving from sitting to quadruped, place the toy on a 9-inch (23-cm) high surface about 15 inches (38 cm) away from him. Place him sitting sideways to the surface rather than facing the surface. With the toy on this surface, it will be at eye level when he is in quadruped so he will move from sitting to quadruped to creep to it.

■ To encourage him to move from sitting to kneeling, place him sitting sideways next to a 6-inch (15-cm) high surface, with a space in between. He will lean and prop on the surface and then move up to kneeling to move to the toy.

*Allow your child's preference to determine whether to help him practice moving from sitting to his stomach, quadruped, or kneeling.* He may choose to move from sitting to his stomach and then pivot or crawl to a toy. He may choose to move from sitting to quadruped and creep to someone he wants. He may choose to move from sitting to kneeling at the sofa to play with a toy. With practice, he will develop the strength needed in his arms, legs, and abdominal muscles to move out of sitting with control.

## Temperament

If your child is **motor driven,** he will love moving out of sitting. He may not want to sit for long and will move to other positions to be active. If he is an **observer,** he may want to sit for a long time and not want to move out of the position. If the choice is between sitting or stomach-lying, he may prefer to sit. When he is able to crawl, creep, kneel, or stand, he will be more motivated to move out of sitting.

## ACTIVITY #12: Moving from Sitting to Stomach-lying

Moving over your child's right side:
1. Place him sitting on the carpet with a toy to the side of his knee (forward lateral diagonal), just out of his reach.
    a. See if he reaches for the toy, begins to weight shift to the side, and props his hands to the side to move to the toy. If not, place both hands on his right side, in between his right hip and knee (closer to his knee).
    b. Wait for him to move down to the floor and provide support for safety, if needed. He may need your support to tolerate practicing this skill. If so, support him at his trunk under his arm (armpit area) and wait for him to bend his elbow to initiate moving down to his stomach. You will guide him as needed to help him land safely on his stomach. You may need to move the toy so he does not bump into it.
    c. With practice, he will lift his head effectively and use his arms to lower himself slowly with control.
    d. If he chooses to move back up to sitting after you place his hands propping on his right side (Step b), then place his hands far to the side so he chooses to move down to his stomach.

e. You can position yourself sitting behind him or in front of him. Use the position that provides the support and motivation your child needs.

2. Repeat the steps above and help your child move over his left side.

## ACTIVITY #13: Moving from Sitting to Quadruped

Only practice this skill when your child is able to creep.
1. Sit on your heels on the floor.
2. Place your child sitting sideways in front of you.
3. To teach your child to move into quadruped over his right side:
   a. Put a toy on a 9-inch (23-cm) high surface about 2 feet (.6 meters) away from him, adjacent to his right side.
   b. Wait and see if he props both hands to his right side, moves to quadruped, and creeps to the toy on the surface. If not, provide the needed support. Place both of his hands to his right side and have him prop on them. Use your left hand to bend his knees and move them together. Place your right hand under his chest and lift it to help him move to hands and knees.
4. Moving into quadruped over his left side: repeat the steps in #3 but assist him in moving over his left side.
5. When your child is familiar with these movements, decrease your support until he can move from sitting to quadruped by himself.

## ACTIVITY #14: Moving from Sitting to Kneeling at a Sofa Cushion

Moving over your child's right side:
1. Place a 5- to 6-inch (12.5 to 15-cm) high sofa cushion on the floor and stabilize it against the wall or furniture to keep it from sliding. Place motivating toys on the cushion.
2. Place your child sitting with his right side next to the cushion, with a 5-inch (12.5-cm) space between him and the cushion.
3. Position yourself sitting on your heels, behind him on his right side.
4. Support his chest with your right hand (with your palm under his armpit) and lean his trunk and arms on the cushion so he is propping on his elbows.
5. With your left hand, support his legs together with his hips and knees bent, and use your thumb and index finger to hold his knees together.

6. Wait for him to lift his pelvis to move up to kneeling. Then place and support his legs so he is stable in kneeling (hips bent and knees together).
7. He can kneel and play, and when he wants to move out of the position, he can move from kneeling to sitting.
8. Repeat the above steps but help him move over his left side.
9. When he is familiar with these movements, decrease your support until he can move from sitting to kneeling at a 5- to 6-inch (12.5- to 15-cm) surface by himself.
10. Then increase the height of the surface. (You child will then be practicing pulling to kneel, and preparing for pulling to stand, which is covered in the next section.)

# Pulling to Kneel

Since your child is familiar with using the kneeling position to play and moving from kneeling to sitting, he is ready to learn how to pull to kneel. He practiced moving to kneeling when climbing and in the last section (Activity #14). He is now ready to practice pulling to kneel in preparation for pulling to stand. He needs to learn to move to kneeling as the intermediate position when pulling to stand. He will learn to pull to kneel from prone, sitting, and quadruped. He will probably learn to pull to kneel from sitting first. Then, later, when he can assume quadruped and creep, he can practice pulling to kneel from quadruped. The ultimate goal is for him to pull to kneel on surfaces of any height.

## Components

The components to focus on are:

1. arm and hand strength to reach, grip, and hold onto the surface when he is pulling to kneel from sitting, prone, and quadruped
2. trunk mobility (side bending and rotation) and strength (abdominals and back muscles) when lifting his pelvis to move to kneel, when moving his knees closer to the surface (knee walking) after he has lifted his pelvis, and to maintain the kneeling position
3. leg strength to hold the knees together with hips in neutral rotation, and to lift the pelvis when kneeling
4. ability to tolerate and initiate weight shifting to begin the move up to kneeling
5. desire to take weight on the legs and choose to use the kneeling position for play

## Tendencies

The tendencies are:

1. to have weak arms and hands or not effectively use his strength to pull to kneel
2. to overuse his back muscles and arch his back, or to have weak abdominals that make it difficult to move into the position and maintain the position
3. to have weak legs or to position his legs in the frog leg posture (hip external rotation) or with a wide base (knees apart) so it is difficult to move to kneeling and maintain kneeling
4. to arch his back and straighten his hips so he slides backwards out of the kneeling position and down to his stomach
5. to be fearful or uncomfortable with weight shifting so he pulls to kneel from sitting by moving through the midline, facing the surface; then he cannot kneel effectively because his legs are locked with his hips in external rotation (frog leg posture)
6. to learn to pull to stand without moving through kneeling by pulling to stand from sitting on the floor, facing the surface; he reaches, holds the surface, and uses arm strength to pull to stand
7. to inadequately bend the knee he is moving over, when moving from sitting to kneeling, and then his legs become tangled and block him from moving to kneeling

## Setup for Learning

To help your child learn to pull to kneel, always start with a low surface. When he is successful at the low surface, you can increase the height, making sure you do it gradually so he is successful. After he has learned to pull to kneel at low surfaces and you are challenging him to pull to kneel at higher surfaces, another strategy is to use a surface with an "edge" he can hold onto. Some examples are: an open drawer, a laundry basket, a toy box, a plastic storage box, a plastic vegetable bin, and crib rails. When he is ready for a higher surface (around 17 inches or 43 cm), he can use the edge of a train table toy. The edge needs to be narrow enough for him to hold easily with his small hands.

If he does not use a surface with an edge, his hands will be on top of a surface, like the sofa or table, and they may slide off as he tries to pull up. Using an edge will enable him to access the arm power he does have since he will be able to hold on and pull. You will need to stabilize some of these surfaces to keep them from moving when he is pulling up on them.

### Pulling to Kneel from Sitting

Pulling to kneel from sitting is generally the best method to begin practicing this transition. You have already familiarized your child with the movements required to move from sitting to kneeling at the 5-inch (12.5-cm) cushion in Activity #14. Now you will set him up sitting sideways to the sofa cushion and toys, with a space in between him and the cushion so that he can weight shift, and wait for him to initiate the weight shift to prop his arms and trunk. You will watch his legs to make sure they are in the best position for moving to kneeling and then wait for him to lift his pelvis to move to kneeling. Once he is in kneeling, you will check his leg position to make sure he is stable. As he is executing this transition, you will anticipate the steps and strategically assist him in succeeding, giving him the least amount of support so he is responsible for completing the skill. When your child can consistently pull to kneel at the 5-inch (12.5-cm) cushion, then the height can be increased until he can pull to kneel at the sofa or coffee table.

### Pulling to Kneel from Prone

The best way to motivate your child to pull to kneel from prone is usually to let him climb up on to your stomach when you are lying on the floor in front of him. You can place his hands on your chest or abdomen and then he will grip your clothes and pull with his arms. He will need to tuck his abdominals to lift his pelvis and bend his hips to move onto his knees. To activate his abdominals, he will need to tuck his head and lean his arms into your chest or abdomen. Once he is on his knees, then he can move each knee one at a time to knee walk closer to you so he is stable in kneeling. You can help him as needed until he is able to do it by himself. When he can pull to kneel onto your belly, then you can lie on your side and see if he can pull to kneel at this higher surface.

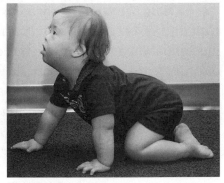

(fig. 4.67)

### Pulling to Kneel from Quadruped

Your child can only pull to kneel from quadruped after he can move into quadruped and creep. He will learn that combining creeping and pulling to kneel from quadruped will provide him with the most efficient way to pull to stand (figs. 4.67, 4.68). To learn this skill, he will need to be setup at a low surface so it is easy to reach up and place one hand on top of the surface. After he places one hand, then he

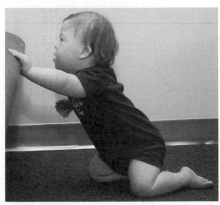

(fig. 4.68)

will place the other and knee walk, moving one knee at a time, to move closer to the surface and be stable enough to play. You may need to place his hand to teach him the skill, or you may need to stabilize his hand after he places it so it does not slip off the surface. When he can pull to kneeling at a low surface, then the height can be increased.

## Guidelines

*Use motivating toys that your child will want to move after.* Place them on top of the surface or hold them at the edge to get his attention and interest. He will know he needs to pull up to play with them. Once he pulls up, encourage him to stay in the kneeling position to play.

*Begin with a surface that is lower than the height of his shoulder (armpit) when in sitting, prone, or quadruped.* Some examples are a sofa cushion placed on the floor, a bottom stair that is carpeted, or a step stool. With lower surfaces, he can lean his trunk over them, and it will be easier to learn the steps and activate his abdominals to move onto his knees. He can use gross movements and move from one position to another. When the surface is higher than shoulder/armpit level, he needs to know the sequence of movements and use arm, leg, and abdominal strength to execute all of the steps of the transition with finesse.

*Know the sequence of steps and the movements needed for this transition and strategically provide support so your child is successful.* Only provide assistance for the part your child cannot do. If you control the transition or provide too much support, he will learn to depend on you to do this skill.

*Play the barricade game to encourage him to pull to kneel.* If your child is not interested in pulling to kneel, make it functional for him. Place sofa cushions or furniture all around him and place him sitting in the center. Place toys on the cushions or outside the barricade and then he will need to figure out how to pull to kneel to play with the toys. With this setup, you can also challenge him to climb out of the barricade or you can use higher surfaces for pulling to kneel.

## Temperament

If your child is **motor driven,** he will like to move from one position to another. He will be challenged by pulling up and moving his legs. If he is an **observer,** he will pull to kneel if the toy is worthwhile and he is motivated to get it.

### ACTIVITY #15: Pulling to Kneel from Sitting

1. Begin with practicing moving from sitting to kneeling (Activity #14) until your child is familiar with the sequence of movements.

Practice until he is comfortable initiating the weight shift to prop his arms and trunk and can pull to kneel at the 5-inch (12.5-cm) surface. If needed, you can provide strategic support and hold his knees together or maximally bend the knee he is moving over.

2. When he is ready to begin pulling to kneel at higher surfaces, try a 7- to 9-inch (18- to 23-cm) high soft surface or use a 9- to 12-inch (23- to 30.5-cm) surface with an edge so he can actively and effectively pull up. If needed, stabilize his hands on the surface. Support his knees together if needed or maximally bend the knee he is moving over.

3. Moving over his right side:

   a. Place your child sitting with his right side in front of the surface, with a 5-inch (12.5-cm) space between him and the surface. (This space is needed for weight shifting.)

   b. Sit on your heels behind him.

   c. Place the toy on top of the surface or at the edge to motivate him to move after it.

   d. See if he will weight shift and place his hands on the surface and try to pull up. If not, place his hands on the edge and wait for him to pull up. (In the beginning, he may need you to put your hand over his hands to help him prop or hold onto the edge.)

   e. After he weight shifts and places his hands, look at his legs and support his knees together, if needed, or maximally bend his right knee. Make sure his legs are in the best position (hips and knees bent, knees together) for moving to kneeling and then wait for him to lift his pelvis to move to kneeling.

   f. Once he is in kneeling, check his leg position to make sure he is stable. Support his knees together if needed.

   g. He will play in kneeling and then can move from kneeling to sitting when he chooses.

4. Moving over his left side: Repeat the steps in #3 but help him move over his left side (figs. 4.69–4.71).

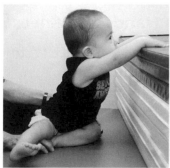
(fig. 4.69)

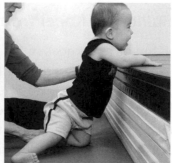
(fig. 4.70)

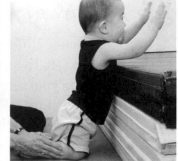
(fig. 4.71)

5. When he is ready, decrease your support and have him pull up to kneel by himself. Make sure that his knees are together or that the knee of the leg he is moving over is fully bent. This will make it easier for him to move over the leg and up to kneeling.

6. When he can pull to kneel on lower surfaces, gradually increase the height until he can pull to kneel on all surfaces.

 ## ACTIVITY #16: Pulling to Kneel from Stomach-lying

1. Place your child on his stomach on the floor.
2. Lie on your back on the floor beside him.
3. Encourage him to pull to kneel on your stomach.
4. Help him by placing his hands on your abdomen and then stabilize his hands as he holds onto your fingers or your clothes.
5. With this hand support, see if he can move up onto his knees. To activate his abdominals to lift his pelvis, he needs to tuck his chin and use his arms to bend his trunk and hips and move onto his knees. Once on his knees, then he needs to knee walk forward to be stable and upright in kneeling. Observe his posture and provide support if needed.
6. Once he has pulled up to kneeling, encourage him to play in the kneeling position, and then move to sitting when he chooses.
7. This skill can also be practiced using a 5-inch (12.5-cm) sofa cushion, placed on the floor. Place his arms on the cushion with his armpits at the edge and hold his chest (supporting his trunk under his armpits) and bend it over the cushion. With this support, he will tuck his chin and activate his abdominals to bend his hips and knees and move onto his knees. Then he will knee-walk forward to kneel at the cushion. With practice, he will learn how to use his arms to pull to kneel by himself, and you can provide strategic support to help him move to kneeling successfully.

## ACTIVITY #17: Pulling to Kneel from Hands and Knees

1. Place your child on hands and knees in front of a low surface (7- to 9-inch (18- to 23-cm) high cushion or surface with an edge).
2. Position yourself behind him with your knees around his knees to stabilize him. (With this support, he will be able to reach up more easily.) Observe his posture. If his trunk is forward over his arms, then support his chest and lean his trunk back over his legs.
3. Place a toy on the surface.

4. See if your child will place his hands on top of the surface or hold the edge of the surface, placing one hand at a time. If not, you place one hand and hold it there, and then wait for him to place his other hand.
5. After your child is holding the edge with both hands, he will need to move his knees forward (knee walk), one at a time, to move to kneeling. Help him if needed.
6. When he is ready, decrease your support and have him pull to kneel by himself.
7. When he can pull to kneel on low surfaces, gradually increase the height so he can pull to kneel on all surfaces.

# Pulling to Stand

During this stage, your child will learn to pull to stand from kneeling. In the last stage, he began practicing pulling to stand from 90/90 sitting holding your thumbs. During this stage, he will do it by holding onto a surface with an edge himself. Through this experience, he will become motivated to move to stand, choose to do it, initiate it, and be responsible for controlling it with your supervision for safety. Using this setup, he will show you his desire to stand and will do it often.

The next goal will be for your child to pull to stand from sitting on the floor. Once he is able to pull to kneel, then he can begin practicing pulling to stand from kneeling. He may begin by leaning his trunk over a low surface and pushing up with both legs. Later, he will use the advanced method by moving through the half-kneel position (see explanation below). As he practices pulling to stand from kneeling, it is very important that he also become competent with moving from standing to sitting on the floor so he can safely move up and down. The goal will be to pull to stand on all surfaces.

## Components
The components to focus on are:
1. arm and hand strength to reach, grip, hold on or prop, and pull to stand
2. trunk strength (abdominal muscle strength) to stabilize the core and assist with moving to stand
3. sufficient leg strength to use both legs to push up to stand, and later to move into the half-kneel position and push up to stand with one leg

4. ability to weight shift the trunk forward to move over his legs and then upward to move to stand; and later, weight shifting to one side to initiate the half-kneel position

5. desire to move up to stand and feel comfortable in this challenging position, and be able to move safely to sitting on the floor

## Tendencies

The tendencies are:

1. to have weak arms and hands or be unable to use his arm strength to hold on and pull to stand

2. to arch his trunk and stiffen his knees for stability, and rely on you to support him

3. to be uncomfortable with weight shifting forward and sideways

4. to sit with his hips in external rotation, facing the surface or you, and hold the edge or your thumbs and pull to stand through the midline

5. to depend on you to assist him with moving to stand rather than trying to figure out how to do it by himself

6. to pull to kneel but not initiate pulling to stand

7. to be afraid of moving from standing to sitting on the floor

## Setup for Learning

### Pulling to Stand from 90/90 Sitting

To practice pulling to stand from 90/90 sitting, your child needs the right setup to feel stable. The bench needs to be the right height (back of his knee to the bottom of his foot) and it needs to be stabilized so it does not move. The surface with the edge (for example, a Rubbermaid storage container) needs to be thin and easy to grasp but rigid so it feels stable to him (fig. 4.72). It needs

to be the right height (approximately 15 to 17 inches or 38 to 43 cm high) so it is easy to reach and grasp. It needs to be about 6 inches in front of your child so he has space to weight shift forward and upward when he moves to stand, and when he stands, he is vertical over his feet. It also needs to be weighted so it does not tip or slide. (I use a 50-pound [23 kg] bag of sandbox sand.)

Before your child pulls up, his feet need to be placed 2 to 3 inches (5 to 7.5 cm) apart, pointing straight, and heels against the bench, and then you place your leg or foot over his feet to stabilize them in this position. Now he is ready

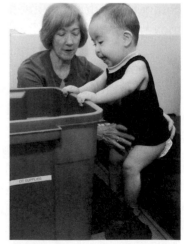

(fig. 4.72)

to pull to stand, and he will be setup to be successful! He will reach and grip the edge, hold it, and pull himself to standing.

When your child is standing, you will check to see if his knees are bent, and you will make sure he holds on to maintain the erect standing position. You can support his chest to prevent him from leaning his trunk against the surface and to keep his buttocks over the bench (to assist mild knee bending). When he is standing, he will maintain the position best if he is watching something rather than trying to touch a toy. At this early stage, he will not be able to maintain his balance with one-hand support and will need to hold on with both hands to be stable in standing. He will need to learn to keep holding onto the edge while standing, and to lower himself to sitting when he is ready to move out of standing.

### Pulling to Stand from Kneeling

Your child will use the method of pulling to stand from 90/90 sitting until he is ready to pull to stand from quadruped or sitting on the floor. To pull to stand from quadruped or sitting on the floor, he first needs to be able to pull to kneel from either position (Activity #15 or 17). When he is able to pull to kneel, he is ready to learn the next step of pulling to stand from kneeling. When he can pull to stand from kneeling, he will be able to put both steps together to pull to stand from sitting on the floor or quadruped.

From kneeling, your child will first move to stand by pushing up on both legs at the same time (figs. 4.73, 4.74). When kneeling at a low surface about 10 to 12 inches (25 to 30.5 cm) high, he will lean his trunk over the surface and then pop up to standing on both feet. This is an easy way to move to stand and is useful to start with so he learns he can move to stand. It is important that he learns to be comfortable in standing, has an easy way to move to stand, and chooses to do it. Otherwise, he will choose to stay in kneeling and will not initiate moving to stand. Once he has the idea and desire to move to

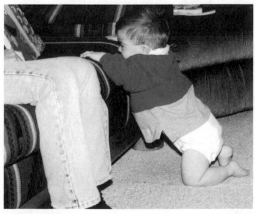

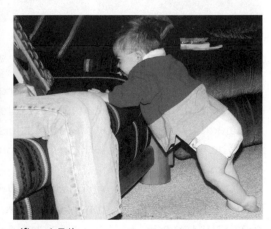

(fig. 4.73)                    (fig. 4.74)

stand from kneeling, then you can teach him the advanced method of using the half-kneel position.

***Half-Kneel Position.*** With practice and if his knees are under his hips (no wider), your child will learn to move into the half-kneel position. The half-kneel position is the kneeling position with one knee on the floor and the other foot on the floor. To move into the half-kneel position from kneeling, he will weight shift and lean his hips to one side, hold that position, and lift his other foot up on the floor. At first, he might move partially into the half-kneel position, with his hip and knee bent and his foot under his hip rather than under his knee. With this partial position, he will be unstable, and he will not be able to push up to stand. You will need to place his foot flat on the floor (and under his knee) so he is stable and can then complete moving to stand.

To move from the half-kneel position to stand, he will weight shift and lean his hips over his foot and then push up to stand (figs. 4.75–4.77). He will learn to use the half-kneel position when pulling to stand if his knees are in the proper position with a narrow base when kneeling, and he has learned to weight shift his hips from side to side.

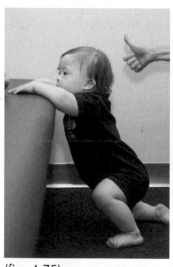 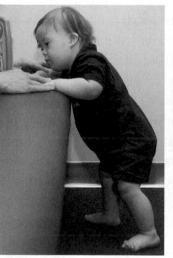

(fig. 4.75)      (fig. 4.76)      (fig. 4.77)

## Guidelines

***Use all kinds of toys to encourage pulling to stand.*** Your child will initially pull to stand because he wants to get the toy you put in front of him. You need to place the toy on top of the surface so he can see it but not reach it until he is standing. He will probably pull to stand to retrieve the toy and then sit down and play with it.

***Use the right height surface to help your child be successful with pulling to stand.*** When pulling to stand from 90/90 sitting, he needs to be able to reach the top edge of the surface from sitting on the bench. The height of the surface should be at chest level once he is standing. When beginning to pull to stand from kneeling, he needs to practice at a low surface (10 inches or 25 cm) so he can lean his trunk over it and easily move to stand. When he is familiar with pulling to stand and motivated to move to stand, then the height of the surface can be increased as tolerated from 12 to 17 inches (30.5 to 43 cm), until he can pull to stand on all surfaces.

*Provide a surface with an edge to help him learn to pull to stand more easily, and he will be able to do the skill earlier than pulling up on the sofa.* In the beginning stages of pulling to stand at lower surfaces, his trunk will lean over the surface, and his arms will do the majority of the work to pull his body weight up to standing. He will use leg strength to maintain standing once he moves to the position. When the height of the surface is increased, he will not be able to use the strategy of leaning his trunk and will need to use arm and leg strength to move up to stand. If he can use a surface with an edge, he will be able to grip the edge and then he will use his arm strength more effectively to pull to stand. If his hands hold the edge, he can balance himself as he pulls his body upward.

At this stage, he will need to use the combined strength of his arms and legs to move to stand. When his leg strength is adequate and he has learned to move through the half-kneel position, he will primarily use his legs to move up to stand, and he will just prop his hands on the surface for balance. When he is at this advanced stage, he can move to stand with his hands propping on top of the sofa or coffee table. When he moves up to stand very easily, he will be able to prop his hands against a vertical surface, such as the wall or refrigerator.

*You need to motivate your child to move up to standing rather than staying in kneeling to play.* After he pulls to kneeling, he will be content to stay in this stable position to play. You will need to show him an easy way to move to stand and have the best motivators to play with when he is standing. That is why we start with the easy way of moving to stand with a low surface by leaning his trunk over the surface and popping up on both feet. Giving him a surface with an edge when he uses a higher surface gives him another easy method of moving to standing. Once he has the motivation to be in standing and wants to move to stand, then we can work on the harder, more advanced method of moving to stand through the half-kneel position. It is important for him to be comfortable in kneeling but only as a temporary position on the way to standing.

*When he can pull to kneel at 10- to 12-inch (25- to 30.5-cm) high surfaces, practice the whole sequence of moving in and out of standing.* He can practice pulling to kneel, moving from kneeling to standing, and from standing to sitting on the floor. By practicing at the low surface, he will feel safer, especially with moving from standing to sitting on the floor (see Activity #20).

*While he is practicing pulling to stand, he will also be practicing climbing up stairs; these skills reinforce each other.* When he is climbing up stairs and moving through the knee, knee, foot, foot sequence, he will be practicing moving from kneeling to the half-kneel position, and then up to standing. By practicing both climbing and pulling to stand, he will have two methods of practicing the components needed for each skill.

---

### How to Determine Bench Height

The height of the bench is determined by measuring your child's leg from the back of the knee to the bottom of the foot when he is seated. This is best measured with your child sitting on a bench with his knees bent 90 degrees and his feet flat on the floor.

---

## Temperament

If your child is **motor driven,** he will be interested in moving up so he will pull up to stand to play with the toy. He may not want to stand for long, but he will like the action of pulling to stand. If he is an **observer,** he will be content to stay in kneeling so will need to be encouraged to move up to stand. If he is motivated by the toy and can only access it if he is standing, then he will move to stand to play with it.

 ## ACTIVITY #18: Pull to Stand and Lower to Sit: from 90/90 Sitting

1. Place your child in 90/90 sitting on a bench or other firm surface with a 90-degree edge so his heels can be placed under his knees. Stabilize the bench against the wall or furniture so it does not move.
2. Place a surface with an edge (like a Rubbermaid container 15 to 17 inches or 38 to 43 cm high) in front of him and place a 50-pound (23 kg) bag of sandbox sand in the bottom so it is stable. Place the surface about 6 inches (15 cm) in front of him so he has space to lean his trunk forward and weight shift as he moves up to standing and so that when he is standing, he is in the optimal position.
3. Place his feet 2 to 3 inches (5 to 7.5 cm) apart, pointing straight, with his heels against the bench. Stabilize his feet in this position with your leg or foot.
4. Put a toy up high so he can see it (by stacking toys inside the container so one is high enough to see) or inside the container so he is curious to find it.

5. Encourage him to lean his trunk forward to reach out, grip, and hold the edge of the surface. If he does not initiate this movement, assist him. Then wait for him to hold onto the edge tightly and pull up to stand. If needed, help him to grip the edge adequately and to maintain his grip while pulling up. You can place your hands over his to stabilize them.

6. After he pulls to stand, check his posture by looking at him from the side. His feet will be properly positioned with your leg/foot support. Make sure his buttocks are back over the bench and his knees are mildly bent (unlocked). Look at his trunk and support his abdomen (to activate his abdominals) if his trunk is excessively arched. If his chest is leaning on the edge of the container, then use your palm to lift his chest up straight so he holds on to stabilize himself in standing rather than leaning. If needed, move the container forward so his trunk is vertical. Since the bench and the surface are stabilized, you will have your hands free to support the areas of your child's body that need to be supported.

7. Encourage him to hold on with both hands and to maintain his grip while standing as you entertain him with the toy or set him up to watch a video. Check his legs and adjust them if needed so he is in the proper standing position.

8. When he wants to move out of standing, wait for him to bend his hips and knees and lower himself to sitting on the bench while holding the edge. Help him lower himself to sitting if needed by gently and slowly moving his pelvis back over the bench.

9. Allow him to sit on the bench and then encourage him to stand up again when he is ready.

10. Continue this activity as long as he likes it.

11. This activity can also be done in the playpen or crib, with your child holding onto the top bar or vertical railing.

## ACTIVITY #19: Pulling to Stand from Kneeling

1. Place your child on his knees, facing the surface he will use to pull to stand, or he can pull to kneel by himself from sitting or quadruped. Use a low (about 10 inches or 25 cm high), flat, soft surface so he can lean his trunk over it.

2. Position yourself sitting on your heels behind him.

3. Place a toy on top of the surface, just out of reach, and encourage your child to move up to stand to play with the toy.

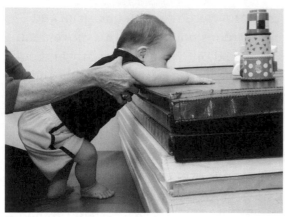 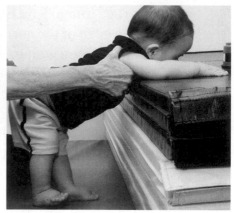

(fig. 4.78)                                    (fig. 4.79)

4. In the beginning, he will lean his trunk over the surface, press in with his elbows and tuck his chin, and this will help him pop up to stand on both feet. If he does not initiate moving up, then place your hands on the sides of his trunk under his arms, and you lean him over the surface and wait for him to move his legs (figs. 4.78, 4.79). With practice, he will learn this easy method of moving to stand.

5. When he can use the method in step #4, then increase the height of the surface from 10 inches to 12 inches (25 to 30.5 cm) and see if he can still move to stand.

6. When he is motivated to move to stand, begin teaching him the method of pulling to stand from kneeling, using a surface with an edge.

   a. Start with a 15-inch (38-cm) high Rubbermaid container and start him in the kneeling position. (You can place him in kneeling or have him pull to kneeling from sitting or quadruped.) From kneeling, see if he will hold on and pull to stand. At first, he may pull up with his arms and push off with his legs to move up to stand.

   b. When your child is confident in his ability to pull to stand and is motivated to stand, then increase the height of the surface with the edge to 17 inches (43 cm). With this increased height, he will probably need to figure out a new method of moving to stand. He will be challenged to figure out how to do it using the half-kneel position.

   c. See if he initiates moving into a partial half-kneel position. If he does, then reposition his foot and stabilize it so it is in the right position with his toes under his knee.

   d. From this revised position, see if he can pull to stand. If not, then support his heel and his opposite armpit, and with this support, he will be able to move to stand.

e. If he does not initiate any movement into the half-kneel position, then weight shift his pelvis slightly to one side and see if he moves the opposite foot into the half-kneel position. (Try to make an educated guess about which leg is dominant or preferred and help him initiate the half-kneel with that foot. Tip: if he has a preference of moving over one side, for example the right side, then he will usually move into the left half-kneel position.) Then provide the foot and armpit support described above to assist moving to stand.

7. Continue to have your child practice using the half-kneel position when pulling to stand using a surface with an edge until the skill is established and he does it spontaneously.

8. The next challenge is for your child to move to stand at the sofa or coffee table, with his hands placed on top of the surface. At this point, he will need to have adequate leg strength and use of the half-kneel position to move to stand, and will only need to use his arms to prop and balance. At first, start with a lower surface (15 inches or 38 cm) and then increase the height as tolerated.

9. The final challenge will be moving to stand with his hands propped against a vertical surface (wall or refrigerator).

## Moving from Standing to Sitting on the Floor

Since your child is working on pulling to stand, he needs to have a way to move safely and comfortably from standing to sitting on the floor. If you do not teach him, he will be scared and upset when he no longer wants to stand, or he will let go and fall and expect you to catch him. The first goal is to teach him the gross movements of moving from standing to sitting on the floor safely. He will stiffen his knees for stability as he moves to sitting on the floor and he will land with a plop. Later, when he is confident in his ability to move safely from standing to sitting on the floor, he can learn to refine his movements using hip and knee bending (fig. 4.80). The goal will be to move from standing to sitting on the floor slowly with control, bending his hips and knees.

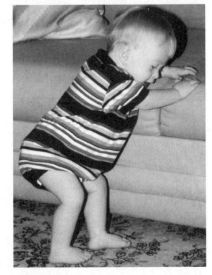

(fig. 4.80)

## Components

The components to focus on are:

1. arm strength to hold onto the edge or prop on the surface and balance himself as he is lowering himself to sitting on the floor
2. trunk strength to tuck abdominals so his trunk leans forward and his hips bend, and then to balance himself as he lowers himself to sitting on the floor
3. leg strength to move toward a squat and lower himself to sitting on the floor
4. ability to initiate weight shifting his pelvis backwards and down to the floor
5. willingness to fall backwards and land in sitting with a plop, and later to lower himself slowly with control

## Tendencies

The tendencies are:

1. to let go with his hands without regard for moving himself out of the position safely
2. to fall like a tower and depend on you to catch him
3. to hold his knees straight and stiff for stability as he moves to sitting on the floor
4. to be afraid as he is lowering himself the long distance to the floor, and to therefore not want to initiate the move or move halfway and then move back up to standing

## Setup for Learning

It is important to start practicing this skill early so your child becomes familiar with it as he is learning to pull to stand from kneeling. After he practices moving from sitting to kneeling and kneeling to standing at a low surface (10 to 12 inches high), then he can move from standing to sitting on the floor. He will tolerate it easily when practicing at this low surface since it is a short distance to sitting on the floor.

At this stage, he will learn the gross movement of moving from standing to sitting on the floor with a plop (4.81, 4.82). He will need to learn how to lean his pelvis back, bend his hips, and fall to sit. He will need to do it consistently to be safe, and he will need

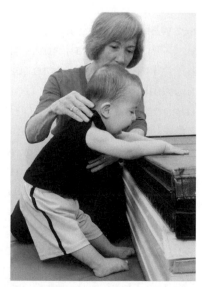

(fig. 4.81)

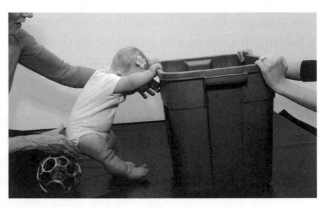

(fig. 4.83)

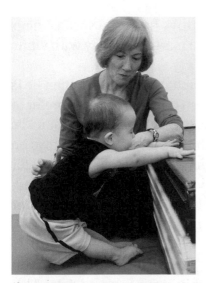

(fig. 4.82)

to feel comfortable with falling and the impact of the plop. If the skill is introduced as part of the moving to stand sequence, he will learn the whole cycle of moving up and down safely. When he practices this sequence, the focus will be on moving up and down from standing. We will not focus on the standing position since the surface will be too low to promote the optimal standing posture.

After your child is comfortable with moving from standing to sitting on the floor at the low surface, you can start practicing at a higher surface, provided you use a surface with an edge (fig. 4.83). You can gradually increase the height of the surface so he feels comfortable with the distance to the floor. As tolerated, you can increase the height of the surface until he can use a 17-inch high surface.

When your child is moving from standing to sitting on the floor with the higher surfaces, allow him to stabilize by straightening and stiffening his knees if he chooses to use this strategy. Since he is also practicing Activity #18 (moving from standing to 90/90 sitting), he is practicing the components of hip and knee bending in an easier skill. With practice, he will feel comfortable with moving down to the floor and will do it safely. He will figure out what method he is most comfortable with and will either move down fast with a plop or he will hold on and lower himself slowly to control the fall to sit.

When your child can lower himself from standing at the 17-inch high surface with an edge, the next challenge will be to lower himself from standing at the sofa or coffee table with his hands propping on top of the surface. When he is confident with lowering himself, he will tolerate learning to bend his hips and knees and lowering himself with control.

## Guidelines

***To encourage your child to move from standing to sitting on the floor, practice this activity when he wants to move out of standing.*** If he likes to stand a lot, you can place favorite toys on the floor to motivate him to move down to the floor. It is best if you remove all the toys from the surface he is standing in front of and put them on the floor. If he has toys to play with while he is standing, he will prefer to keep standing.

*Continue to encourage knee bending as much as possible.* When he is comfortable with moving from standing to sitting on the floor, he may prefer to keep his knees straight and "plop" on his buttocks to change positions quickly. You can encourage knee bending by having him bend down to pick up toys on the floor and move from standing to 90/90 sitting. If he continues to prefer keeping his knees straight, he will learn the components of hip and knee bending in the next stage when he practices moving from plantigrade to stand or when he practices squatting to play with toys (on the floor) when walking.

### Temperament

If your child is **motor driven,** he will probably move fast and "plop" his buttocks on the floor to move to sitting on the floor. When he is first learning, he will be a little slower until he knows what to do. Once he is familiar with how to do it, he will go fast and will enjoy the feeling of falling. If he is an **observer,** he will lower himself slowly and carefully. He may stop halfway down and then move back up to standing. Once he understands how far he needs to go and feels confident lowering himself the whole distance, he will lower himself faster.

 ### ACTIVITY #20: Moving from Standing at Low, Soft Surface to Sitting on the Floor

1. To move over his right side from sitting to standing (or reverse the instructions and move over his left side):
   a. Place him sitting on the floor with his right side in front of a 12-inch high soft surface (stacked sofa cushions or mats). Leave a 5-inch space between him and the surface.
   b. Sit on your heels behind him.
   c. Place motivating toys up on the surface, out of his reach until he stands at the surface.
   d. He will move from sitting to kneeling. Then he will lean his trunk over the surface and pop up to stand.
2. To move from standing to sitting:
   a. After he stands for a few seconds and reaches the toy, he will want to drop the toy on the floor and then sit on the floor and play with it. See if he initiates leaning his pelvis backwards to plop to sitting on the floor. If not, assist him to show him how to do it.

b. If he does not drop the toy on the floor, let him play for a few seconds and then you place the toy on the floor to encourage him to change positions.

## Activity #21: Moving from Standing at Surface with an Edge to Sitting

1. Start with your child standing at a 15-inch high surface with an edge, holding on to maintain the position.
2. Sit on your heels behind him.
3. Place a toy on the floor and encourage him to move down to the floor to get it.
4. Let him figure out how to do it safely, using a method that he is comfortable with. If he does not initiate moving down to the floor, assist him.
5. When he can lower himself to the floor consistently, then increase the height of the surface.

## Activity #22: Moving from Standing with Hands Propped on a Surface to Sitting

1. Start with your child standing at a sofa or coffee table with his hands propped on top of the surface.
2. Follow steps 2-5 above in Activity 21.
3. When your child can move from standing to sitting on the floor, the next challenge is for him to lower himself slowly with control while bending his hips and knees. If he needs support to bend his knees, then cue him by tapping with your thumb and index finger behind his knees when he is moving to sitting on the floor.
4. If he is fearful, place a sofa cushion behind his legs and he can learn to move down to sit on it. Gradually decrease the height of the pillow until he learns to move to sitting on the floor with knee bending.

# Standing Holding On

In this stage, your child will learn to pull to stand from sitting on the floor. When he can do this skill, he will use whatever standing posture he has practiced and is comfortable with. At this point, you will not really be able to change how he stands because he will be in control of moving to stand when he wants to.

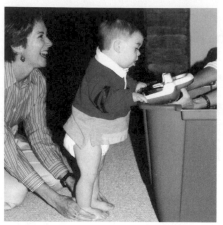

(fig. 4.84)

The goal for this interim period, between Stage 3 and before he pulls to stand on his own, will be to work on every detail of the components needed to establish the optimal standing posture. You will support every part of his body—his feet, knees, hips, pelvis, trunk, and arms—until he learns how to hold and move each part (fig. 4.84). Once he can stand with this desired posture, then the time in standing can be increased. As he stands for longer periods, his strength will improve, and he will also work on balance and movement in the position. He will start with two-hand support and then learn to balance with one-hand support. He will experiment with weight shifting through his feet, rising up on tiptoes, and weight shifting from side to side (fig. 4.85). He will also practice dancing and bouncing with his hips and knees bending.

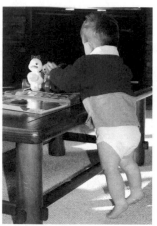

(fig. 4.85)

## Components

The components to focus on are:
1. hips in neutral rotation so your child's knees and feet point straight ahead
2. knees unlocked and mildly bent
3. feet 2 to 3 inches apart (narrow base), pointing straight ahead, and heels against the bench
4. pelvis in a neutral tilt, with buttocks over the bench
5. trunk straight but not arched, so the front and back muscles are activated in a balanced way
6. arms active and strong to hold onto a surface with an edge or to prop on top of a flat surface, and continued activation to maintain the position
7. arm strength to hold on while pulling up to stand and when lowering to sitting on the bench or floor
8. the ability to add dynamic action to the above components to bounce in standing, rise up on tiptoes, and weight shift to each side over each foot

## Tendencies

The tendencies are:

1. to position the hips in external rotation so the knees and feet point outward
2. to lock the knees and hold them stiff and straight (fig. 3.29)
3. to position the feet wide apart (wide base), with the toes turned outward and the inside borders of the feet collapsed toward the floor
4. to arch the trunk and tilt the top of the pelvis forward (overusing the back muscles and not using the abdominals)
5. to lean the pelvis back over the heels with the knees stiff and the toes lifted off the floor
6. to lean the trunk over or against the surface, and use both hands to play with toys
7. to use the strategy of maintaining standing using the static position of a leaning tower with a wide base, knees locked, and trunk leaning rather than being dynamic with optimal alignment, balance, and weight shifting

## Setup for Learning

When your child practices standing, he will need strategic support to learn how to position his feet, knees, hips, pelvis, trunk, and arms. You will need to prioritize which components to focus on first. You will also need to *use a bench* to set him up to pull to stand, to help him be successful when standing, and to allow him to move from standing to sitting when he chooses to move out of standing. (The height of the bench is critical and the edge needs to be at the crease behind his knee.) *The standing surface* needs to be at the level of his chest (nipple level to 2 inches below). It is best to use a surface with an edge until he has learned the optimal standing posture.

It is best to position his feet and stabilize them before he pulls to stand. You will place them 2 to 3 inches apart (narrow base), pointing straight ahead, with heels against the bench. Then you can place your leg over his feet to maintain them in this position when he pulls to stand. If you place the surface with an edge in front of him, then he will grip the edge, hold on, and pull to stand.

While your child is standing, you will check his feet and reposition them if he moves them. You will watch his foot position to see how stable he is. Some children have too much ligamentous laxity, so their arches collapse and their toes turn outward. Some children feel unstable, and compensate by excessively using peroneal muscles on the outsides of their lower legs (see figs. 4.86, 4.87). This causes their arches to flatten and toes to turn outward (fig. 4.93). If these

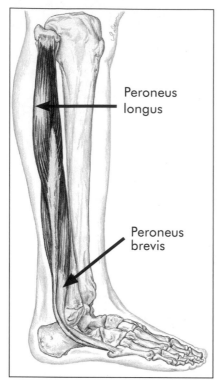

Peroneus longus

Peroneus brevis

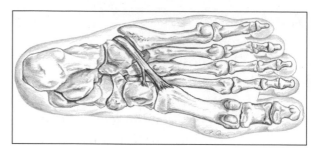

*left* (fig. 4.86); *top* (fig. 4.87)
Used with permission from Andrew R. Biel, and Robin Dorn, illustrator, *Trail Guide to the Body* (Boulder, CO: Books of Discovery, 2010), 376.

abnormal foot positions persist, check with your physical therapist to see if foot support is needed. (See the box on "Foot Support" on pp. 184-85.)

After his foot posture is stable in the desired position in standing, observe his knees from the side to see if they are "unlocked" (mildly bent). If they are locked, you need to figure out the easiest method to unlock them. From the side view, see if his heels are against the bench, and, if not, place them there. Then look at his trunk to see if it is arched. If so, he may lock his knees in combination with arching his trunk. If you place your hand on the front of his pelvis (below his navel) and gently and slowly move his pelvis back so his buttocks are over the bench, his knees will unlock against the edge of the bench. By providing this support, his posture will change from being stiff with hips and knees straight and trunk arched with an upward lift, to being relaxed with his hips and knees mildly bent and with his trunk straight.

After your child is comfortable with his feet and knees in the desired position, then you can focus on his trunk posture. The goal is to stand with his trunk straight, with his back and abdominal muscles in balance. The height of the surface is critical. If it is too low, he will bend forward and lean over the surface. Even if the surface is the right height, he may try to lean his trunk against the surface, which you should discourage. If needed, place your thumb and index finger against his upper chest to cue him to hold his trunk up straight and also make sure he does not lean against your hand. With his trunk up straight and with his knees unlocked, his pelvis will be relaxed with buttocks over the bench, in a neutral tilt.

While he has been practicing the foot, knee, hip, trunk, and pelvis posture, you have been working on the goal of having him hold on to a surface with an edge to maintain the standing position. After he has mastered the desired posture, you can challenge him by having him prop his hands on a surface and maintain the position. While he needs two-hand support, he will need to be entertained with toys since he cannot balance with only one hand.

When he is ready, you can teach him to hold on with one-hand support. It will be easier to balance if he is holding a surface with an edge. You may need to put your hand over his to stabilize it adequately. With practice, he will develop better strength and balance, and learn to do it on his own. When practicing, it is best to have him hold a lightweight toy like the stick of the xylophone, and he can hit the keys as you hold the xylophone. He can also play with push button toys if the buttons are easy to activate. You will need to stabilize the toys and place them in the best position for him to be successful.

Once your child has developed the components of standing, then he is ready to be dynamic in the position. He will be able to combine proper alignment with balance, bouncing, rising up on tiptoes, and weight shifting over the outer edges of each foot (so that he lifts the inner edges into an arch). As long as he has a narrow base, his feet are pointing straight, and he is barefoot, he will spontaneously use these foot movements while playing in standing. When he hears music, he will dance by bouncing or weight shifting to sway. These movements will set him up to be able to master the skills in Stage 5—in particular, cruising and balancing in standing.

## Guidelines

*When your child is first standing with two-hand support, use toys he can watch so he can use both hands to hold on for balance.* Some examples of toys are: spinning toys, music box or other musical toys, and DVDs. You can also sing songs, whistle, or encourage him to dance.

*When he is practicing standing with one-hand support, use lightweight toys that are easy to play with.* Some examples are: xylophone, reading books and pointing to pictures, push button sound books or toys, iPad, soap bubbles to pop, knocking over a block tower, putting toys into a container, and shaking interesting rattles, bells, or musical instruments. Place the toys in front of him initially. As he gains strength and balance, he will be able to reach to the side.

*The height of the surface needs to be between nipple level to 2 inches below his nipples.* If the height is too short he will lean over the surface. When the height is correct, his trunk will be up straight when he is holding on with his hands.

*The height of the bench is critical to promote mild knee bending and unlocking his knees.* The top edge of the bench needs to be at the crease behind his knee and at a 90-degree angle. His heels need to be against the bench,

## Foot Support

As discussed in the Introduction, children with Down syndrome have ligamentous laxity. Because of this laxity, they are at risk for heel and foot alignment problems. (See Foot Management section in Chapter 6.)

When you look at the bones of the foot (see figure 4.88—4.90), it is easier to understand what is happening. The heel bone (calcaneus) is large, and when there is ligamentous laxity, the top of the heel bone tilts inward. Then the bone that sits on top of the heel bone (talus) follows, as do the five bones (midfoot) in close proximity to the calcaneus and talus, since they are all in close contact. Depending on the degree of ligamentous laxity, there could be increased tilt in the heel bone. If so, there is increased shifting of the bones so that the inside border of the foot falls downward and collapses to the ground.

There are three potential alignment problems when the heel bone has tilted inward: at the heel, at the inside arch area, and with the long bones of the foot. You can observe the tilt of the heel bone if you look at your child's foot while standing behind him (see fig. 4.91. If you look at your child's foot from the front or side, you can observe the collapse of the arch area (see fig. 4.92). The third area to look at is the toes, looking to see if they point straight ahead or turn outward ("toe out").

### Bones of the Right Foot

Top View

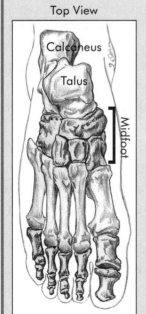

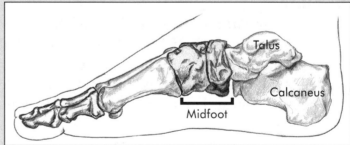

Medial View (Inside Border)

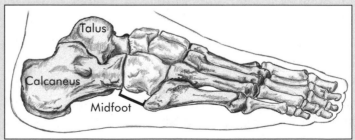

Lateral View (Outside Border)

left (fig. 4.88); top right (fig. 4.89); bottom right (fig. 4.90) Used by permission from Andrew R. Biel and Robin Dorn, illustrator, *Trail Guide to the Body: A Hands-on Guide to Locating Muscles, Bones, and More* (Boulder, CO: Books of Discovery, 2010), 346 and 355.

After your child pulls to stand, wants to stand often, and plays while standing, his foot posture needs to be evaluated to determine if he can stand barefoot or if he needs support. It will be important to position his feet in the desired posture (heels in line with hips or narrow base, feet pointing straight) and then look at his foot align-

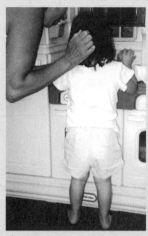

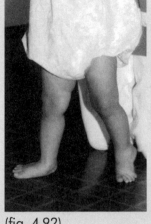

(fig. 4.91)  (fig. 4.92)

ment to see the influence of ligamentous laxity. If he is allowed to stand with a wide base with his feet turned outward, you will exaggerate the heel tilt, medial collapse, and toeing out. In this case you will see the combined influence of poor positioning and ligamentous laxity.

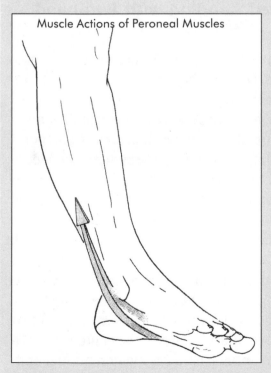

Muscle Actions of Peroneal Muscles

(fig. 4.93) Used by permission from Blandine Calais-Germain, *Anatomy of Movement* (Seattle, WA: Eastland Press, 2007), 288.

There are a variety of types of shoe inserts, arch supports, and orthoses that can provide the support needed to hold a child's feet, particularly his heels, in optimal alignment so that he feels more stable. If he feels more stable in his ankles, he may not need to compensate by locking his knees or overusing his peroneal muscles (see fig. 4.93). The foot support will also align his legs and feet so that he will develop strength using optimal movement patterns. His joints will be lined up properly so he can use his strength more efficiently. Types of support and shoes to use with the support are discussed in Chapter 6.

and his buttocks need to be back over the bench (side view). When he learns to use the support of the bench, he will relax his knees and unlock them.

*Have your child go barefoot when he is practicing standing, if possible.* If he wears shoes, his feet and ankles will be held stiffly, and he will not learn to move his ankles when weight shifting or to assist with balance. With his ankles stiff, he will tend to hold his knees stiff. If he is barefoot, he has access to developing strength, balance, and freedom of movement in his feet and knees. It's OK for him to wear socks on the carpet when you are not observing his foot position.

### Temperament

If your child is **motor driven,** he will stand as long as the toys are motivating enough to play with. Since he prefers to move, he will stand to play but then will get down to the floor to creep and move around. When he can cruise (see Stage 5), he will enjoy standing and cruising to move around. If your child is an **observer,** he will love to stand as long as he can. He will love to play with toys in standing and will stand to look out a window. He will get down from standing when he is tired or if he decides to do something else.

 ### ACTIVITY #23: Supported Standing with Two-hand Support

1. Place your child sitting on a bench about 6 (15 cm) inches away from a surface with an edge. (Follow the steps for Activity #18.)
2. Encourage him to pull up to stand.
3. Once your child is standing, focus on having him maintain standing, using the desired posture of feet, knees, hips, trunk and pelvis, and arms. While he is standing, provide support where needed and have him hold on to the edge with both hands to maintain the standing position. Let him choose when he wants to move to sitting, and have him hold on and lower himself with control.
4. Entertain him while he is standing and encourage him to maintain his balance.
5. When he feels comfortable maintaining his balance with two-hand support, encourage knee bending and bouncing in standing by providing music and having him dance. If he leans to either side or backwards, see if he can move himself back to the centered standing position. If not, help him until he can. Also watch his feet and if they are positioned under his hips and pointing straight, see how he moves his feet when weight shifting over each side. (Reposition his feet if needed so he can use the desired movements.)

6. When your child stands well with two-hand support holding a surface with an edge, begin using a flat surface without an edge. He can place his hands on top of the surface and stand with his trunk up straight. Watch him and if he tends to lean his chest or trunk against the surface, use the pads of your thumb and index finger to cue his chest to stay upright.

7. When you are initially teaching your child to rise up on tiptoes, he will need to lean his trunk against the surface so he feels stable. If you place a toy in front of him, just out of his reach, see if he will push up on tiptoes to get the toy. If he does not try to push off on his toes, then support his feet to show him the movement. Once he knows how to move onto his toes (weight shift forward) and then push up on tiptoes, he will repeat the movement. At first, he will feel more stable and it will take less strength if he can lean over the surface. With practice, he will start rising up on tiptoes with his hands on top of the surface, without leaning his trunk.

## ACTIVITY #24: Supported Standing with One-hand Support

1. Place your child in standing and have him hold onto a surface with an edge.
2. Position his legs with his feet under his hips and his toes pointing straight ahead.
3. Place a bench behind his legs and stabilize it against furniture. He will use the support of the bench to bend his knees slightly and to sit down when he is ready.
4. Encourage him to play with lightweight toys with one hand and see if he can balance himself by holding onto the edge with his other hand. See "Guidelines" in this section for examples of toys to use. If needed, place your hand over your child's to assist his grip and help him be successful.
5. Encourage him to maintain his balance while playing as long as tolerated.
6. When he consistently maintains his balance, encourage him to reach for toys to his side and behind him.
7. When he stands well with one-hand support holding a surface with an edge, begin using a flat surface without an edge. He can place his hand on top of a surface such as the sofa or a table.

## MOTOR MILESTONE CHECKLIST

### Crawling

- ☐ He can do 1-2 pulls with his arms to move his body forward
- ☐ He moves forward 5 feet (1.5 meters), using any method
- ☐ He moves forward 10 feet (3 meters)
- ☐ He uses a fast and efficient pattern, moving opposite arm and leg simultaneously (reciprocal pattern)

### Climbing Up

- ☐ He climbs up onto a sofa cushion placed on the floor
- ☐ He climbs up the top 2 stairs of the flight, onto the landing
- ☐ He climbs up onto the sofa (with cushion removed)

### Climbing Down (with Support)

- ☐ Climbing down off the sofa or your lap: he tolerates being moved to his stomach and sliding down until his feet touch the floor

### Moving into Quadruped

- ☐ He assumes the hands and knees position by himself, and maintains it
- ☐ While on hands and knees, he rocks forward and back on his own

### Creeping

- ☐ He moves forward 2-4 steps
- ☐ He creeps 5 feet (1.5 meters)
- ☐ He creeps 10 feet (3 meters)
- ☐ He creeps quickly and efficiently using a reciprocal pattern

### Scooting (in Sitting)

- ☐ He scoots using his own method for 5-10 feet (1.5–3 meters) (optional)

### Moving to Sit

- ☐ He moves to sit from kneeling
- ☐ He moves to sit from stomach-lying
- ☐ He moves to sit from hands and knees
- ☐ He moves to sit using his own method (optional)

*(continued on next page)*

### Moving Out of Sitting

❑ He moves from sitting to stomach-lying with control

❑ He moves from sitting to kneeling at a 5- to 6-inch (12.5- to 15-cm) high cushion

❑ He moves from sitting to quadruped

### Pulling to Kneel

❑ He pulls to kneel from sitting using a low surface (9-12 inches or 23-30.5 cm high) with an edge

❑ He pulls to kneel from sitting using a flat, low surface

❑ He pulls to kneel from sitting using a high surface (15-17 inches or 38-43 cm high) with an edge

❑ He pulls to kneel from sitting using a flat, high surface

❑ He pulls to kneel from stomach-lying by climbing onto your stomach as you lie on the floor

❑ He pulls to kneel from quadruped using a low surface (9-10 inches; 23-25 cm high) with an edge

❑ He pulls to kneel from quadruped using a flat, low surface

❑ He pulls to kneel from quadruped using a high surface (15-17 inches; 38-43 cm high) with an edge

❑ He pulls to kneel from quadruped using a flat, high surface

### Pulling to Stand

❑ He pulls to stand from 90/90 sitting using a surface with an edge

❑ At a 10- to 12-inch high surface, he moves from kneeling to standing, pushing up on both legs simultaneously

❑ He moves into the half-kneel position when pulling to stand from kneeling using a surface with an edge

❑ He pulls to stand using any height surface, moving through the half-kneel position

### Moving from Standing to Sitting on the Floor

❑ He moves from standing to 90/90 sitting by himself using a surface with an edge

❑ He holds onto a surface with an edge and moves to sitting on the floor with a plop—with his knees straight

❑ He holds onto a surface with an edge and moves to sitting on the floor with a plop—with his knees mildly bent

❑ He moves from standing to sitting on the floor using any surface, lowering himself with control, with his knees mildly bent

(continued on next page)

### *Standing Holding On*

Using a surface with an edge:
- ❏ He stands holding on with both hands
- ❏ He bounces in standing, with hips and knees bending (dancing)
- ❏ He stands holding on with one hand

Using a flat surface:
- ❏ He stands propping on both hands
- ❏ He bounces in standing, with hips and knees bending (dancing)
- ❏ He rises up on tiptoes
- ❏ He stands propping on one hand

# 5

# Stage 5: Standing, Cruising, Climbing, and Walking

## Introduction

Your child is now independent in her environment. She can move from one place to another by crawling or creeping; move from one position to another; use the positions of sitting, quadruped, kneeling, and standing; and she has begun climbing. During this stage, she will make the transition from mainly being on the floor to mainly standing up. She will want to play in standing, and then will learn to step sideways (cruise) to move to the toys. When she is practicing stepping sideways, she will also be ready to learn to step forward with support. The focus of this stage is learning to walk.

### Motor Skills

The motor skills to focus on during this fifth stage of development are:

1. cruising
2. walking with and without support
3. climbing off the sofa and up and down stairs
4. plantigrade and moving from plantigrade to stand
5. standing balance

### Components

The components to focus on are:

1. stepping movements with the legs, sideways and forward, and later endurance
2. strength and coordinated use of the arms, legs, and abdominals through climbing and walking

3. effective and efficient use of the abdominals in each position (standing balance, moving from plantigrade to stand, walking, cruising, and climbing)
4. experimenting with moving from one position to another—from quadruped to plantigrade, from plantigrade to stand, and from stand to plantigrade
5. strength in trunk and legs to balance in standing, and proficient balance reactions to maintain balance while walking

## *Tendencies*

The tendencies are:
1. to resist practicing stepping and prefer to use her familiar and established method of mobility (crawling, creeping, bear walking, or scooting in sitting) since it is fast and efficient, and she is independent with it
2. to initially step with an awkward, stiff, and uncoordinated pattern
3. to love climbing and have this become her focus
4. to practice stepping for a few steps and then want to move to the floor to move independently
5. (for us) to wait for her to show us when she is ready to practice stepping…it will never happen, or if it does, it will occur later than when she is physically ready

You will need to be strategic about practicing the skills of this stage. Now that your child can pull to stand and is motivated to stand, your first priorities are to teach her **cruising and stepping.** You will need to set her up to learn the leg stepping movements because she will not initiate them on her own. She will only be able to learn them with your support and with a motivating setup to make each skill fun and valuable to practice. When she is done practicing cruising and stepping, then practice **climbing.** On her own, she will experiment and figure out how to move to **plantigrade** (hands and feet). When she is able to take independent steps, she will need to learn how to move to stand in the middle of the floor and then you will teach her to move from **plantigrade to stand.** While she practices independent steps, she will learn **standing balance.**

Each skill of this stage has many steps to learn, so the chapter will be divided into five sections. This way each skill can be considered individually. Although these skills will be discussed separately, you will practice the skills your child is ready to learn in the sequence described above. If your child shows an interest in learning a skill such as standing balance or moving to stand before she is taking independent steps, it is fine to practice it. But **make**

**sure your first priority is practicing walking** and then you can practice the skill she wants to do.

## Guidelines

*When you are practicing gross motor skills, focus on what your child needs your help to practice.* If your child can cruise along the sofa, then practice stepping together with her and let her cruise during her own playtime.

*During this stage, your time is best utilized if you practice stepping.* Your child needs your help to improve her stepping pattern and it will only improve with practice. She cannot practice this on her own and she needs your support to practice, so anytime you have a spare minute, practice stepping. By practicing it often and playfully throughout the day, it will become a familiar game and habit, and she will look forward to doing the "walking game" with you.

*Practice for brief periods, several times a day.* Most children at this stage want to be independent, so your child will participate best if you practice for five minutes and then let her do what she wants.

*Label what you are going to do so your child is Setup for the activity you are going to practice.* If you are going to practice walking, sign and say "walk." If you want her to stand up, sign and say "stand." Say key words like "up" and "down" when practicing climbing. She will be more engaged in the activity if she knows the "game" you are playing together.

*You need to lead your child to learn walking, so start it at the right time.* If you practice it at the right time and frequency, then your child will be open to practicing it, and it will become familiar and part of her movement repertoire. If you wait, she will become overly proficient and independent in her other method of mobility (for example, creeping), and then she will be more resistant to learning something new like walking.

*During this time your child is going to master many different skills.* Life will be very active for both of you. You will need to spend more time chasing, managing, and supervising her.

# Cruising

Cruising is stepping sideways while holding onto furniture. It is generally how a child learns to take her first steps with support. Your child will be ready to learn this skill after she can pull to stand from sitting on the floor. Since she can pull to stand and is comfortable in standing, she will be motivated to spend more time in standing, and she will want to be able to move to toys while in standing. She will need support to learn how to cruise since her tendency will be to maintain her stable balanced standing position. The goal will be for your child to cruise along furniture and from one piece of furniture to another.

Cruising is an example of a gross motor skill that a child with Down syndrome learns differently than a child without Down syndrome. For a child without Down syndrome, Lois Bly (1994) gives an excellent description of how cruising is learned. A simple turning of the head cues the body to learn to cruise:

When cruising along the furniture, the child starts from the position of facing the sofa. Interest in a toy (placed to the side) causes the baby to rotate her head, trunk, and pelvis. The baby then shifts her weight to the face-side leg. Next, she transfers her weight to the face-side leg and *"steps in"* with the back leg. Then she shifts her weight to the back leg, which frees up the face-side leg to *"step out."*

In other words, when a child has normal tone and tightness of the ligaments, rotating her neck causes rotation in the trunk and pelvis, which produces the weight shift onto the face-side leg. However, in a child with Down syndrome with hypotonia and ligamentous laxity, rotating the neck would not produce the trunk and pelvic rotation to facilitate a weight shift. Also, she would be standing with her heels wider than her hips and her feet turned outward, so that leg posture would block weight shifting. To teach cruising in a child with Down syndrome, I therefore use the strategy of provoking a balance reaction (staggering reaction) in order to teach her the idea of "stepping out" with one leg to catch her balance, and then "stepping in" with her other leg.

## Components

There are three levels of cruising: early cruising by eliciting a staggering reaction, typical cruising, and advanced cruising. The components to focus on for each level will be described:

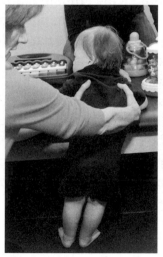
(fig. 5.1)

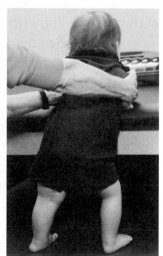
(fig. 5.2)

1. **Early cruising** (figs. 5.1, 5.2):
   a. leaning her trunk forward over a lower surface (at the level of 2-3 inches or 5-7.5 cm below the nipples) so her elbows can prop on the surface
   b. placing her feet with heels together and pointing straight

   c. supporting her trunk forward, and then leaning it to the side
   d. pausing to wait for her to "step out" (using a staggering reaction) with the foot on the side she is leaning toward, and then "step in" with her other foot

**2. *Typical cruising*** (figs. 5.3, 5.4):
   a. propping her hands on the surface (1-2 inches or 2.5-5 cm below nipple level) to maintain balance, and then moving her hands along the surface as she steps sideways
   b. activating her trunk (front and back muscles) to hold it erect and balanced so she steps sideways with control, with her trunk facing the surface
   c. stepping sideways to move to the toy (by "stepping out" with the leg in the direction she is traveling toward, and "stepping in" with her other leg)
   d. being able to step the length of the sofa, in both directions

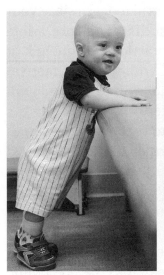 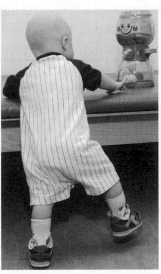 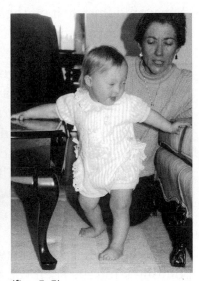

(fig. 5.3)          (fig. 5.4)          (fig. 5.5)

**3. *Advanced cruising*** (fig. 5.5):
   a. activating abdominals while propping on a coffee table or ottoman to cruise around the corners of the furniture
   b. using hands to prop and balance, rotating the trunk, weight shifting through the feet, and stepping, in order to cruise between two surfaces (fig. 5.5)
   c. using hands to prop and balance while cruising with hands against the wall

## Tendencies

The tendencies are:

1. to learn to stand with a wide base (feet wide apart) for stability so your child does not initiate weight shifting to the side
2. to feel off balance when leaned to the side and become afraid and resistant and want to move to the floor
3. to move to the floor and creep closer to the toy and then pull to stand to play with it
4. to stand with her knees and feet turned outward (hip external rotation), which blocks weight shifting to the side
5. to stiffen her knees for stability in standing, which makes it hard to step
6. to lean her trunk too far to the side in order to reach the toy and need you to assist her balance

## Setup for Learning

Children with Down syndrome need to be taught cruising earlier than they would initiate it on their own. It is a challenging skill to learn since your child will learn to do it by being tipped to the side so she is off balance, while in standing. You will need to be strategic when you practice it by doing it at the right time, with the right setup and support, and with the right motivators. The focus will be to have her move her legs so her arms and trunk will be supported so she can learn to activate her legs to step.

To learn the **early cruising** pattern, she needs to practice while standing at a low surface so she can lean her trunk forward over the surface and prop on her elbows. This will help her feel stable in the position. If you set her up at a higher surface, she will be afraid and stiffen her body and will not be able to step. To entice her to move, you will place a motivator to the side, just out of her reach.

To elicit the step, you will place her heels and feet together and her feet pointing straight. Then you will hold her trunk and lean it to the side (while maintaining her trunk forward over the surface). You will pause and wait for her to step out with her face-side leg. Because she is off balance, she will "step out" with her foot to regain her balance (this is a staggering reaction). After she "steps out" with one foot, see if she will "step in" with her other foot. The most important movement is the "stepping out." If she does not step out, then slightly lift her trunk on the face side, and see if she can then step with that leg. Also practice the early cruising pattern in each direction to determine if it is easier in a particular direction, and then practice to that side first. Through practicing cruising in this fashion, she will learn the sideways stepping pattern. Then she will be ready to learn the typical cruising pattern.

When she consistently steps side-ways, you can experiment with providing the least amount of support to assist cruising. Use the best possible motivator so she is dying to step to get it, even if she does it in a way that you have to help her balance. You can support her arms by:

- moving them to the side to lean her trunk,
- supporting her under the arm (armpit) on her face-side to prevent leaning too far,
- having her hold a surface with an edge or your fingers, or
- placing your hands over hers to help her feel stable.

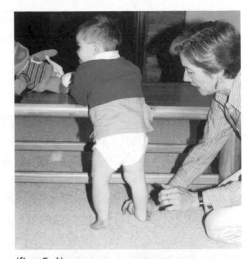

(fig. 5.6)

You can also assist her to step if you place her heel (on the skull-side) next to the face-side heel (fig. 5.6, 5.7). She will not want to stand with such a narrow base and will "step out" with the face-side heel (fig. 5.8). By providing minimal strategic support, she will learn to do the stepping movements and eventually be able to do them without your support. She will progress to the **typical cruising** pattern and step sideways on her own using a marching pattern (hips and knees bending), her arms will prop and move sideways to maintain her balance, and she will use controlled trunk movements to lean and balance.

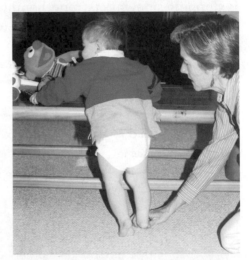

(fig. 5.7)

Through cruising, your child will learn to weight shift in standing, step with one leg at a time, and balance herself while stepping using her arms and trunk muscles. With practice, she will be able to cruise from one end of a table or sofa to the other end, and learn to do it in both directions. Later, she will practice

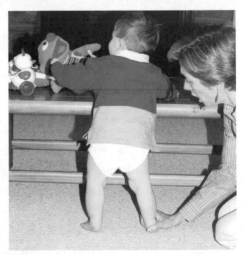

(fig. 5.8)

**advanced cruising** and cruise from one piece of furniture to another. She will learn to cruise along the wall and will be able to move through the house and cruise when and where she wants to. The more she cruises, the stronger her legs will become and the more motivated she will be to use stepping for mobility. Cruising can be practiced until she has another way to step independently in the house, such as by stepping with a push toy.

I recommend practicing cruising and stepping forward with support (see Walking, below) simultaneously in order to teach the leg stepping pattern. Your child may prefer one skill more than the other, and then you can practice the preferred skill more often or for longer distances. It is important to develop both skills since they use different muscles. This will help the hips become strong in all directions and improve pelvic and hip stability. In both skills, your child is practicing weight shifting in standing, but in cruising she is stepping sideways (strengthening the muscles used for stepping in and out) and in walking she is stepping forward (strengthening the muscles used for stepping forward and backwards).

---

### Steps in Learning to Cruise

Your child will learn all levels of cruising by practicing the following sequence of activities:

1. take the first 1-2 steps ("stepping out" and "stepping in")
2. take 3-4 steps
3. cruise along the length of the table or sofa in one direction
4. cruise in both directions
5. cruise around the "corner" of the table
6. cruise from one piece of furniture to another, with the surfaces next to each other
7. cruise from one piece of furniture to another with the surfaces parallel to each other; for example, from the sofa to the coffee table
8. cruise with hands against the wall

---

## Guidelines

*To motivate your child to cruise, pick the perfect motivator and place it just out of her reach.* She will need to figure out a way to move to it to play with it. After she is familiar with cruising, use toys to motivate her to cruise longer distances or between pieces of furniture.

*Remember that the height of the surface is critical in early cruising.* It needs to be approximately 3 inches (7.5 cm) below the level of her nipples so she can lean her trunk over the surface and prop on her forearms (fig. 5.9). When she can use the typical cruising pattern, then she will be able to cruise using a surface of any height.

*In early cruising, cruise barefoot.* It will be easier for your child to move her feet sideways with bare feet since each foot will slide along the surface. With bare feet, she will also feel the weight shifting through her feet and activate the muscles on the inner and outer borders of her feet. Once she is able to use the typical cruising pattern, she will bend her knees and march sideways and then she will be able to cruise with shoes.

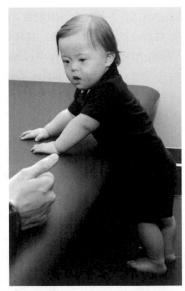

(fig. 5.9)

*Early cruising can be a scary experience, so experiment to find the support that will help your child feel comfortable enough to practice it.* Experiment with the height of the surface and with how you provide arm or trunk support. You can also kneel (with your hips straight) behind your child's pelvis and legs so she feels more stable. You need to find the right setup for her so she is willing to think about how to move and "step out" with her face-side leg rather than stiffening up and freezing with fear.

*When she is able to cruise, she will automatically use a narrower base in standing.* Her cruising experiences will make her want to move when standing and will help her feel stable with her heels closer together.

*Support her arms or trunk and have her learn to step with her legs.* The most difficult part of cruising is learning to take the first one or two steps. If you support her arms or trunk, she will feel stable enough to move her legs. If she does not initiate moving her legs, as a last resort, you may need to move her legs, one at a time, in the beginning. However, when possible, move toward supporting her arms or trunk and having her actively move her legs.

*As she learns to cruise, gradually reduce the amount of arm support that she uses.* There will be four types of arm support used:

- leaning over the surface and propping on her elbows;
- "holding on" to your fingers or a surface with an "edge";
- propping her hands *on top of* a surface;
- propping her hands *against* a surface.

She will probably take her first cruising steps by leaning over the surface and propping on her elbows. She will need to feel secure and adequately stable to initiate stepping out with her leading leg. When she is able to step with each leg, she will hold on to a surface with an "edge" and use her arms and stomach muscles to balance herself. With this support, she will develop trunk and leg strength and hold her body upright as she cruises along the surface. She will not need to lean her body against the surface for support. With practice, she will learn to prop her hands *on top of* a surface like a table or the seat of the sofa. Later, she will be able to cruise with her hands propping *against* a surface, like the wall or refrigerator. As she learns to cruise with her hands propped *on top of* or *against* surfaces, her trunk muscles will work harder to maintain her balance. As she uses her arms less for support, her trunk muscles will be primarily responsible for controlling her balance.

*Make sure her trunk and hips are parallel to the surface she is cruising along.* She needs to practice "stepping *out*" and "stepping *in*" to strengthen specific hip muscles. This is the primary skill in which your child uses these muscles and, by strengthening them, she will develop better hip stability for standing balance and stepping. To help her keep her hips parallel to the surface, keep her arms forward on the surface. If you are at her side, do not encourage her to hold one or both of your fingers because then she will turn her trunk and hips to face you. She will then step forward with her legs rather than stepping sideways.

*Encourage her to cruise in both directions to see if it is easier for her to move in one direction.* If she prefers moving in one direction, let her practice that direction first. When she masters cruising in the favored direction, she will be ready to learn to cruise in the other direction.

### Temperament

If your child is an **observer,** early cruising will probably be scary because she will feel out of control. She will be standing and tilted off balance. This will be a challenge for her, so you need to watch her and see her reaction. Since she is *careful* in her approach to learning new skills, she may want more support in the beginning. Once she is familiar with cruising, knows how to do it and understands how she can move to toys, she will be happy and motivated to do it.

If your child is **motor driven,** she will be *more daring* when she is learning to cruise. She may lean her trunk too far and not use her hands to hold on to keep her balance. She will be motivated to move to the toy without regard for doing it safely. You will need to supervise her to make sure she is safe. When she learns how to do it, she will cruise with control and balance.

### ACTIVITY #1: Early Cruising

1. Stand your child at a soft surface like the sofa. Make sure it is low enough that she can lean her trunk over it and prop on her elbows. The height of the surface should be 2-3 inches (5-7.5 cm) below nipple level.

2. Place a favorite motivator to her side, just out of her reach.

3. Place her heels together with her feet pointing straight ahead.

4. Place your hands on the sides of her trunk (under her arms) and lean her trunk sideways, keeping her armpits level, while maintaining her trunk forward over the surface.

5. Pause in this position and wait for her to "step out" with her face-side leg.

6. Keep motivating her with the toy. If she does not step after 10 seconds, then lift the armpit on her face-side (the side facing the motivator). See if this helps her free her foot to "step out." Also check her feet and make sure her heels are together and her other foot is planted so it frees up her face-side leg to step. If she tries to move down to the floor, kneel up tall behind her to support her pelvis and trunk so she will feel more stable in standing.

7. After she "steps out" with the face-side leg, then see if she will "step in" with her other leg.

8. Once she takes a step to move to the toy, let her play with the toy to reward her.

9. Practice the above steps in each direction to see if it is easier to step with a particular foot. If she has a preferred direction, continue to practice that way until she can cruise on her own and then practice in the opposite direction.

10. After she can "step out" and "step in" consistently with maximal trunk support, then practice with less support. Follow steps 1–3 above and then experiment to determine the least arm or trunk support needed to elicit "stepping out."

   a. Lean her trunk to the side and support her forearms and then see if she will take a step.

   b. She may try to reach for the toy, lean her trunk too far, and lose her balance. If this happens, place your finger under her armpit (on the side she is leaning toward) to support her. Lift upward and see if she will step with her leading leg.

   c. Place her hands to the side and then place your hands over hers to help her feel stable. With this support, she will step.

   d. Let her hold your fingers (with your fingers placed on the surface in front of her) or hold onto a surface with an edge and try to step sideways.

11. When she can do #10, experiment with supporting one foot. Follow steps 1–2 and then place the heel on her back foot right next to the face-side heel. Since she wants to move to the motivator, she will "step out" with the face-side foot.

12. With lots of practice, she will learn how to "step out" and "step in" with her legs, move her arms, lean her trunk, and maintain her balance to cruise (fig. 5.10).

13. When she can cruise three to four steps easily, she can practice cruising the length of the surface, like the length of the sofa. Encourage her to cruise longer distances, with a variety of surface heights, and in both directions.

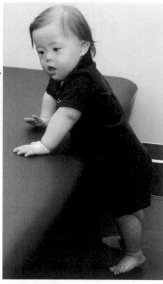

(fig. 5.10)

## ACTIVITY #2: Cruising with Hands on Top of a Surface and around Corners

1. When your child can cruise well along lower surfaces and at a surface with an edge, in both directions, then she is ready to learn to cruise with her hands on top of surfaces with her trunk erect. Try a variety of surfaces and gradually increase the height. Examples include: coffee table or other types of tables, sofa, bed, chairs lined up together, rectangular storage box, or the bathtub.

2. Have her pull to stand at the surface and then place toys about 2 feet away from her. Encourage her to cruise to the toys. With practice, increase the distance until she cruises along the length of the surface.

3. When she is able to cruise along the length of the furniture, you can further challenge her by encouraging her to walk around the corner of the coffee table. This will be more difficult, and you will need to help her learn how to move around the corner. Use a motivating toy and initially give her hand support to help her balance as she steps around the corner.

4. As she learns what she needs to do, decrease your support until she can do it by herself.

## ACTIVITY #3: Cruising from One Piece of Furniture to Another

1. Arrange your furniture so that one piece of furniture is next to another. For example, place a table next to the sofa. Or, place one dining room chair next to another. The surfaces should be approxi-

mately the same height. They need to be setup in a line and need to be stable so they do not slide or move. Begin with a small space between the surfaces.

2. Encourage your child to cruise from one piece of furniture to another. To do this, she will need to let go of the furniture with one hand and balance herself while she places her first hand on the next piece of furniture. From this position, she will either do a cruising step or move her second hand to the next piece of furniture. She may feel more stable if you place your hand over her first hand.

3. As she becomes motivated to cruise from one piece of furniture to another, increase the distance between the two pieces of furniture. This will further challenge her balance and control in cruising.

4. When she can cruise well between two surfaces placed next to each other, then place the surfaces parallel to each other. For example, place the coffee table in front of the sofa or place a Rubbermaid container (weighted so it does not move) in front of the sofa.

    a. Place her standing at the sofa and put a toy behind her on the coffee table (or in the Rubbermaid container). She will need to turn her trunk to see the toy while standing at the sofa.

    b. Encourage her to cruise from the sofa to the table or Rubbermaid container. Begin with the surfaces close together so it is easy to prop her hand on the table or hold the edge of the Rubbermaid container. If needed, place her hand on the table or edge of the container and stabilize it by placing your hand on top of hers. With this support, it will be easier to cruise to the next surface.

    c. After her hand is placed on the next surface, she will need to step sideways with each foot and then move her second hand to the next surface. While practicing this step, she will weight shift through her feet and balance herself.

    d. When she knows how to cruise between these two surfaces, then increase the distance as tolerated to challenge her further.

    e. When first setup to practice this skill, your child may try to move to the floor and then pull to stand at the next surface rather than cruise between the surfaces. If so, kneel behind her to block her from moving to the floor, and stabilize her hands to help her continue standing and learn the cruising method.

**ACTIVITY #4: Cruising with Hands against a Surface**

1. Use surfaces that your child will prop her hands *against,* for example, the wall, refrigerator, or cupboards.
2. Encourage her to step sideways and maintain her balance with her hands against the surface. Use magnets or Colorforms and place them to her side, just out of reach.
3. If she cannot step sideways with this support, encourage her to stand in the position and play with one-hand support. After she is comfortable in this position, she may take one step sideways to get a toy.
4. When she is comfortable with cruising with her hands against surfaces, she will be able to walk around the kitchen with her hands against the cupboards and walk around the house with her hands against the walls. This will give her a way to step independently within the house rather than creeping or crawling.

# Walking

During this stage, your child will begin by learning the leg stepping pattern with maximal support, and by the end of the stage, she will learn to walk by herself. To walk, she will need to develop strength in her trunk and leg muscles, endurance, and balance. However, the key to developing walking will be her motivation to walk. To help her develop walking skills, you will need to focus on motivating her and setting up walking as fun. When she is motivated to take steps, then you can help her build the component parts needed for walking. Walking will be the hardest gross motor skill for her to learn.

## Components

The components to focus on are:

1. an automatic stepping pattern in the legs by weight shifting over one leg and stepping with the other, and progressing to stepping with an efficient pattern over long distances
2. trunk control to be able to step with two-hand support, with the trunk leaning forward, and with hands held in front of the trunk or holding a push toy
3. the habit of walking with support within the daily routine so the activity becomes expected and valued, and the ability to do it several times a day for long distances to build endurance
4. trunk control to walk with one-hand support using the waddle pattern, with trunk erect and leaning from side to side

5. balance and perseverance to work on independent steps, and then determination and motivation to walk longer distances, progressing to wanting to walk all of the time.

## Tendencies

The tendencies are:
1. to wait for your child to indicate when she wants to practice stepping and to only practice as long as she wants to (for short distances)
2. to lift her legs up (hips bent and knees straight) to avoid walking when you stand behind her and encourage her to step with hand support
3. to use an uncoordinated or immature stepping pattern (wide base, knees and feet turned out, big step with one leg and short step with the other, stiff knees, inside borders of the feet collapsing)
4. to avoid walking or be reluctant to practice walking because she would rather be independent using her established method of mobility (for example, creeping)
5. to have unstable ankles and need foot support
6. to resist when she is challenged with the next level skill in the progression of walking, and for her walking pattern to initially regress with each new challenge because she will use compensations to feel stable

## Setup for Learning

When your child is practicing cruising, you will also practice stepping forward, and she will probably do best with trunk support. Since it is a new movement and you are controlling her, she may resist since she would rather be independent and be in control, moving where she wants to go. You will need to start with short distances so she feels comfortable with the new movements and ensure that she walks to motivating toys at the endpoint. As long as she is motivated by the toys, she will tolerate being supported to step for a short distance to them. You will need to provide whatever support she needs to help her be successful with stepping with her legs. Once she reaches the endpoint, clap for her and reward her by letting her play with the toy. With this setup, she will understand the game, know what she has to do, and learn that stepping is valuable since it leads to playing with the toy and receiving your praise. It is also helpful to sign and say "walk" to label the game.

Your child may tolerate the above setup and easily practice stepping with support. Or, your child may resist stepping, lifting her legs up to stop the game and showing you that she does not want to do it. *The focus now is to figure out how to encourage your child to practice stepping, since she is ready to learn the skill.* Do not wait for her to show you that she wants to practice walking because her preference will be to continue to use her easy and independent method of creeping. The longer you wait to practice walking, the more established and efficient her creeping will be, and the more resistant she will be to start the new method of walking, which requires her to give up her independence. The sooner you familiarize her with walking, the easier it will be for her to tolerate using stepping as another method of mobility.

Once she is familiar with the stepping pattern over short distances and tolerates practicing several times a day, then you will increase the distance. Between now and when she walks independently, your goal will be to develop leg strength and endurance to prepare her to walk all of the time. To give you an idea of how much walking a new walker does, consider Karen Adolph's research (Adolph, 2002).

Karen Adolph used a "step counter diary" method to quantify infants' walking steps. She studied three 14-month-old toddlers and found they walked between 500 and 1500 steps per hour, traveling the lengths of 29 football fields (2700 meters) and taking 9000 walking steps.

If this is the distance that a typical toddler walks, then we need to start working toward this level of endurance with children with Down syndrome, and begin early on. We can practice endurance from the time the child can walk 30 feet, by focusing on increasing the distance and frequency of walking on a daily basis. In my experience, if a child has worked on endurance between the time she could walk with two-hand support and the time she learned to walk independently for 15 feet, then she will progress to walking all of the time more quickly.

When your child is comfortable with stepping for long distances with trunk support, then she will be ready to be challenged to walk with less support. You can support her hands and provide **two-hand support,** with her hands at the level of her shoulders (not higher). When she is comfortable with this support, you can continue to focus on doing it several times a day for long distances, and to make it fun, you can go fast. The next challenge will be to learn the waddle pattern and walk with **one hand support**. Once your child is familiar with the waddle, she will be ready to practice taking an **independent step.**

As she is challenged to walk with less support, she will use compensatory patterns to try to feel stable. At this point, do not focus on the quality of the walking. If you nag her to walk with quality when she is learning to walk, walking will be laborious and she will resist practicing it. Practice and repetition over long distances will improve her stepping pattern, and through this experience, she will figure out how to balance her body to walk. You will focus on refining the quality of her walking pattern after she is able to walk all of the time (on level surfaces) and is a confident and competent walker.

---

## Steps in Learning to Walk

Your child will need to practice the following steps to learn to walk by herself. They are listed in the order they develop.

1. Walking with trunk support, with you standing behind her using your legs to support her back
2. Walking with two-hand support
3. Walking pushing a standing toy, push toy, or posterior walker (Kaye or Nimbo)
4. Lunging steps to a horizontal surface
5. Walking with one-hand support, using the waddle pattern
6. Independent steps, from taking the first step to walking 15 feet
7. Walking long distances in the house (level surface)
8. Walking all of the time in the house (level surface)

---

## *Walking with Trunk Support*

The first goal is to teach the stepping pattern of the legs. Then, once your child is familiar and comfortable with stepping, do it several times each day for brief practice periods. You will test what support your child likes best and set her up to step short distances to toys placed on a raised surface, like the sofa. She will want to move to the toys quickly, so give her the support she needs to help her step fast.

In the beginning, you just want her to tolerate practicing stepping so it needs to feel easy to her, and be rewarding. To help her step, you will need to weight shift her (sideways movement) over one leg so her other leg has no weight on it and is free to move. She will feel most stable if you stand behind her with your feet on the sides of her feet and her trunk leaning and stabilized against your legs. Then you will hold the sides of her trunk (either just below her armpits, or if needed, lower and around the front of her abdomen) and weight shift her, and see if she steps. Generally, she will step after you weight shift her. If not, you can assist her in taking a step by swinging her trunk forward on that side, or assisting her leg. She will begin to learn the stepping pattern if you provide maximal support and make it fun and easy. Practice for short distances and step fast to an endpoint with a great motivator. The more she practices during the day, the more automatic her pattern will become.

If your child resists stepping by lifting her legs and feet when you are standing behind her, then use an alternative strategy. Set her up with her trunk leaning forward over a stable surface like a cube chair (14.5 inches or 36 cm high) or a standing toy. You can prop her elbows on the surface and knee walk behind her. Place your arms against the sides of her trunk (under her armpits), with your hands on the surface, and then you can push it forward and control the speed and direction. She will step with this support, and your arms can guide weight shifting if needed to assist stepping. By kneeling behind her you will give her pelvic support and also block her from sitting down.

When first learning the leg stepping pattern, your child's movements may be stiff, awkward, and uncoordinated, and she may step with a wide base. Just keep practicing stepping, and with experience, her pattern will improve. The goal now is to establish an automatic and consistent leg stepping pattern. Once she knows this movement with her legs, she can learn to use it with two-hand support.

## ACTIVITY #5: Walking with Trunk Support

1. Place a motivating toy on a table or the sofa in front of her, about 3–4 feet away.
2. Place your child standing in front of you, facing away from you. Stand with your feet on the outsides of her feet. Lean her trunk against your legs, and hold her on the sides of her trunk under her armpits. (If she needs more support, place your hands on her abdomen.)
3. Sign and say "walk." You can also sing a walking song if useful to motivate her to walk (and distract her). Some children like you to count the steps.
4. Then you weight shift onto one foot and she will feel this movement and then step forward with her other foot. If she does not step, then pause after the weight shift and wait for her to step. After she steps, then repeat with weight shifting over your other foot and wait for her to step. Test to see if it is easier for her to step with a particular leg. If so, then assist the leg that has difficulty, as needed, to keep the stepping going.
5. Continue with stepping until she steps to the endpoint. Then clap for her and praise her, and give her time to play with her toy.

### *Walking with Two-Hand Support*

Now that your child knows the leg stepping pattern, the next goal is to use it with two-hand support (fig. 5.11). Since she is familiar with you walking behind her, you can let her lean her trunk against your legs so she feels stable and test if she can step with two-hand support. Have her hold your index fingers and position her hands in front of her chest, at the level of her shoulders. You will need to lean your trunk over her to position her arms and trunk properly. You want to teach her to hold your fingers, while you hold her wrists with your hands so she feels stable. When she is familiar with walking with two-hand support, you can lessen your support at her wrists and have her hold onto your index fingers to learn to hold on and balance herself. She needs to learn to be responsible for controlling her own balance. If you hold her, she will not have to balance herself and will depend on you to do that for her.

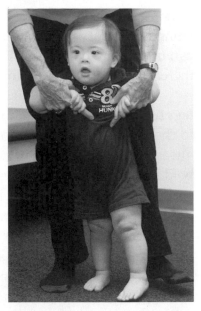

Her hands need to be at shoulder level or lower and in front of her chest to enable her to activate her abdominal muscles when stepping. If her arms are supported with her elbows straight and her hands above her head, she will learn to walk by arching her back and primarily using her back muscles. You also need to watch her elbows. It is best to have her elbows slightly bent and forward of her trunk (side view). If she excessively bends her elbows and

(fig. 5.11)

pulls them back even with her trunk or behind her trunk (side view), then help her learn to walk with her elbows forward. By pulling her elbows back, she is pinching her shoulder blades together and arching her trunk, primarily using her back muscles to walk. It is important to support her in the most strategic way to trigger use of the abdominals when she is learning to walk since she will need to know how to use them to ultimately take independent steps.

With your child's arms in the optimal position and her hands actively holding your fingers, you are ready to practice stepping short distances to an endpoint with motivating toys. Start with short distances to make it easy and rewarding until she is comfortable with this game. As you are supporting her, read her cues to determine if she likes stepping and leans forward, eager to move to the endpoint or if she is reluctant and trying to stop, putting on the brakes. If she is trying to stop, you need to figure out how you can engage her to help her feel safe and to make it fun. When she is familiar with the game and actively participates, then you can increase the distance. You can start with 5 feet, then increase to 10 feet, 20 feet, 50 feet, and 100 feet. When stepping for longer distances, make it fun by chasing siblings, kicking a ball and chasing it, or moving fast. If your house has a circular path, then move around the circle for several repetitions. You can also watch your child and when she starts creeping somewhere quickly, then stand her up and walk her to that endpoint.

**Strategies for Reluctant Walkers.** *If she is reluctant to practice stepping*, you can sit her on a bench, have her hold your thumbs (and you hold her wrists), and have her take 2 steps to you sitting (or kneeling) in front of her. You may be the best motivator and she may feel more confident moving to you in the beginning. When you are guiding her to step to you, weight shift her to assist her with being successful with stepping. When she is comfortable with stepping, then you can use the method of standing behind her and walking 3- to 4-foot distances, increasing the distance in small increments until she is accustomed to walking.

When you are practicing walking for longer distances, *if she lifts her legs to quit,* then you need to use strategies to keep her standing and stepping to the endpoint. You want to structure the game of walking so she learns to always walk to the endpoint. So if she quits midway and lifts her legs, do not hold her by her hands and wrists if her legs have gone limp. This is too much strain on her shoulders with her lax ligaments. The best strategy is to quickly catch her trunk with your knees and tell her "stand up" and "more walking" to label the game. If she does not take weight on her legs, then hold her trunk and bounce her in standing, and with this fun way of distracting her, she will take weight on her legs again.

*If she frequently lifts her legs to quit walking,* then use the alternative strategy discussed under "Walking with Trunk Support" (her trunk leaning forward over a stable surface like a cube chair or standing toy with you knee walking behind her). With the supporting surface in front of her, she cannot lift her legs to quit. You need to figure out why she is quitting, and then test what will help her step the distance. Experiment with giving her more support (maybe trunk support), moving faster, or using a better motivator. With frequent practice and your resourcefulness in figuring out how to support her and make walking fun, she will become comfortable with walking, and it will be one of the games she loves to play with you!

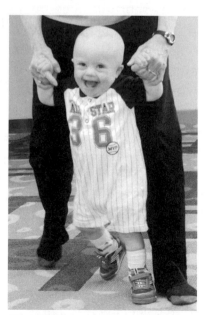

Practice walking with two-hand support as one of your walking activities until she is walking independently all of the time. It will be the best method to improve her endurance in walking, working toward walking 29 football fields a day! When it is easy for her, you will walk long distances several times a day and walking will become her habit for moving in her environment. She will be motivated to do it and enjoy playing this game with you. You can test if she walks longer distances inside or outside the home (see fig. 5.12). You can also test speed, and do fast stepping. You can also see if she walks better with her arms in the high guard position, since she will need to use this arm position for balance when she takes independent steps.

(fig. 5.12)

## ACTIVITY #6: Walking with Two-Hand Support

1. Setup the endpoint by placing a motivating toy on a table or the sofa in front of her, about 3-5 feet away.

2. Place your child standing in front of you, facing away from you. Stand with your feet on the outsides of her feet. Lean her trunk against your legs, have her hold your index fingers, and you hold her wrists (fig. 5.13). Place her hands forward in front of her chest, with her hands at the level of her shoulders. You will need to lean your trunk forward to keep her trunk upright and her arms forward.

3. Sign and say "walk." You can also sing a walking song if useful to motivate her to walk (and distract her). Some children like you to count the steps.

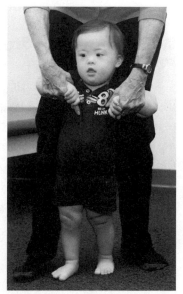

(fig. 5.13)

4. Then weight shift her and wait for her to step. Repeat so she steps with her other leg. Continue with stepping until she steps to the endpoint. Then clap for her and praise her, and give her time to play with her toy.

5. Increase the distance when she is ready. Begin with stepping for 3-5 foot distances and then work toward walking 5-10 feet. Keep increasing the distance as tolerated. Also have her practice walking several times a day as part of her daily routine—e.g., walking to the high chair to eat or walking to the bathtub to take a bath. Always create a fun experience and use the best motivators.

6. If she resists stepping for 3-foot distances with you standing behind her, try this method:
    a. Place her sitting on a bench, facing you.
    b. Sit on the floor (or kneel, sitting on your heels) approximately two feet away from her.
    c. Say and sign "stand up" and have her pull up to stand holding onto your thumbs.
    d. Then say and sign "walk" and give her extra support by holding her wrists while she holds your thumbs. With the hand support, weight shift her to one side and wait for her to step. Then repeat to the other side. Encourage her to take 2 steps

to you. If she needs extra support in the beginning, support her trunk so she feels comfortable and learns the game.

e. When she reaches you, praise her, hug her, clap for her, and show your excitement.

## Walking with a Standing Toy, a Push Toy, or a Posterior Walker

Since the goal is for your child to be motivated to walk and to walk long distances, you will use whatever setup accomplishes that goal. Some children practice walking better if they feel they are in control. If they are propping on a piano (stationary standing toy) and you stabilize and move it slowly so they feel in control, they may tolerate practicing walking more easily. If your child tolerates stepping better with this experience than when you hold her hands, it is the method to use.

### Using a Standing Toy or Push Toy

Once your child knows the leg stepping pattern, you can test her readiness and interest in stepping with a standing toy or push toy. Your child will probably prefer the standing toy first because she will feel more stable and in control. She may feel that the push toy is wobbly and moves too fast. To help her understand how to walk with this equipment, have her hold the handle, prop on the surface, or lean her trunk over the surface and then place your arms on the sides of her trunk for stability and your hands on the handle or top of the surface to control the speed and move it forward. You will knee walk behind her to provide pelvic support (if needed) and to prevent sitting down. Just like walking with hand or trunk support, you want to setup the endpoint so she knows where she is going, and is motivated to get there.

When choosing a standing toy or surface to push, look for one that has a minimum width of approximately 14 inches (35.5 centimeters) so she can prop her hands or lean her trunk over it, and it will be stable. It is best if it is soft if she is leaning her trunk against it. You can also use a Rubbermaid container with the lid (fig. 5.14), or without the lid, and she can hold the edge. It needs to slide easily on the carpet (or whatever surface it is placed on). It is helpful if it is entertaining (like a piano) because the music will distract her while she is stepping. If it is just a surface like a cube chair or ottoman, you can place a toy on it or have the motivator at the endpoint.

Pick the push toy that will work best for your child. The **height** of the handle needs to be at chest level so her trunk is vertical when she is standing and holding the handle (fig. 5.15). If it is too low, she will lean her trunk too far forward and then it will move too fast. The **handle** needs to be wide so her hands are in front of her shoulders, and then she will feel more stable. If it is

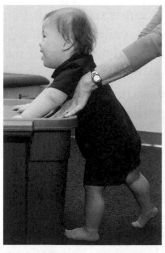 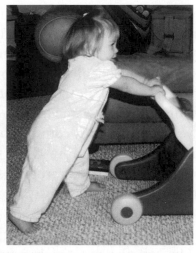 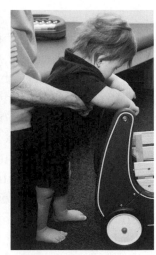

(fig. 5.14)                    (fig. 5.15)                    (fig. 5.16)

too narrow, she will feel wobbly when weight shifting. The diameter of the handle needs to be small so she can grasp it easily with her small hands and short fingers. The **width** of the base needs to be broad so it is stable, and does not tip over, and her feet can step in between the wheels, without hitting them.

Since toy manufacturers change the types and designs of push toys often, I recommend that you test the models available when your child is ready to use one. If your child is tall, the Radio Flyer classic walker wagon (fig. 5.16) and the Little Tykes shopping cart may work. As an alternative, you can use a wagon such as the Radio Flyer wagon or the Little Tikes 2 in 1 wagon, because they have an edge to hold onto. Generally, lightweight baby strollers and shopping carts do not work well since they tip over easily.

When your child is first learning to walk with the push toy, she will lean her trunk forward. She will be working on stepping and holding the handle, and you will need to hold the push toy and move it forward, controlling the speed and the distance between her and the push toy, and keeping it stable. Make sure that the push toy is not too far forward, causing her to lean her trunk forward excessively, because this will make her less stable and unable to step. With practice, she will learn to stand tall with her trunk more vertical. Then she will be able to control the speed and work on her balance. At this point, you can try letting go of the push toy so she can try to push it by herself with control.

You also need to test what external support your child needs so that she feels safe with the push toy, and it does not move too quickly. If she does not need you to hold the handle and knee walk behind her, then you can position yourself in front of her and place your hand on the front of the push toy to control the speed. You can also try weighting the push toy to see if this helps your child. Just make sure the additional weight does not cause her to lean her trunk forward in order to push it to the endpoint. How much support is needed depends on the type of push toy and the surface it is used on. If you are moving on a thick rug, less support is needed than if walking on a hardwood floor. Therefore, you need to test the support needed depending on the push toy, the surface she is walking on, and her temperament. If she is careful and wants to be in control, she will want more support to feel stable; if she is a risk taker, she will not mind having to step quickly to keep up.

Test what surface your child is most comfortable using. She will probably prefer a carpeted surface in the beginning. If you try it on tile or hardwood floors, the push toy will slip and slide in all directions and your child may feel unstable and uncomfortable. On a carpeted surface, the only direction the push toy will move is forward.

In the beginning, it is best to practice walking in a wide-open space so steering is not needed. She can also practice in a hallway where there is no furniture. Keep the skill as easy as possible until she is motivated to do it. Later, when she wants to do it on her own, then you can teach her how to steer. It is best to teach steering when it is functional for her—for instance, when she is stuck. Have her hold the handle and then you hold her forearms and rotate her trunk to slide the push toy sideways to an open area. Help her stand tall and then make it a big movement so she feels it and then learns to imitate it. When you assist her, you can give her the verbal cue "turn."

Later, when your child loves stepping with hand support, she may like walking with a push toy because she can walk independently, spontaneously initiating walking on her own, and realize the value of walking in her environment. She can choose when she wants to practice walking rather than only doing it when you practice it with her. She can also use the push toy outside to walk for long distances. With the push toy, she can work on endurance by increasing the distance and frequency of walking. To be independent walking with the push toy, she will need to learn to pull to stand at the push toy. To teach her this, you will need to stabilize the push toy and have her pull to stand. With practice, she will learn to do it on her own.

### Using a Posterior Walker (Kaye or Nimbo)

If your child is tall and the push toys are too low for her to stand with her trunk up straight, an alternative is to use the Kaye Products Posture Control Walker (www.kayeproducts.com) or the Nimbo Lightweight Gait Trainer (fig. 5.17) by Wenzelite Re/hab and available through Drive Medical (www.drivemedical.com). In my experience, children with Down syndrome easily learn to walk with this equipment once they are familiar with it. It is best if you use the following specifications: 4 wheels, front swivel wheels, and rear ratcheted wheels. The front swivel wheels are initially locked to track straight. Then, when your child is comfortable with the walker, they can be unlocked so she can learn to steer and balance herself when steering. The one-way ratchet rear wheels prevent the walker from sliding backwards.

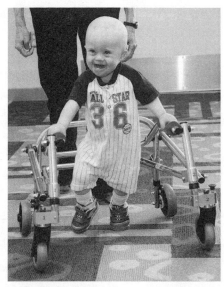

The walker is placed behind the child and she holds the handles. You need to adjust the height of the walker so her elbows are mildly bent. The back pelvic bar of the walker will be approximately at your child's waist. This is higher than how the walker is usually fitted because you want to adjust it for the optimal arm position. Since children with Down syndrome have short arms (in proportion to the trunk), the walker height will be higher so the child stands holding on, with the elbows

(fig. 15.17)

mildly bent (about 25 degrees). With the walker properly adjusted, you can stand her in the walker with the back of the walker against the wall. She will feel stable with this support and can become familiar with how it feels to stand in the walker. If she tolerates standing, then you can sit on the floor in front of her and see if she will tolerate stepping while you move the walker forward.

Initially, she may feel unstable with stepping because she will feel the bar behind her waist pushing her forward, and she may feel as if she is going to fall. She will learn that she needs to stand with her trunk up straight (not leaning forward), hold on and use her arms and hands for balance, and step with this posture and support. To make it easier for her, you can set her up to walk a couple of steps to a motivating endpoint. You can knee walk behind her, supporting her pelvis against the walker and weight shifting her to help her step. If you give her this support so she feels stable as she learns how to use the equipment, she will learn to like stepping with it. Once she is used to stepping with you holding her pelvis, you can lessen your support and just hold the walker. You will stabilize it when she is standing and move it forward after she takes a step. You will keep the pelvic bar against her waist while she is standing and stepping.

With practice, she will learn how to step and balance herself while you manage the walker. Then she will need to learn how to push the walker and step on her own. She may want ongoing support as you increase the distance. If so, you can support her with a scarf or belt around her chest and under her armpits. Gradually you will increase the distance, and when she is confident, add steering. To adjust the walker for steering, you will unlock the front swivel wheels. When she can steer, you can have her walk with it in the community so she builds endurance. She will also like practicing fast stepping with it, running with her siblings and friends. When she can do this, she will want to walk all of the time.

She will need to learn to pull to stand and lower to the floor safely to be independent with the walker. To pull to stand, she will creep into the walker, and hold the pelvic bar or red handles to pull to stand from kneeling. Once standing, she will need to learn to turn around so she is facing forward to step (with the pelvic bar behind her). To lower from standing to the floor, she will bend her knees to lower herself to the ground, moving to hands and knees or hands and feet.

 ## ACTIVITY #7: Walking with a Standing Toy, a Push Toy, or a Posterior Walker

1. Determine if your child prefers a standing toy (cube chair, piano, ottoman, or Rubbermaid container) or a push toy, and place it on the carpet. Place her standing at the toy and either lean her trunk over the surface or have her hold the handle (of the push toy) or the edge of the Rubbermaid container. Kneel behind her and place your arms on the sides of her trunk (to stabilize her) and your hands on the surface (or handle).

2. Set her up to walk 3 feet to an endpoint with a motivating toy. Sign and say "walk."

3. Push the toy or surface forward and knee walk behind your child with your hips close to hers to prevent sitting down. Assist her with stepping to the endpoint. When she reaches it, praise her, clap for her, and show your excitement.

4. When she is familiar with this game and is cooperative with stepping, then reduce your support and only stabilize her hands on the surface (with your hands over her hands). Continue moving it forward and controlling the speed. Increase the distance as tolerated.

5. When she likes walking, then position yourself in front of her and just support the surface, moving it forward and controlling the speed. Have her hold the handle or edge, or control propping her hands on the surface, while stepping. Increase the distance as tolerated.

6. If she prefers the standing toy at first, test her to see when she is ready to use the push toy, while you control the speed and move it forward.

7. When ready, focus on walking with the push toy to help her gain confidence walking with this type of support. Place your hands on the front of the push toy to stabilize it and slowly move it forward. Your job is to keep it stable, move it forward at the right speed, and keep it the right distance in front of her. Her job is to hold on and step forward.

8. Begin with 3-5 foot distances, and keep increasing the distance as tolerated while walking inside the house.
9. When she is familiar with walking with the push toy and is motivated to use it, encourage her to pull up to stand, holding the bar. You stabilize the push toy to keep it from moving so she learns how to pull to stand at it. Later, have her pull to stand by herself.
10. When she is comfortable, confident, and experienced with walking with the push toy, let go and see if she can control it by herself. Provide intermittent support if needed and see if she will figure out how to maintain her own balance. She will need to learn to hold her trunk up straight to be successful.
11. After she has mastered walking with the push toy without your support, teach her to steer it around furniture. Help her when she is stuck against furniture and wants your help. Have her learn to grip the handle while you support her forearms and turn her trunk to slide the push toy sideways. As you do this exaggerated movement, say "turn." From this experience, she will learn how to slide the push toy on the floor to maneuver it around furniture. (It is easier to do if the push toy is light and easy to slide.)
12. Since the goal is walking long distances, if your child has difficulty learning how to steer, assist her to encourage walking.
13. If she resists stepping and even has difficulty with the standing toy, try using two people. Have one person in front of her supporting her hands and motivating her, and the other person behind her, holding and moving her legs. Practice for a short distance and then praise her. Sometimes, a child is fearful and does not know what to do and initially needs maximal support to learn the movements.
14. If she has difficulty stepping with one leg, assist that leg to help her be successful.
15. If she uses a posterior walker (Kaye or Nimbo), the biggest difficulty will be when she is initially learning how to step with it. See the above section, "Using a Posterior Walker (Kaye or Nimbo)," for tips on teaching her how to step with it, providing support, increasing the distance, learning to steer, and pulling to stand and lowering to the floor.

## *Lunging Steps to a Horizontal Surface*

While your child is practicing walking with two-hand support, you can test when she is ready to try taking lunging steps to a horizontal surface such as a sofa (figs. 5.18–5.20). Some children practice this skill very early, and it may be the first way they take steps with support, particularly if they resist stepping with hand support. Others like to be familiar with the leg stepping pattern and

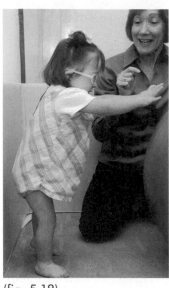 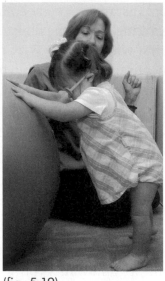 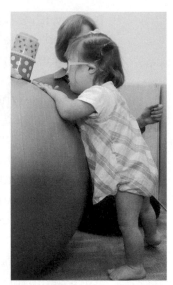

(fig. 5.18)          (fig. 5.19)          (fig. 5.20)

then feel more comfortable practicing the skill. This skill is important because it prepares your child for the risk of "falling" forward when taking her first step. From a supported standing position, she will choose to lean her trunk forward away from your support and fall forward until she props on the sofa.

When you practice this skill, the setup and timing of movements are crucial. You need to quickly move her to standing, only providing support by kneeling behind her, and then focus her attention on the motivator on the sofa so she chooses to move to it. If the setup is prolonged or she holds your hands, then she will probably be distracted and may resist taking the lunging steps.

She needs to be setup for safety. It is best if she practices lunging steps to a soft surface like the sofa or a padded chair. If you use a table or firm surface, she may fall or bump into it. You also need to watch her hands to make sure she figures out how to prop effectively. After she props, you want her to take two steps to bring her feet closer to the sofa, so wait for her to do it rather than do it for her. Since she will be leaning forward against the surface with her feet behind her, she will feel off balance and will spontaneously move her feet to stand vertically.

## ACTIVITY #8: Lunging Steps to a Horizontal Surface

1. Select a soft surface (sofa or padded chair) your child will walk to and place a motivator on the surface.
2. Sit on your heels in front of the surface with your knees approximately 15-18 inches (38-46 cm) away from the surface. Place your child sitting on your lap with her feet on the floor. Playfully hold her lower legs and pat her feet against the floor. Then place her feet 2-3 inches (5-7.5 cm) apart and pointing straight.

3. Support her lower legs and then move to tall kneeling, and she will move to standing. Let go of her legs and quickly stabilize her trunk against your abdomen. Avoid holding her hands or letting her grasp your hands. (When you are in tall kneeling, you are tucking your abdominals so that she has a balanced place to rest in standing. When you do this, your buttocks are over the middle calf areas of your legs.)

4. Firmly tap her abdomen 3 times with the pads of your fingers (to activate her abdominals).

5. Sign and say "walk." Wait for her to choose to move to the motivator. Do not help her move forward by leaning your body forward. Keep her attention on the motivator, and if it is something she really wants, she will move to it.

6. Anticipate that she will lean her trunk forward, prop on the surface, and then take 2 steps to stand (vertically) at the surface. Watch these movements and spot her as needed for safety.

7. When she reaches the toy, praise her, clap for her, and show your excitement.

8. When she is comfortable with this activity, you can start her in the standing position, with you tall kneeling behind her (step 3).

## Walking with One-Hand Support

When your child can walk well with two-hand support for long distances, is confident and motivated to walk with support, and is familiar with walking several times daily, then you can see whether she is ready to work on the next challenging walking skill—walking with one-hand support (fig. 5.21). To

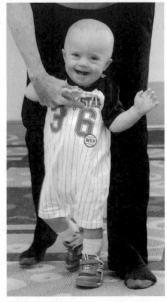

walk with one-hand support, she will need to learn the waddle pattern, which is holding her trunk up straight and leaning it from side to side to weight shift. As she weight shifts to each side, she uses her abdominals to control her balance and take steps. She needs to learn the waddle pattern in order to take independent steps with control.

Up until now, your child has learned to step with hand support with her trunk leaning forward and has become competent with the leg stepping pattern with her trunk in this position. Now that the leg stepping pattern is established, she needs to learn a new method of holding and controlling her trunk and legs to take balanced steps. She will not be able to take independent steps with her trunk in the old position. To take balanced steps,

(fig. 5.21)

she needs to learn to hold her trunk up straight, lean it from side to side (wad-dle), and activate her abdominals. At first, you will teach the waddle pattern with maximal support. Then, when you feel her using this new pattern, you will decrease your support.

To introduce this new method of walking, she will need maximal sup-port as described in Activity #10, below. When you first practice walking with one-hand support, she will want two-hand support, since this has been her habit, and she feels more stable with this support. She may resist walking with one-hand support and move to the floor. If she is resistant, then be strategic about how you set her up to practice, and work to find a way to engage her in practicing the skill. Provide whatever support is needed, practice for a very short distance, and select the very best motivator. Practice with each hand to determine if it is easier for her to walk with a particular hand supported.

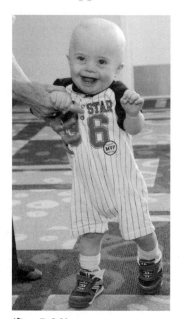

(fig. 5.22)

After she is comfortable with walking with one-hand support with maximal support with you standing behind her, then try a new method with less support. As described in Activity #10, start her sitting on a bench and position yourself at her side. Provide 3 points of support by having her hold your index finger, then you hold her wrist with one hand, while your other hand holds her trunk under her armpit (fig. 5.22). As she tolerates one-handed walking with this support, increase the distance. When she can walk easily with this support, then you can gradually decrease your support, by first eliminating the trunk support and later the wrist support.

When practicing walking with one-hand support, the first focus is learning the waddle pat-tern, which is holding the trunk vertical, and lean-ing it from side to side to elicit the stepping pattern. When your child tries this new challenging skill, she will compensate to feel stable and may stiffen her knees, widen her base, or take big steps with one leg and small steps with the other. Do not focus on the leg posture and the quality of her stepping pattern at this point. They will improve with practice, as she becomes comfortable with walking with one-hand support, and after the waddle pattern is auto-matic. She will lift each leg after her trunk is weight shifted and learn to walk with her hips and knees bending and full sole weight bearing.

When you help her walk with one-hand support, avoid the two common mistakes: 1) holding her hand forward and above her head (with her elbow straight), and 2) leaning her trunk forward. This support is frequently provided to help a child step forward faster. If you support your child in this way, however, she will not learn the waddle pattern and will just continue to use the trunk posture used when walking with two-hand support and doing lunging steps. With her trunk supported leaning forward, you will need to balance her, and she will not learn how to use her abdominals to balance herself now, and prepare her for taking independent steps later. This is the strategic time to teach her the trunk posture needed for independent steps. She will learn it if you mold, model, and guide her trunk movements while providing the right kind of hand support with her arm in the optimal position.

When you first practice walking with one-hand support, test to see if it is easier with a particular hand supported. Usually, there is a preference, and you want to practice with the preferred hand until your child is cooperative and comfortable with one-handed walking. She will feel more stable using a particular hand, either because it is her stronger arm or because holding that hand assists her weaker leg. When walking with one-hand support, it is more difficult to step with the opposite leg. So if her right leg is weaker, supporting her right hand will assist stepping with the right leg. Once she can walk long distances with her preferred hand supported, you will need to practice walking with her other hand supported. She needs to learn to use her abdominals on both sides in order to take independent steps with each leg.

If practiced properly, walking with one-hand support will strengthen the core (trunk) muscles and teach the posture needed for independent steps. To walk with one-hand support, she will need to hold her trunk up straight (not leaning forward), lean it from side to side to weight shift, stabilize it and balance both sides of her trunk while stepping with each leg, with only one side (hand) supported. It will be easier to step with the leg on the supported side. When she steps with that leg, she will be balanced in the center by her other leg and the supported hand. However, when she steps with her leg on the unsupported side, her weight will be leaning over the supported side, and it will be harder to keep her balance in the center and step. So, when she steps with that leg, she may spin in a circle and fall. With practice, she will learn how to use her abdominals to stabilize and balance her trunk as she steps with the leg on the unsupported side.

### Setting Your Child Up for Success

To teach your child to walk with one-hand support, the setup is critical. You need to provide the **right support to the preferred hand**, and you need to **position yourself** so she is working on how to balance herself while doing the waddle pattern.

- In the beginning, when you need to provide maximal support, you will stand behind her.

- When she is ready to practice with three points of support, you will be kneeling at her side, facing her, as she steps for 2-3 foot distances to the endpoint.
- When she is practicing for 2-3 steps, you could also be sitting on your heels on the floor, facing her, with her standing at the sofa and then encourage her to take a couple of steps to you. If she holds your thumb (positioned vertically), then you can place your fingers under her forearm to provide additional support, and then you can guide the waddle pattern to assist her with stepping to you.
- When she is ready to step for 3-5 foot distances and more, then you will need to stand at her side and step sideways to the endpoint (Activities #11 and #12).

### Increasing the Distance

Practice one-handed walking as much as tolerated until your child becomes familiar with using it most of the time. The more she uses the trunk and arm posture of the waddle pattern through one-handed walking, the easier the transition to taking independent steps. When she can walk 10 feet with one-hand support, just holding your index finger, she will be ready to practice taking an independent step.

As you are increasing the distance using one-hand support, alternate between providing two-hand and one-hand support. You can begin the walk with two-hand support and then let go of one hand and have her walk to the endpoint with only one hand supported. Since walking with one-hand support will be at a slower pace, you can alternate it with fast stepping with two-hand support so she experiences the fun of a faster pace. When she is comfortable with walking with one-hand support, you can challenge her by having her hold your finger and balance herself without any assistance from you. You can also hold her arm in the high guard position (fig. 5.23), since she will use this posture for balance when she takes independent steps. When she is walking with this minimal support, you can walk behind her to

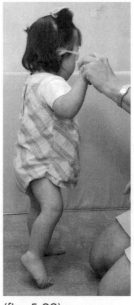
(fig. 5.23)

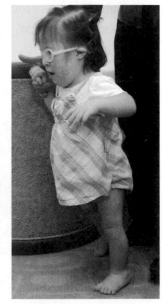
(fig. 5.24)

keep her centered in the midline (fig. 5.24). I do not recommend walking beside her while holding her hand, since the tendency will be to lean her sideways toward you, and then she will be off balance.

### ACTIVITY #9: Walking with One-Hand Support, Maximally Supported

1. Stand behind your child, with her legs in between your legs, and your feet on the sides of her feet. (It is best if you are not wearing shoes.) Her trunk will lean back against your legs.
2. Have her hold your index finger while you hold her wrist. Then place your index finger against her chest to cue her to hold her trunk up straight and rest it back against your legs. (Test each hand to see if she has a preference, and if so, use the preferred hand.)
3. With her body in this supported and optimal position, weight shift (lean) to one side and wait for her to step with her other leg. After she steps, then repeat and weight shift to the other side, waiting for her to step. Continue to guide this waddle stepping pattern, moving a short distance (3-4 feet or .9 to 1.2 meters) to the motivator and endpoint.
4. When she reaches the endpoint, praise her, clap for her, and show your excitement.
5. As tolerated, increase the distance with this support until she is comfortable with this new walking pattern and steps quickly and easily.
6. If she is nervous and needs more support when first practicing the skill, bend your hips and knees and use your legs to hug her trunk to give her more support.

### Activity #10: One-handed Walking for 3-5 Feet (.9-1.5 Meters) with Less Support

(The examples in A and B are with right-hand support. If your child prefers left- hand support, reverse how you support her.)

*A. At her right side, providing 3 points of support:*
1. Setup the endpoint with a motivator about 3 feet in front of her.
2. Place your child sitting on a bench with her feet on the floor. Kneel at her right side, facing her.
3. Provide 3 points of support by having her hold your right index finger with her right hand, while you hold her (right) wrist, and your

left hand holds the right side of her trunk under her armpit (your thumb on her chest and your fingers on her back). Support her right hand in front of her chest at the level of her shoulder.

4. Say and sign "stand up" and have her stand up on her own or with your assistance.

5. Say and sign "walk" and encourage her to step to the endpoint. Initiate the waddle by supporting her trunk up straight and then lean it to each side, and wait for her to step. Then continue the weight shift and waddle stepping pattern to the endpoint. While you are moving her trunk, support her arm and hand to move with her trunk so she feels stable and balanced.

6. When she reaches the endpoint, praise her, clap for her, and show your excitement.

7. Test each hand to see if she has a preference, and if so, use the preferred hand until she is comfortable and steps quickly and easily. Then practice with 3 points of support to her other side.

8. As she tolerates one-handed walking with this support, then increase the distance.

*B. With you in front of her:*

1. Place your child standing at furniture or standing with her back against the furniture. You sit on your heels on the floor, in front of her, facing her. Position yourself about 2-3 steps away from her, and she will be motivated to step to you. Position your knees wide apart so your knees do not block her from stepping to you.

2. Say and sign "walk" and encourage her to step to you (the endpoint).

3. Place your left thumb vertically in front of her right hand and encourage her to hold it. Position her hand in front of her chest at the level of her shoulder. Use your fingers to hold (and stabilize) her wrist and forearm.

4. With the hand support, initiate the waddle by supporting her trunk up straight and then lean it to each side and wait for her to step. Guide the waddle pattern and assist her in stepping to you.

5. When she steps to you, praise her, clap for her, and show your excitement.

6. Test each hand to see if she has a preference, and if so, use the preferred hand until she is comfortable and steps quickly and easily. Then practice by supporting her other hand.

7. As she tolerates one-handed walking with this support, increase the distance.

# Activity #11: Increasing the Distance Walking with One-Hand Support

*A. Three points of support:*

Follow steps 1-8 in Activity #10A with the following exceptions:

1. Set her up to walk 5-foot (1.5-meter) distances to the endpoint (and increase as tolerated).
2. Stand at her side and step sideways to the endpoint.
3. When providing 3 points of support, continue to have her hold your right index finger with her right hand and support her wrist in the same way, but the trunk support will be different. Your left hand will hold the right side of her trunk under her armpit with your thumb on her back and your fingers on her chest. The hand supporting her trunk will guide the waddle pattern (trunk vertical and leaning side to side), and she will balance herself with the hand support. You need to face her and step sideways to the endpoint in order to keep her trunk upright, promote the waddle, and have her experience stepping and balancing herself.

*B. Two points of support:*

1. When your child can walk easily with three points of support, let go of her trunk and continue with her holding your index finger while you hold her wrist (fig. 5.25).
2. Stand at her side and step sideways to the endpoint.

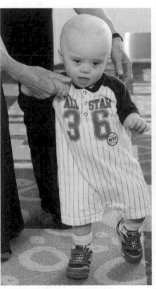
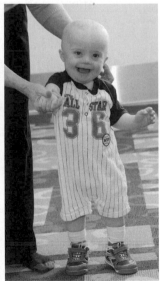

(fig. 5.25)          (fig. 5.26)

*C. One point of support:*

1. When she can walk easily with two points of support and you feel her doing the waddle pattern, let go of her wrist and have her hold your index finger and step to the endpoint. At first, position your hand with your palm up as she holds your index finger; this will give her a little extra support.

2. She will hold your finger with her hand at the level of her shoulder (and in front of her chest) and with her elbow mildly bent. It will be critical for her to learn to hold your finger and balance herself, rather than you holding her hand and having her depend on you to control her balance.

3. If she needs additional support to walk longer distances, you can hold the sleeve of her shirt (over her opposite shoulder or upper arm), and this may help her feel more stable (fig. 5.26).

 ## Activity #12: Walking Long Distances with One-Hand Support

Once the waddle pattern is established, your child is ready to learn to use it for long distances.

1. Have your child hold your index finger, with her arm in the high guard position, and balance herself without any assistance from you. Walk behind her or at her side, whichever is more comfortable for both of you. You want to move with the same waddle rhythm, and let her lead, and you follow. Also make sure she is centered in the midline and balanced, and you are not encouraging her to rely on you for balance.

2. If helpful, have her hold a small, lightweight toy in her unsupported hand.

3. Make it fun by changing the pace. Alternate between providing one-hand and two-hand support. You can begin the walk with one-hand support and then provide two-hand support and fast step.

---

### Hand Preference

As your child is progressing through the levels of support while stepping with one-hand support, test each hand to see if it is easier to balance and step when holding on with a particular hand. If she has a preference, let her use the preferred hand until she is comfortable and steps quickly and easily. To help her cooperate with one-handed walking, place a lightweight toy in her unsupported hand. When she is confident with one hand, then practice with her other hand. She will need to be competent using each hand in order to take independent steps.

---

## Independent Steps, from Taking the First Step to Walking 15 Feet

When your child is comfortable walking with one-hand support (with just one point of support) and doing the waddle, she will be ready to learn to take an independent step (fig. 5.27). From practicing lunging steps to a horizontal surface, she will be prepared for the risky movement of "falling" forward to move to another surface. To take a step, she will need to combine what she has learned from these two skills. She will need to be willing to risk moving forward without support and keep her trunk erect and use the waddle to step to the supporting surface.

In my experience and from my data, I have found that the skills of walking 10 feet with one-hand support (just holding my index finger) and taking 1-2 independent steps occur at the same time. Therefore, if your child can walk with one-hand support, she is ready to learn to take 1-2 independent steps, and it is our job to figure out how to elicit this new skill. Some children are easily motivated to work on taking independent steps, and it is a fun game for them. Other children are not interested because they already have an established method of moving that is automatic and effortless. Since learning to walk seems laborious to them, you will need to:

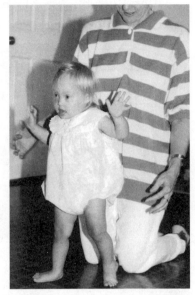

(fig. 5.27)

- build the skill step-by-step,
- use the best motivators to make it fun, and
- show your child the value of walking.

The goal will be to walk 15 feet consistently, and this is the criterion that I use to give credit for the skill of walking.

Progressing from taking one step to walking in the house all of the time will be a gradual process and can take months to develop. (I am specifying walking in the house to mean walking on a firm, level surface.) Your child will start with taking one step, and then you will need to practice each distance until she masters it, and then you can move on to the next distance. When she can walk distances of 15 feet consistently, then she will be ready to learn to walk long distances in the house. When she has adequate endurance, then she will be ready to learn to walk all of the time in the house.

Your child will learn to use her abdominals for balance while practicing independent steps. She does not need to be able to balance in standing before practicing independent steps. Through practicing walking with one-hand support, she learned to use her abdominals in the context of doing the waddle. To take independent steps, she will learn to activate her abdominals in an effective and timely way while taking each step. Even if she has strong abdominals in other positions, she will need to learn how to use them within the skill of taking independent steps.

## Setting Your Child Up for Success

In practicing independent steps, the setup is critical for your child to be successful. Remember, this is the hardest gross motor skill your child will need to learn so we need to set her up in the most strategic way. Follow these guidelines:

1. *Walk to a high, soft surface approximately 21-24 inches (53-61 cm) high* (figs. 5.28–5.31). Examples of surfaces are: large ball, 24-inch wide (60 cm) mat placed vertically against the wall, kitchen set, parent in

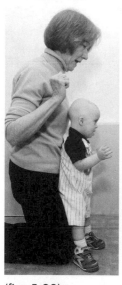
(fig. 5.28)

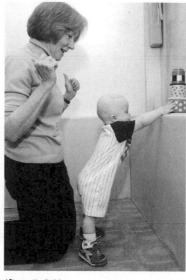
(fig. 5.29)

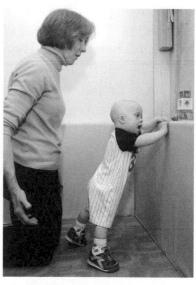
(fig. 5.30)

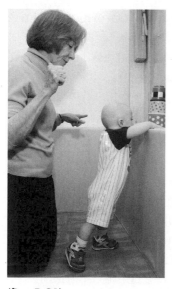
(fig. 5.31)

tall kneeling or sitting on heels, with knees wide apart. **Place a motivating toy on the surface at her eye level.** With this setup, when she looks forward at the toy, her head will be erect, and this will promote holding her trunk up straight. She will hold her arms up to prepare for playing with the toy and to prop her hands against the surface, which will also encourage her to hold her trunk up straight. **Keeping her head and trunk up straight are the key elements in taking independent steps.** If her head or trunk lean forward or her eyes gaze downward (causing her head and trunk to lean forward), she will go down to the floor. With this setup, she is also learning to raise her arms, which she will later need to use for balance in the high guard position when taking independent steps.

2. *Start her in standing, while you are in tall kneeling behind her, without hand support.* This is the same way that you supported her when you

practiced lunging steps (Activity #8, step 3). It is important to place her in the standing position quickly, without hand support and have her balance against you. Place her about 18 inches (46 cm) away from the surface.

3. *Place one foot forward to set her up to take a step with her other foot.* If you place both feet in line with each other, she will probably just do a lunging step by leaning her trunk forward, propping, and then taking a couple of steps. If you place one foot forward, she will just step with her other foot to move to the surface. Set her up to take a step with her preferred leg. If she has shown a preference to move through the half kneel position with a specific leg, then set her up to step with that leg by placing the other foot forward.

4. *Do 3 firm taps to the abdomen (with the pads of your fingers) to activate her abdominals.*

5. *Give the verbal cues and sign "walk" or "more walking" or say "1,2,3, go," if that motivates her.* Then wait for her to choose when to step to the surface. She will initiate activating her abdominals, balancing herself, initiating the first weight shift to step, and taking a step forward—and she needs to be in control of this.

6. *Walk to the endpoint.* Setup the game with the expectation that she always walks to the endpoint.

7. *Set her up to learn to prop against the endpoint, or against your body if she is walking to you.* If you hold your hands out, she will reach for your hands and lunge to you (leaning her trunk forward), expecting you to catch her. If she learns to prop against you and all endpoints, she will learn to keep her trunk up straight and balance herself until she reaches the endpoint. If she is stepping to you, place your hands to pat the area you want her to move toward. For example, if you are tall kneeling, pat your belly; if you are sitting on the floor or on your heels, pat your upper chest area. This will let her know where to prop her hands.

8. *When practicing independent steps, have her wear a onesie.* She will be more free to move and balance, and will not be limited by the stiffness of the pants or shirt.

9. *Test if it is easier to take independent steps when barefoot or wearing orthoses and shoes.* If she has not needed orthoses, she will practice independent steps barefoot. If she has used orthoses and shoes, see whether she can take independent steps better when barefoot or with the orthoses and shoes. Some children prefer the stability of the orthoses and shoes and learn to take independent steps with this support. Other children who have used orthoses and shoes to walk with support take independent steps better when barefoot. The added stiffness and weight of the orthoses and shoes may make it harder to weight shift and step,

and the rubber soles of the shoes may catch on the floor and cause the child to trip. Once independent steps are established, then the child will resume wearing the orthoses and shoes all of the time. While practicing independent steps barefoot, they will continue to use the orthoses and shoes when walking long distances with support.

10. ***Practice walking on firm, level surfaces.*** Try a variety of surfaces such as carpet, tile, linoleum, and hardwood floors to see if she prefers one surface to another. Use the preferred surface consistently to teach her to take independent steps. If she walks in the same place, it will be familiar, and she will feel secure. She will also learn this is where she practices the game of walking. Later, when walking is easy and automatic, she will be able to experiment with walking on a variety of surfaces.

11. ***When she is taking steps, make sure the area is clear of obstacles that she could trip over, bump into, or be distracted by.*** If you are kneeling on the floor or sitting on your heels and she is walking to you, make sure your legs are out of her way so she does not trip over them. Keep her focused on the endpoint and motivator at eye level to her. Avoid distractions, because they will limit her performance.

12. ***Avoid falls, especially if your child has the careful (observer) type temperament.*** Your child will stop practicing independent steps if she is afraid due to a fall.

### Increasing the Distance

After your child can take two independent steps, she will be ready to start working on distance. You will assess her progress by measuring the distance, rather than counting her steps. Her step length will vary, so distance is the best measure of her progress. You can set her up to take steps from standing, or sitting on a bench, depending on which method she likes best and motivates her to take the most steps. Some children prefer sitting on the bench as the starting position because they want to initiate walking on their own, rather than being placed in standing to walk.

When she is working on walking two-foot distances, the next big challenge is to learn to initiate the first weight shift to one side to begin the waddle. She may have the perfect posture, but she will not be able to take a step if she is not comfortable starting the first movement of leaning her trunk to one side. You need to determine if any hesitancy is due to fear or because she just cannot figure out how to do it. You can be playful and model the movement with your arms in the high guard position, tilt your trunk from side to side, and say "waddle, waddle" and then see if she will imitate you. If you are kneeling behind her, you can lean her to start the weight shift. If you are in front of her, she can hold your finger to start the first step and then you can let go. You will

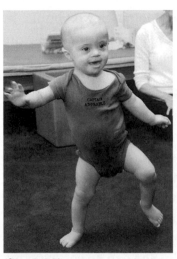 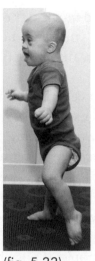 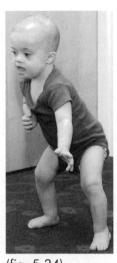 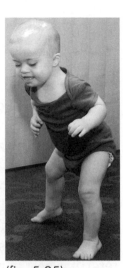

(fig. 5.32)          (fig. 5.33)          (fig. 5.34)          (fig. 5.35)

need to experiment with methods to help her learn how to start the waddle. For many children, this is the hardest part, and once initiated, stepping is easy.

Your child's first steps will look like this: She will learn to walk like other toddlers, with a top-heavy trunk. It may be even more difficult, since her trunk is long in proportion to her short legs. She will learn to use the waddle pattern, keeping her balance by moving her trunk from side to side over her base (width of her feet), and keeping her trunk up straight to move within her center of gravity (figs. 5.32–5.35). The side-to-side movements of her trunk will also elicit stepping movements. She will move her trunk and pelvis as a unit and take short steps. She will use this pattern until she can walk long distances at home. Later, with practice, her pattern will advance to the marching pattern with trunk erect, hips and knees bending, and full-sole weight bearing.

Once she is comfortable with taking steps for two-foot (60-cm) distances, you will systematically set her up to learn how to walk longer distances. Most children who are learning to walk up to five feet (1.5 meters) notice each inch that you add to the distance. They will quit if they think the distance is too far, so it is better to increase the distance in small increments at the beginning. While practicing distances, your child will show you what distance she is comfortable with. When setup to walk that distance, she will immediately step to the endpoint. Once you know the distance she is comfortable with, then test whether she can go one or two inches further if you use a superb motivator.

When a child will consistently walk for a specific distance, I have realized that this means that **visually**, when they see that distance, they **know** they can walk that distance, and they automatically do it. The child is showing you that she "visually knows" she can walk that distance. If we work to expand the distance in small increments, while building confidence and competence through repetitions, then she will "visually know" that she can walk longer distances. I do not recommend moving the endpoint—for example, by having your child walk to you while you keep moving backwards. You want her to "visually know" that she can walk 3 feet (90 cm) to you (if that is the distance you usually are from her).

You will need to practice distances until your child walks 15 to 20 feet (4.5 to 6 meters) consistently. In my experience, after a child walks this distance, she will spontaneously start walking long distances on level surfaces. A child without Down syndrome quickly progresses from taking two to three independent steps to walking all of the time. A child with Down syndrome will usually need to be taught to walk 15 feet (4.5 meters), and then she will progress to walking all of the time when she has adequate endurance.

When she is practicing walking distances of 4 to 5 feet (1.2 to 1.5 meters), it is best to practice with two people, if possible. She can be setup standing with her back against the wall or furniture, one adult or older sibling can be at the endpoint with a motivator, and another adult can position himself at her side about 3.5 feet (one meter) away. With this setup, the second adult can make sure she is safe and spot her, if needed, to prevent falls, and can keep her looking up and at the endpoint. If only one person is available, he or she should be beside the child, because the focus is for the child to be safe and to prevent falls, while moving to the motivating endpoint. Another idea when practicing this distance is to setup three pieces of furniture about 3 to 4 feet (.9 to 1.5 meters) away from each other. Your child can decide when to move from one piece of furniture to another, to go to the toy she chooses. You can position yourself in front of her, at the endpoint she is walking to. When she is comfortable with this setup and game, then you can increase the distance between the pieces of furniture.

You will keep increasing the distance in small increments as tolerated and build her confidence so she "visually knows" she can walk increasingly longer distances. When she is practicing 5- to 7-foot (1.5- to 2.1-meter) distances, you will position yourself at her side, about 2 feet from the endpoint, making sure she keeps her head and trunk upright, as she moves to the endpoint. You will need to sit on your heels so you are at her eye level. You will direct her attention to the endpoint because if you direct her attention to yourself, she will walk to you and walk a shorter distance.

When your child is practicing walking distances of 7 to 15 feet (2.1 to 4.5 meters), it is ideal if you can do this in a hallway, so there are no distractions, and there is only one focal point. It is best if the endpoint is large so it catches her attention, and it needs to be a superb motivator. For example, she may love to walk to a kitchen set, and it is great if a brother or sister is playing there to entice her. If a parent is there, he or she can talk to her and encourage her, as well as make sure she keeps looking forward (not down). I like to position myself walking behind the child, with a space in between us, and I follow her lead and walk with the same foot that she does, so we are in the same waddle rhythm. With this setup, I can keep her walking all the way to the endpoint, spotting her as needed. I can catch her if she begins to fall forward, or I can step closer to let her lean against me to regain her balance if she starts falling back. By practicing in this way, she becomes comfortable seeing this distance and walking it, even if she needs intermittent support along the walk. Eventually, she will walk it by herself.

As your child is practicing walking independently, you will need to use the best toys, people, or even snacks to motivate her. You need to convince her of the value of walking. In the beginning, you will need to distract her to engage her in walking since her preference will be to use other easier methods of mobility. She may like you to sing a walking song, to count, to say "1, 2, 3, go," or to keep saying and signing "walking" or "more walking." You also need to build her competence by making sure she is successful when practicing independent steps. Practice each distance until she is confident and has mastered it for many repetitions before increasing the distance. If you practice in this way and focus on building her confidence, she will have the support needed to succeed.

To walk 15-20 foot (4.5-6 meter) distances, your child will need to be motivated to walk, figure out how to maintain her balance over the distance, and have the perseverance and persistence to keep walking. You will begin practicing walking as a game, but then it needs to become spontaneous for her so that she spontaneously walks on her own rather than always needing you to set her up to do it. Over time, she will become competent and confident, and her motivation to walk will become automatic.

As you practice walking independently for longer distances, your child will enjoy alternating that challenge with fast stepping with two-hand support (fig. 5.36). It will be fun to have a change of pace and move at a fast speed and need to respond by moving her legs quickly to keep up with you. It will teach her how to step faster and use coordinated leg movements, and this will help her with independent steps, especially when she is losing her balance and needs to step quickly to stagger and recover her balance. It will also improve her endurance, which she will need to progress to walking all of the time.

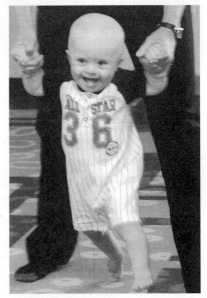

(fig. 5.36)

---

### General Strategies for Practicing Independent Walking

If your child is ready to walk longer distances and resists, you need to try to figure out why. It could be because she is afraid, or not motivated, or unable to figure out how to initiate the waddle, or because it is harder to step with one leg, or because she just wants to walk with support. Since she is ready to progress, we need to figure out the best way to practice the skill so she learns that she can do it, and it becomes part of her walking repertoire.

**The first strategy is to use the best motivators.** If you use the best motivator, your child will be dying to get to the endpoint. She will probably just go quickly and step to it, and won't pause and think about it. If you use an average motivator, she will pause and take time to decide whether she feels like challenging herself to step to it.

**The next strategy is to set her up to be successful.** Practice when she is at her physical best, and with the best setup to be successful. It is best to practice in a hallway free of distractions or in a new environment that is not familiar to her. If you practice in a familiar environment (like her bedroom or play room), she already has "habits" of what she does in that space and may not want to walk there. She may prefer to creep and play with toys or read books. Once you establish a place to walk, she will develop the habit that this is where you do the walking game. You also may need to do brief walking warm-up activities that are easy and fun, or start by walking shorter distances to start stepping activities.

Once she is warmed-up with stepping, then you can begin challenging her, using the best motivator. Start with small challenges and go slowly. With each successful practice, praise her and show huge excitement, and do something that she loves (like tickling her belly or throwing her up in the air). With this response, she will be happy and proud, and walking will be a fun event.

**The final strategy is to know when to stop practicing.** Keep the practices fun and stop before she becomes bored or tired or fussy. If she becomes physically tired, she may feel unstable and fall. If she gets tired of the activity or the challenge, but you keep practicing, she will get mad or upset. Therefore, when you see signs of diminished interest or she no longer is demonstrating her best performance, stop practicing independent steps.

### Possible Reactions When Learning to Walk Longer Distances

As you help your child learn to walk from 5 to 15 feet (1.5 to 4.5 meters), watch how she responds to walking and try to see what she needs to help her move to the next level. Possible examples are:

1. Some children are motivated to walk and keep increasing the distance spontaneously. You can help by using the best motivators and increasing the distance when ready.

2. Some children need incentives to keep increasing the distance. You can help by figuring out what is needed. You can experiment with trying different motivators, practicing briefly and giving breaks in between walks, giving her more visual or verbal cues to keep her attention, showing more excitement, changing the pace by alternating independent steps with fast stepping with two-hand support, or changing the sequence of how you usually practice walking.

3. Some children learn to sit down after taking steps for 3-5 feet (.9 to 1.5 meters). Now they know how to stop walking, and they choose when they want to. Before they learned to sit down, they thought the only way to stop walking was to walk to the endpoint. You can help increase the distance by using a better motivator to see if your child will not pay attention to the distance and keep stepping to get the motivator. If that does not help, you can walk behind her and keep her standing and stepping to the endpoint. You can help her to take a standing break and then continue stepping to the motivator.

4. Some children need to work on improving their balance and increasing their endurance in order to walk independently for longer distances. A boy named Michael and his father taught me this. Michael could walk independently for 7-10 feet (2.1-3 meters) and seemed stuck at that distance. He loved to walk and preferred two-hand support. His father started having him practice walking with one-hand support every night when he came home from work. They would walk down their street to a tree that Michael loved, and Michael would pick a leaf off the tree. They would take a break and then walk back to their house. Michael was motivated to walk to the tree and back home to see his brother and mother. In the beginning, it took a long time to walk the distance. With practice, Michael gained the strength and control to do it faster. Within a short time, he was walking by himself in the house.

5. Some children need more practice to use walking within the daily routine so it becomes a familiar method for mobility. They need to walk with and without support as much as possible to build the strength and balance needed to walk longer distances without support.

6. Some children need more praise or a more outrageous motivator. You need to be creative and keep thinking of possibilities!

Your child *will* learn to walk 15 feet (4.5 meters), and she will show you when she is ready to do it. As long as you regularly practice it, you are building the components needed for her to do it. You will need to be patient and wait for her to have that "aha" moment to want to walk. It will be her surprise gift to you and to herself. Just keep motivating her to walk and giving her opportunities to walk. With practice, she will take more steps and develop the best method she knows for her body and learning style.

---

## The Eleven Essential Steps for Walking Activities

Whenever practicing independent steps with your child, whether she is taking one step or walking independently for 15 feet, follow these guidelines:

1. Have your child walk to a surface that is 21-24 inches (53-61 cm). Examples include: large ball, mat placed vertically against the wall, kitchen set, sofa with 2 cushions stacked for increased height, parent in tall kneeling or sitting on heels (with knees wide apart).
2. Use the best motivators, and place them at eye level.
3. Always encourage head up, trunk up, and arms in high guard and discourage looking down at the floor (fig. 5.37).
4. Sign and say "walk" so the game is labeled (or use other verbal cues like "1, 2, 3, go").
5. Set your child up to walk all the way to the endpoint and prop against it when reaching it (fig. 5.38). (If she is walking to you, place your hands and pat the area where you want your child to prop against you.)
6. Have her wear only a onesie.

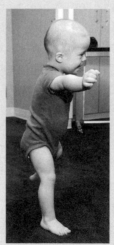
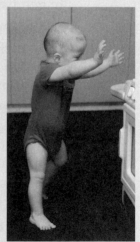

(fig. 5.37)          (fig. 5.38)

7. Decide whether to walk barefoot or in shoes and orthoses.
8. Avoid falls.
9. Practice each distance until your child has mastered it and is confident.
10. Practice where there are no distractions.
11. Use a firm, level surface so she feels stable.

## Activity #13: Taking 1-2 Independent Steps to a High Surface

1. Place a favorite toy or other motivator on a soft surface such as a couch.
2. Place your child in standing, 15-18 inches (38-46 cm) away from the surface, with her back against you (tall kneeling behind her). Make sure she is facing whatever she is walking toward.
3. Place one foot forward and then place your knee behind that foot. Set her up so she will step with her preferred leg, so place her non-dominant leg forward.
4. Tap her abdominals 3 times with the pads of your fingers (to activate her abdominals).
5. Say and sign "walk."
6. Wait for her to choose to take a step and move to the surface and motivator.
7. Provide assistance if needed for safety when she steps.
8. After she moves to the surface, clap and praise her and show your excitement.
9. This activity can also be done between two persons, with both of you kneeling up tall and straight. Place your child standing in front of one person with her back supported against the person's legs. The other person can encourage her to take a step to him/her. Place the motivator at eye level to your child. Place your hands and pat the area where you would expect her to prop against. The person she is stepping toward could also sit on his/her heels with knees wide apart so he/she is at eye level to the child.

## Activity #14: Walking 2- to 4-Foot Distances to a High Surface

When practicing walking 2-4 feet (60-120 centimeters):
- Measure the distance and increase in 1-inch (2.5-cm) increments.
- Make sure her whole body is facing the surface that she is walking toward (figs. 5.39, 5.40). It would be too difficult to take a step if she is standing with her side facing the surface.
- Remember, there are many ways to help your child learn to take her first steps and progress to walking longer distances. Try these setups and see what she likes best, and also use them to give her a variety of ways to practice walking.
- See if she will self-initiate walking during her own play.

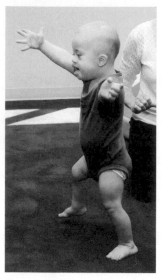 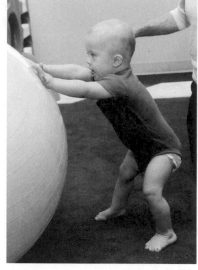

(fig. 5.39)        (fig. 5.40)

*A. Walking to You:*

1. Position your child in standing with her back supported against furniture or the wall. If your child can stand without support, place her standing in the middle of the floor.
2. Position yourself two feet in front of her, with you or the motivator at eye level to her. Depending on your height, you can sit on the floor or sit on your heels. Make sure your legs are wide apart so she has room to step all the way to you.
3. Place the motivator in your hands (or pat the area) where you anticipate she will prop against you. You can have her give you a kiss, touch your nose, or find a toy or a pen in your shirt pocket.
4. Sign "walk" and encourage her to walk to you. If she has difficulty initiating the waddle, assist her. You can also give her the verbal cue "waddle, waddle" (and have her imitate you, with your hands up in the high guard position, leaning your trunk from side to side playfully).
5. After she takes independent steps to you, praise her, clap for her, and show your excitement and pride.
6. As tolerated, increase the distance in one-inch (2.5-cm) increments and have her learn ("visually know") that she can walk each distance.
7. If needed, catch her to avoid falls.

*B. Walking to the Sofa:*

1. Position your child standing 2 feet (60 cm) in front of the sofa, and kneel up tall behind her. Stack 2 cushions to make a high surface

for her to walk toward. You could also stand her with her back against furniture that is stabilized.

2. Place a motivator on the sofa and encourage her to step to it. Say and sign "walk" or whatever verbal cue she likes.

3. Follow Activity #14A, steps 5, 6, and 7 above.

4. When she is ready to walk 3-4 foot (.9-1.2 meter) distances, it is best if you stand her with her back against furniture (stabilized so it does not move) while you position yourself to her side at the endpoint in order to assist her as needed for her own safety.

*C. Walking from One Piece of Furniture to Another:*

1. Arrange your furniture so two pieces are facing each other, 2 feet apart. For example, place a padded chair in front of the sofa.

2. Position your child standing with her back against the chair.

3. Position yourself at her side (at the endpoint) to assist her as needed for her own safety.

4. Place a motivator on the sofa and encourage her to walk to it. Follow Activity #14A, steps 5, 6, and 7 above.

*D. Walking from One Person to Another:*

1. Have two people kneel on the floor, facing each other and 2 feet apart. Each person needs to kneel up tall and straight.

2. Place your child standing in front of one person with her back supported against the person's legs. The other person can encourage her to take a step to him/her. Place the motivator at eye level to the child. Place your hands and pat the area where you would expect her to prop. The person she is stepping toward could also sit on his/her heels with knees wide apart so he/she is at eye level to the child.

3. Follow Activity #14A, steps 5, 6, and 7 above.

*E. Moving from Sitting on a Bench to Standing and Then Walking:*

The height of the bench should be 1-2 inches (2.5-5 cm) higher than the distance from the back of your child's knee to the bottom of her heel, so that when she is sitting on the bench, her buttocks are higher than her knees. The bench needs to be stabilized so that it does not slide.

1. Place your child sitting on a bench, with her feet on the floor. Stabilize the bench so it does not move while sitting and when she moves to standing.

2. Position yourself at her side (at the endpoint) to assist her as needed for her own safety.

3. Place a motivator on a high surface, 2 feet (60 cm) in front of her, and encourage her to stand up and walk to it. (Sign and say "stand up" and "walk."

4. Follow Activity 14A, steps 5, 6, and 7 above.

## Activity #15: Walking 5- to 7-Foot Distances

Use the setups in Activity #14A–E and work on 5- to 7-foot (1.5- to 2.1-meter) distances.

1. Place her with her back against the wall, furniture, or sitting on the bench.

2. Position yourself at her side, about 2 feet (60 cm) from the endpoint, so you can keep her looking up and focused on the endpoint, and you can catch her, if needed, to prevent falls.

3. Encourage her to walk to a high surface with a great motivator placed at eye level. Sign and say "walk." Keep giving her verbal and visual cues to keep her looking up throughout the duration of the walk. You can also snap your fingers, clap your hands, and make funny gestures and faces to keep her walking by distracting her (from thinking about whether she wants to walk or not).

4. Follow Activity #14A, steps 5, 6, and 7 above.

## Activity #16: Walking Distances of 7-15 Feet

1. Pick an area in your home that is 7-15 feet (2.1-4.5 meters) long and free of furniture, obstacles, and distractions. Rearrange the furniture if needed. An ideal area is a hallway. (If a particular location works well, keep practicing there as you increase the distance.)

2. It is best if you have two people to practice this skill. One person stands behind the child for the starting position and the other person is at the endpoint.

3. Set your child up to walk to a high surface with a large motivating endpoint (like a kitchen set with siblings playing there, a mirror, a large ball, etc.).

4. Sign and say "walk" or "1, 2, 3, go."

5. Wait for her to choose when to start walking. You walk behind her, with a space in between both of you. Use the waddle pattern, following her and stepping with the same foot so you have the same waddle rhythm. As you step, your goal is to keep her walking all the way to the endpoint. Catch her if she starts to fall forward, and if she leans back, step closer so she can lean against you and regain her balance.

6. If minimal support is needed for her to participate more easily and feel stable, hold her shirt either at the back of her neck or on top of her shoulders (figs. 5.41, 5.42). If she feels this support, she may relax and step longer distances, knowing you are there and helping her.

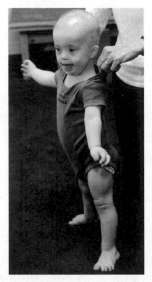 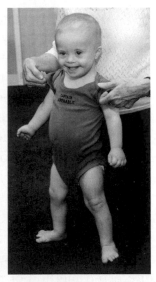

(fig. 5.41)          (fig. 5.42)

7. When she reaches the endpoint, celebrate this huge accomplishment! Do something fun like vigorously tickling her belly, clapping her hands firmly, saying "hurrah" and raising your hands above your head, or throwing her up in the air and catching her! She needs to know that this is a big deal, and you are very happy and proud of her!

8. Practice these long distances for many repetitions. After she reaches the endpoint, then move her back to the starting position in a fun way. She can fast walk with two-hand support back to the starting position, or you can hold her trunk (under her arms) and slide her backwards to the starting position. She will enjoy feeling her feet slide along the surface, and then you can place her in standing by bouncing her on her feet. Then you can sign and say "more walking" and have her do it again.

9. When she can consistently walk independently for 15 to 20 feet (4.5 to 6 meters) in her favorite location, then you can generalize to other locations.

10. Watch to see if she self-initiates walking to move between furniture within a room of the house, or from one room to another.

## Walking on Level Surfaces

When your child is able to walk independently on level surfaces for distances of 15-20 feet (4.5-6 meters) consistently, the remaining goals to achieve are:

1. to walk long distances in the home on level surfaces; and
2. to walk all of the time in the home on level surfaces.

You have taught your child to visually know that she can walk 15-20 feet (4.5-6 meters) by systematically increasing the distances. Through this practice, she has learned by experience how to maintain her balance and persevere to walk long distances. Now, you will need to expand her experience to walk for even longer distances, from one room to another within the house. Once she has adequate endurance in walking, she will ultimately realize that she can walk everywhere in the house and walk all of the time. You will rarely see her creep in the house any more; she will mostly walk. Once she can walk everywhere in the house, you can increase the distance and generalize this skill to other settings with level surfaces—in a mall, in a gym, in church or school hallways, and everyplace else you go.

While working on these goals, she will need to practice on level surfaces until walking is mastered, and she chooses to consistently use walking as her preferred method of mobility. To consolidate the skill, continue to practice walking on level surfaces for about a month. With this strategic practice of focusing her attention on walking on level surfaces, your child will emerge a confident, motivated, competent, and exploring walker. It will become automatic and easy for her to walk on level surfaces.

To help her experience the feeling of walking independently for long distances, you will need to give her minimal support without holding her hand, as described in Activity #17. You need to make sure you are giving her the least support possible and make sure you are not leaning her off balance, depending on where you are positioning yourself while walking with her. She will challenge herself because she will feel more secure having you involved, even though your support is minimal.

While she is practicing walking independently for longer distances, it is best to walk in a straight line toward an endpoint. She can stop and pause in her walk, regain her balance, and then continue walking again. As she improves her balance and confidence in walking, she will figure out how to turn to walk in a new direction while maintaining her balance. Eventually, she will learn to turn in a circle, and walk in any direction.

Since she is focusing on walking longer distances, it is best to set her up to walk on the same surface, rather than from one surface to another, such as from the carpet to the hardwood floor. As her competence improves, then she can explore walking on different types of level surfaces (tile, linoleum, hardwood floors, and carpets with different types of padding), and from one surface to another. Be sensitive to her reaction to the various types of surfaces, and set her up to be successful. If she initially needs support to walk on the surface or from one surface to another, provide it until she is familiar and comfortable on the surface and then wean your support. When she first starts walking on a new surface, supervise her until she is familiar with it and is safe. It is easy to fall, and she needs to learn to catch herself effectively with her hands to be safe.

When children with Down syndrome are learning to walk from one surface to another, a frequent strategy is to move from standing to plantigrade (hands and feet), then use the plantigrade position to move (climb) onto the new surface, then stand up and walk on the new surface. Your child will do this to be safe and will figure out this climbing strategy because she does not know if the surfaces are the same height. With practice, she will learn that the surfaces are the same height and then will proceed with walking from one surface to another by herself. She will develop depth perception through walking experiences.

Through practicing walking on level surfaces over time, your child will develop better balance strategies. She will hold her arms in the high guard position to balance herself when walking at her regular pace and at faster speeds. She will learn to fall to the floor safely, either falling downward to sitting or falling forward to plantigrade. When falling forward to plantigrade, she will need to "catch" herself with her hands. She will need to learn to move her arms quickly to catch herself, and her arms will need to be strong enough to stop her from falling forward and bumping her face. It is best for her to practice this on a padded surface such as a mat or carpet. Her ability to catch herself with her hands will depend on the speed of the fall. If she falls slowly, it will be easier. If she falls fast and with momentum, she will need to react quickly and use more arm strength to stop the fall in order to be effective. She will need to practice both situations in order to be safe on all surfaces, especially to prepare her for walking on concrete sidewalks.

To be a functional walker, she will need to be able to move to stand from the middle of the floor, instead of pulling to stand on furniture. She will not choose to walk all of the time if she needs to creep to furniture in order to stand up and walk. When she can take independent steps and can balance in standing, then moving to stand from plantigrade will be practiced. When she is practicing moving to stand from plantigrade, she can also practice falling forward to plantigrade and catching with her hands. This can be a playful up/down game with siblings to familiarize her with these necessary movements, which will make her independent and safe with walking.

She will begin walking using the "new walker waddle pattern" and with practice, her pattern will mature to the marching pattern. To use the marching pattern, she will hold her trunk erect rather than leaning it from side to side, and she will bend her hips and knees to step with full-sole weight bearing. Her arms will be in the high guard position, and she will move her trunk and pelvis together as a unit, taking short steps. For balance, she will probably use a wide base with heels wider than hips (what you see if you are behind her), and her feet turned outward (what you see if you are in front of her). After she is a confident and motivated walker, her pattern will be refined through foot management and practicing post-walking skills (see next chapter). The refined pattern will consist of a narrow base (heels in line with hips), feet pointing straight, trunk erect and pelvic rotation, arms at her sides, and weight shifting through her feet, from her heels to the balls of her feet.

When your child is learning to walk long distances on level surfaces, continue to have her walk with the foot support that makes walking easiest for her. Test whether she can walk longer distances while barefoot or in orthoses and shoes (if she already has them). The goal now is to increase the distance. After she can walk all of the time, she can be evaluated to determine whether foot support would help improve her walking pattern. If she already has orthoses and shoes, then she will resume using them and learn to walk with them. If she has been walking barefoot, then it will be determined what foot support and shoes are needed. Types of support and shoes will be discussed in Chapter 6.

When she is working on walking all of the time on level surfaces, she will be more motivated to walk if we let her explore and choose where she wants to walk. When I practice this skill in the PT clinic area of the hospital, I find that the children love to walk in the long hallways, and then they look into each of the rooms or walk to where they hear other children. They also love to wave and say "hi" to everyone they see in the hallway. They walk long distances because they are entertained and motivated to keep walking by socializing, being independent, choosing where they want to go, and having the joy of exploring. With these distractions, they walk further and more often. The practice and repetition improves their speed and balance, and, over time, they trip less often.

## ACTIVITY #17: Walking Long Distances on Even Surfaces

1. Pick an area 15-20 feet (4.5-6 meters) long with a consistent, level surface and minimal distractions (for example, a hallway).
2. Setup a motivator at the endpoint and encourage her to walk the whole distance to it. If possible, have one person at the endpoint cheering her on. You walk behind her and keep your attention on her so you can intervene as needed. If she sits or falls, pick her up and place her in standing, and then encourage her to continue walking again. Try to prevent her from sitting or falling by catching her before she moves to the floor, and keep her standing so she can continue walking. Your goal is to keep her walking all the way to the endpoint, even if she pauses in standing while walking.

3. Continue to practice until she can walk the distance consistently. Provide minimal support if it makes walking easier. Put a belt or scarf around her chest (under her arms) and hold the ends together at her upper back (at the level of her shoulder blades). Or hold her shirt above her shoulders and walk behind her, or have her hold the handle of a toy hammer or jump rope while you walk beside her.
4.  When she reaches the endpoint, celebrate and clap for her!
5. Within the same area, increase the distance to 25-30 feet (7.6-9 meters). Encourage her to practice walking this distance until she can do it well. Continue to increase the distance when tolerated.
6. When she has mastered walking long distances in one area, then generalize this skill to other areas. Either use another type of floor surface (tile, hardwood floor, linoleum, or carpet) or use the same type surface as above but in another location. Practice walking in each area until she is comfortable and competent.
7. Practice walking on a variety of types of level floor surfaces in a variety of locations. Do this until she is able to walk on all types of level surfaces.
8. Practice walking distances several times a day until she shows the endurance and motivation to walk all of the time on level surfaces.
9. When she chooses to walk all of the time, then practice walking from one type of surface to another. If needed, let her hold your finger until she is familiar with walking between these surfaces.
10. As she practices walking, guard her when she falls forward to make sure she does not bump her head. Watch and see if she can catch herself effectively with her hands (with quickness in her arm movements and strength to sustain her body weight) when she falls slowly or quickly. Assist her as needed when she trips and falls.
11. While practicing this walking skill, use whatever foot support is easiest for walking long distances. After she chooses to walk all of the time and has mastered this skill, then optimal foot support will be used.

## Guidelines

*Walking is the hardest gross motor skill that your child will ever have to learn.* She will have to transition from moving with 4 points of support (hands and knees or hands and feet) to 2 points of support (feet). To make it even harder, her two points of support are very small, since children with Down syndrome have very small feet. She will not ease into walking through a natural flow, and then spontaneously progress into walking independently. *It will take a major transformation to transition from moving on the floor to standing erect and stepping with balance and control.* Therefore, simple, usual methods, and just waiting for walking to happen, will not be effective. Your child will be physically ready to do it before she chooses to do it.

The goal here is not to accelerate her rate of learning to walk, it is to use the window when she is ready to learn the skill and give her the tools and support to see that she can do it. You will guide her to do it when she is physically ready rather than wait for her to do it at a much later time. *You will need to provoke it, and wean your support during the process so she learns to do it by herself.* You will need to work within your child's temperament and learning style, challenging her with what she is ready to learn.

*It may take boot camp rigor and systematic progression to help her learn the next steps.* The key will be to figure out when she is ready to progress to the next level, and how to help her practice the next skill so she tolerates practicing it. You will need to be wilder, crazier, and more creative with games in order to make it fun and to motivate her. She will be out of her comfort zone and will need to be willing to be risky to experiment with taking independent steps. It will be a leap for her, and you need to set her up to be successful and then go for it. If you approach walking timidly, so will she. You need to use everything you have learned about her learning style to engage her in walking.

Your PT can help provoke walking with your child, but the key will be how you practice at home so that she learns to generalize it there rather than just doing it in the PT setting. If she does not practice it at home, she will just continue doing her habitual method such as creeping or bear walking. To change her habit, walking needs to be structured into her daily routine at home. Having it be part of her repertoire at home will have her own it, realize the value of it, and be motivated to use it at home.

*Remember that children vary as to HOW motivated they are to walk and WHEN they are motivated to walk.* Each child's readiness needs to be understood and respected so we do not discourage them, scare them, overwhelm them, or make them avoid walking. Possible reactions to walking are:

1. She may want to step and easily be motivated to do stepping. She may even creep over to you, pull up to stand, and indicate she wants you to walk her around the house.
2. She may feel very independent at this stage in her life and want to be independent, doing what she chooses to do. Therefore, she will not be interested in walking, since it requires her to be dependent on someone, and she may even feel forced to walk and dominated when walking.

3. She may be efficient in creeping and be able to go wherever she wants to go. To her, creeping or bear walking is fast and efficient, well established, automatic, and known. She may resist walking because it is new, she is unstable and unbalanced, she cannot do it by herself, and she does not see the value in it.
4. She may fluctuate between wanting to walk sometimes and not wanting to walk other times.

Your child will choose walking when it has value to her, and she is motivated to persevere with doing it. For example, even though Patrick had mastered the physical skills necessary for walking for some time, he did not decide it was a worthwhile endeavor until he figured out it was the only way he could carry a book to his mother so she could read to him.

***Consider it your job to turn on your child to the world of walking.*** It will be different for her to be stepping rather than moving on hands and knees. It will take time for her to learn to walk with support and feel comfortable with it. Motivators can help to keep her interest. Even if she is not interested in walking, she will want to move to the motivator! Once she uses walking to move to the motivator, she will begin using walking to move from one place to another.

To help her discover the value of walking, make walking activities very familiar to her. Show her what she can do by being able to walk and how she can play. When she is familiar with walking, she will be more cooperative about practicing it. As she practices it, she will do it better and become more motivated to walk. If she is motivated to walk, she will walk more often and her strength, balance, and endurance will improve. By walking more often, she will become confident in her ability to walk. When she is confident, she will be willing to challenge herself. You need to move at her pace and be responsive to her temperament to be successful.

***Use a variety of motivators or games to encourage your child to walk.*** You can use special new toys, favorite toys, or setup a game. Make the toys and games fun so she wants to play, and she will walk to play with them.

Some examples of creative games are:

1. She can walk to the computer or TV, walk to a favorite room like the bathroom or a sibling's room, or walk to a book.
2. She can walk to a door and knock on it or open and close it.
3. She can walk to a baby doll and feed the baby, put on its clothes or shoes, or show you the baby's nose.
4. She can walk to her mom or dad and give a kiss.
5. She can play "chase" games and try to catch her mom, sister, the cat, or dog.

6. She can play the game "Where is mom?" and walk to find her.
7. You can sit on the floor in front of her and partially hide a small toy in your shirt pocket or under the collar of your shirt and have her come and find it.
8. You can hide a toy in the sofa cushion and have her find it.
9. You can use a favorite food (goldfish cracker, veggie stick, pretzel) that she would eat for a snack anyway, and have her walk to get it. Make sure the snack is small and bite sized so she is not eating large amounts. She could also walk to get a sip of a drink.

After your child completes the walk to the endpoint, give her some time to play with the motivator; don't just take the toy away. When she is ready to walk again, move her back to the starting position in a fun way. I setup the game by saying "bye bye," and then I step backwards and slide the child's feet on the floor as I move her back to the starting position. I bounce her in standing to give her a playful sensory experience to setup the next walk, and I sign and say "more walking" or a fun verbal cue that she is used to. When you are sliding her back, she will enjoy feeling her feet. This will entertain her and make the transition easy since she is distracted.

For some children, the best motivator of all is clapping for them when they finish a walk. When they reach the endpoint, they look at you and wait for you to clap, or they may clap too since they know they have done something great! They will see your enthusiasm and excitement and will feel proud and happy and want to do it again. They will enjoy celebrating their walking successes with you.

***Only do walking activities you can motivate your child to do.*** As you practice each new skill that she is ready to learn, observe how she responds. If she dislikes practicing a particular walking activity, try distracting her by using a great motivator or gently tossing her up in the air or tickling her belly. She might forget what she was resisting and then practice the skill. If she continues to resist it, skip it and try it again later or the next day. If an activity consistently makes her not want to walk and she sits down, discontinue it temporarily. You cannot force her to practice it because she will only resist it more. There is a fine line between challenging her to progress to a new skill that she is ready to learn, and being counterproductive because it discourages walking and kills her motivation to walk.

For example, Sammy enjoyed walking with two-hand support, but every time I let go of one hand, he would sit down and refuse to walk. Even if I used great motivators, he would not walk with one-hand support. I continued to practice walking with two-hand support and walking with the push toy so he would be motivated to walk and continue walking. If I had insisted on using one-hand support at that time, I would have decreased his motivation to walk at all, even with two-hand support. I periodically tested if he would tolerate one-handed walking, and one day he did.

***Provide verbal and visual cues.*** When you practice walking, you need to label the game and give your child a verbal cue so she knows what you are going to do together. Sign and say "walk" or "more walking." She may like you to sign and say "1, 2, 3, go." When she is walking long distances, she may keep walking if you keep repeating the word "walk" or make up a song about walking with your child's name. Bridget would spontaneously walk (march) with her siblings when her mother sang "The Ants Go Marching" song.

Use a visual cue to have her look forward and to motivate her while she is walking to the endpoint. The visual cue needs to keep her looking forward at eye level so she keeps her trunk erect and balanced. If it is above eye level, when she tilts her head back to look at it, she will fall backwards. If she looks down to the floor, her trunk will tilt forward and she will go down to the floor.

When she is practicing walking for long distances, you can walk in front of her or beside her and exaggerate your walking pattern so she looks at your legs and imitates you. For example, you can do marching steps and she will focus on your legs and try to march, too.

***When practicing walking, help your child develop good movement patterns or habits.*** You want to give her the support she needs so she feels comfortable taking steps and develops the strength and balance needed to progress to walking alone. Sometimes, when she is first practicing a new skill, you may need to compromise good habits in order to motivate her to practice the skill. If this happens, resume the good habits as soon as she tolerates the skill. For example, when she is walking with two-hand support, the good movement pattern is to have her hands at shoulder level or lower. However, when you first start practicing this skill, you may need to hold her hands higher to help motivate her to walk. Once she will take steps and shows some motivation to walk, lower her hands to shoulder level.

***When she is learning to walk, focus on having her learn the leg stepping pattern.*** The quality of her stepping pattern will improve with practice, repetition, and walking for increased distances. The quality of her walking pattern will be refined after she is a confident and competent walker. When taking her first steps, her knees may be stiff, her feet may be wider than her hips, and one foot may step better than the other. Since walking is new, she will use compensations to feel more stable. She will need to figure out how to balance herself with her tone, ligamentous laxity, strength, and balance. With practice, her pattern will improve. If you focus on changing how she moves her legs, she will feel nagged and controlled, her walking will be interrupted and slow, and she will lose her motivation to walk. As walking becomes easier and familiar to her, the compensations will decrease, she will be more relaxed with the skill, and her joint movements will flow more easily. After she walks independently and is confident in her ability to walk, then her walking pattern can be refined through providing foot support and practicing post walking skills. (See Chapter 6.)

*Practice walking on a firm, flat, level surface.* The surface needs to be consistent and level so your child is familiar with the feeling of the surface and learns by experience how to walk on it. A carpeted surface is best if it is not too padded. If it is very padded, she will feel unstable because her feet will rock on the soft surface. Her feet will be more stable on a firm, carpeted surface. You can use hardwood, tile, or linoleum floors if they are not slippery.

Walking will be more complicated and confusing to her if she needs to walk from one surface to another—from a hardwood floor to a rug. With this setup, she will need to pay attention to the changes in the surface, plan to step up and down, and plan how to walk on the new surface. Needing to pay attention to the surfaces will challenge her walking skills too much in the beginning.

When she is ready to practice walking longer distances, use an environment with a level surface and a lot of space, like a gym floor, long hallways in a church or school, or the mall. Go at a time when it is less busy. Pick an area that is relatively quiet. She will get to choose what she is motivated to walk to and can walk from one area to another. Your job will be to keep her standing so she uses walking to explore everything.

*Practice walking skills for short periods, several times a day.* If you assist her to walk often in her daily routine, it will become a habit and a familiar method of moving from one place to another or doing a favorite activity like taking a bath. She will cooperate best if you practice for 1-5 minutes, many times a day. Be sure to stop if you start to see signs of fatigue or resistance. Common signs of fatigue are: fussiness, rhythmical tongue sucking movements, clumsiness when stepping, and resistance to stepping. The biggest mistake is to keep going when she is done practicing because she will become upset or may fall.

*Increase the distance your child walks when she is ready.* Start with short distances as a warm-up and keep increasing the distance to see how far she can step. When she is practicing walking, setup an endpoint or destination so she knows where she is going. If she sits or falls down before she reaches the end point, quickly stand her up and help her keep walking to the endpoint and motivator. By setting her up with an endpoint, she learns how far she can walk. Remember, do not move the endpoint as she is walking toward it. She will be frustrated with the game since she is not setup to win. When she can consistently walk each distance, increase it.

*Simultaneously work on all of the walking skills your child is able to do.* To practice the stepping pattern, speed, and endurance, walk with two-hand support for long distances and do fast stepping. To practice independent walking with support, have her walk with the push toy or posterior walker. To work on balance, practice one-handed walking and the waddle pattern. When she is ready to practice independent steps, do it when she is at her physical best.

The sequence of practice is important to set her up to be successful. Start with a brief, easy activity to warm her up and then move to the most challenging skill so she practices it when she is at her strongest. If she needs a change of pace, practice a walking activity with more support at a faster speed for fun. Then see if she will do the most challenging skill again. When she is done with the challenging skill, practice easier walking skills to improve distance, speed, strength, leg coordination, balance, and endurance. Each walking skill contributes to the ultimate goal of walking all of the time. You can also increase the frequency of walking and how long she will continue to practice walking skills within one practice period.

*Practice walking in a wide open space.* If the area is open and free of distractions and obstacles, she will be setup to be successful. When she is walking for 5 feet or more, clear out the area so she is safe and will not bump into furniture or toys and potentially hurt herself. You may need to rearrange furniture so she can practice walking longer distances of 7-15 feet, or she can practice walking down a hallway.

If she does fall, watch your reaction. You want to calm and soothe her so she is comforted and reassured. Make sure you do not overreact, verbally or non-verbally. If you do, this will upset her more and she may be afraid to try again.

*Be patient and remember that timing is everything. Also rule out medical issues that could be interfering with walking.* The age range in which children with Down syndrome learn to walk is very wide. There are many reasons why some children walk earlier and some later. Their physical skills, temperament, and motivation all play a role. Be proactive if medical issues are influencing your child's ability to walk. If she has visual limitations, she may be more careful or scared when working on independent steps. If she has fluid in her ears, she may feel off balance and not feel confident to take independent steps. Remember, once your child walks, the remaining gross motor skills will be easy.

*If you have access to a pool, your child can practice walking there.* You can practice all of the walking skills in a pool. Ideally, the water should come up to mid-trunk level—from approximately your child's navel to her nipples. Your child can walk with hand support and the buoyancy of the water will help her balance to take independent steps. Walking in the water will also improve strength and endurance.

*Pay attention to the walking skills that occur together, and if she is practicing one skill, help her learn the other.* You can guide your child to learn a skill when she is physically ready even if she is not showing an interest in it yet. By knowing what skills emerge at the same time, you can figure out a way to practice the other skill. In my experience with children with Down syndrome, the walking skills that occur together are:

1. Cruising and walking with two-hand support; and
2. Walking with one-hand support for 10 feet and taking 1-2 independent steps.

### Temperament

If your child is an **observer,** she will want to feel secure and balanced. She will learn to move to stand from plantigrade and then will take steps. She will step carefully and balance herself with each step. She will resist changes in the type of support provided; for example, progressing from walking with two-hand support to walking with one-hand support. She will not like falling and will work to control her balance so she does not fall. She will notice changes in the floor surfaces and will carefully adjust to each type. To help her learn to walk, focus on:

1. moving at her pace,
2. increasing the distance as tolerated,
3. avoiding falls,
4. praising her,
5. building motivation and confidence.

By understanding how she feels about walking, you can help her develop walking skills in a way that works best for her.

If your child is **motor driven,** she will want to move and generally want to step. She may initially resist walking because it will be slower than her fast method of creeping. Once she is motivated to walk, she will boldly take steps, whether she is balanced or not. She will step and fall and will not mind falling. She will step first and learn to control her balance later. She will take risks in order to step, and you will need to supervise her for safety. She will not be concerned about details such as the type of surface she is walking on. You will need to point out obstacles on the floor, or she might trip over them. When she wants to walk all the time, she will learn to move from plantigrade to stand. To help her learn to walk, focus on:

1. stepping quickly,
2. developing balance through walking activities by decreasing the support,
3. supervising her for safety,
4. praising her,
5. building motivation and confidence.

By understanding her desire to move, you can help her develop walking skills in a way that works best for her.

# Climbing

Your child will learn to love climbing during this stage. She will figure out what she can do and where she can go using climbing. If she is able to creep or bear walk but not yet able to walk by herself, climbing will be her source of adventure and exploration. She will need to be supervised closely because she will not have the judgment needed for safety. In the last stage, climbing up onto the sofa (without the seat cushion) and up a couple of stairs was focused on. During this stage, the goal will be for her to learn to climb safely off the sofa, and up and down the flight of stairs. You can encourage her to practice climbing after she has practiced standing, cruising, and walking skills.

## Components

The components to focus on are:

1. arm, abdominal, leg, and foot strength to climb up and down
2. learning each step and performing the sequence of steps needed for climbing up and down
3. learning the motor plan for safety by always climbing up to the top of the surface (sofa or landing for the flight of stairs) or down to the floor
4. becoming aware of her body and the space around her (recognizing when she is at the edge and could fall)
5. climbing competently and safely on a consistent basis

## Tendencies

The tendencies are:

1. to place her hip, knee, or foot in such a way that it slides off the surface
2. to lose motivation to climb to the top of the stairs or become distracted, and then stop and try to sit on the stair, causing her to fall
3. to choose to climb off the sofa or down the stairs, head first, because she sees what she wants and does not realize she is unsafe
4. to keep her hips bent after she moves to her stomach when climbing down from the sofa or down stairs, and to then push with her arms and fall backwards.
5. to be unaware that she is close to the edge of a surface and then fall off it

## Climbing Up Stairs

During Stage 4, your child learned to climb from the second stair (from the top of the flight) to the landing. During this stage, you will keep

## Steps in Learning to Climb

Your child will learn to:
1. climb up a flight of stairs,
2. climb off a sofa by herself,
3. climb down a flight of stairs,
4. do other climbing.

You can practice climbing off the sofa and climbing up the stairs at the same time, but you should wait to practice climbing down stairs until your child has mastered the first two skills.

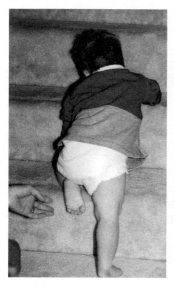

(fig. 5.43)

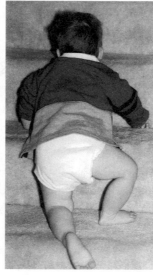

(fig. 5.44)

increasing the number of stairs when she is ready, until she can climb up the whole flight of stairs. At first, she will execute the climbing sequence using four steps by moving one knee, then the other, then moving one foot to the half kneel position, and then moving onto her other foot. With practice, she will develop the advanced method using the sequence of two steps, by moving one knee and then the other foot (half kneel) (figs. 5.43, 5.44. Through practicing climbing, she will strengthen her arms with the actions of pulling, propping, and alternating them as she moves up the flight of stairs. Her leg and foot strength will improve through the actions of moving each knee and foot, and pushing off on tiptoes.

As she is learning to climb, the best way for you to assist her is to anticipate the steps and be ready to support her knee or foot after she places it. If she forgets the sequence, you can assist her with moving her knee or foot to help her be successful with climbing to the top. I do not recommend supporting her pelvis because it teaches her to lean her pelvis back, and it is better to assist her knee or foot to keep her moving forward and upward. It is best if you kneel behind her. From this position, you can lean forward to move the toy and then you can lean back and help her as needed. You can also stop her from trying to sit back on the stair.

With practice, climbing up will become automatic for her and she will competently plan how to move up the whole flight of stairs. She may surprise you the first time she climbs up the whole flight by herself, moving after her brother or sister. She will have achieved the goal of climbing up a flight of stairs when she can do it safely on a consistent basis. If she develops the method of climbing up on her hands and feet, let her go as long as her method is safe.

## Climbing Off the Sofa

During Stage 4, you familiarized your child with the actions of moving down off your lap when she wanted to move down to the floor. During this stage, you will teach her each step and assist her until she has the judgment to consistently execute the plan to move down safely by herself.

To climb off the sofa by herself, your child will need to:

1. roll over onto her stomach (fig. 5.45)
2. straighten her legs, especially her hips
3. maintain her trunk over the surface and push with her arms to control sliding down to the floor (fig. 5.46)
4. continue to slide down until her feet touch the floor, and then catch with her feet and land in standing. Once in standing, she can choose to stay in standing or move to sitting on the floor.

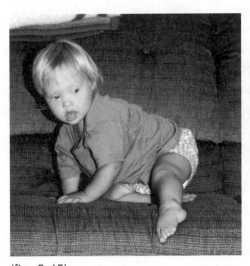
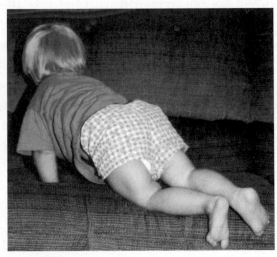

(fig. 5.45)                    (fig. 5.46)

It is important to use verbal cues to help your child learn the sequence, especially the first step of turning over. Test what verbal cue works best for your child. For the first step, I have used the following verbal cues: "on your belly," "turn over," or "over." The most challenging parts to learn are to turn over onto her belly, and to straighten her legs, especially her hips. If her hips and knees are bent after she rolls to her stomach and she begins pushing with her arms, she will fall backwards off the sofa.

Once she knows the steps, she needs to learn how to do the sequence of steps safely by herself. If she is sitting on the sofa and you place a toy on the floor and say "down," observe her to see if she will move to her stomach and climb off the sofa feet first, or if she will move after the toy head first because she wants it so much and does not stop to plan how to climb off safely. She will need to learn to use judgment and inhibit her impulse to move forward to quickly get what she sees and wants. Once she starts climbing off feet first by herself, you will still need to watch her because she will sometimes forget and climb down head first. With practice, climbing off safely will become automatic and she will do it consistently.

When your child has mastered climbing off the sofa, then you can practice climbing off other furniture such as a chair or bed. Watch the height of the furniture and supervise her until she feels comfortable climbing down. Use a variety of surfaces so she learns to climb down all types and heights.

### Climbing Down Stairs

Your child will be ready to begin learning the skill of climbing down stairs after she can climb off the sofa and climb up the flight of stairs by herself. You will teach her the easiest method, which will be sliding down on her belly ("prone slide"), the same way she learned to climb off the sofa. Climbing down stairs is more difficult because she has to focus on executing the skill, and then persevere with using the method while moving down the whole flight of stairs. She cannot raise her head and trunk up to look behind to see where she is going, or she will lose her balance and fall backwards. She needs to keep her head looking forward and can occasionally turn it to glance back, while she moves her body down several stairs. Once she reaches the bottom of the stairs, she will finally be able to sit and play.

To climb down the stairs, she will use one of three methods:

1. Sliding down on her stomach (prone slide);
2. Climbing down on her hands and knees or hands and feet;
3. Sitting on the stair, facing forward, and "bumping" down on her buttocks.

You will teach her the easiest method, which is sliding down on her stomach. Later, after practicing stairs for awhile and before she can walk down the stairs, she may figure out how to do methods 2 or 3 listed above. They are optional methods, and you do not need to teach them. If your child initiates them, just observe her to make sure she can execute them in a safe way.

To **slide down the stairs on her stomach** (figs. 5.47, 5.48), she will need to:

1. straighten her hips and knees so she can slide down each stair
2. keep her head and trunk leaning forward over the stair

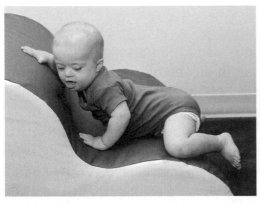
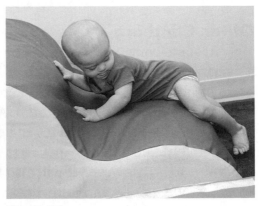

(fig. 5.47)                              (fig. 5.48)

3. push off with her hands to push her body down the stairs
4. use her feet to touch each stair and stop herself if needed, to maintain control while descending the stairs
5. move to her stomach to prepare to climb down feet first (when she is ready to climb down from the top of the flight)

To begin practicing climbing down stairs, it is best to limit the number of stairs and start on the 4th stair from the bottom of the flight. When she is ready, you can increase the number of stairs until she can climb down the whole flight. Be patient as you help her learn to move down the whole flight of stairs. She will need to learn how to do it safely and keep her attention focused on repeating the steps until she reaches the floor at the bottom of the stairs. She will need to be motivated and determined in order to carry it out safely. Keep practicing it until she shows you she is ready to do it independently and consistently.

She may prefer to **climb down feet first on her hands and knees or hands and feet.** To climb down, she will lean her trunk over the stair her arms are on and stabilize herself; then she will slide each knee or foot down to the next stair. With her knees or feet stable on the next stair, she will move her hands down to the stair above her knees. She will repeat this sequence to move down the flight of stairs.

**Sitting and "bumping"** down the stairs is generally used when children are taller, during the post walking period of development. At this time, the child wants to see where she is going, but is not tall enough to walk down the stairs holding the railing, so she discovers the method of sitting on the stair and sliding down the stairs on her buttocks, or "bumping" down the stairs. In order to use this method, her legs need to be long enough for her heels to reach the edge of the next stair. Then she hooks her heels over the edge and bends her knees to move her buttocks down to that stair. As long as she holds her trunk up straight and leans it back against the stair behind her, she will maintain her balance and be safe. If she leans her trunk forward, then she is at risk for falling forward down the flight.

## Other Climbing

At some point, your child will be motivated to climb and will want to do it everywhere, all of the time. She will climb on and off the sofa, on and off benches, foot stools/ottomans, and chairs, and up and down stairs. She may try to climb in or out of the bathtub. Anywhere she can figure out how to do it, she will! You will be proud to see her maneuver her whole body and climb so effectively. You will be happy to see her explore, be active, and get where she wants to go. However, it will also be a challenge to keep up with her and keep her safe. For example, Michael wanted to get a cookie from the cookie jar on the kitchen counter. He noticed that the dishwasher door was open, so he climbed onto it to reach the cookie jar. That's where his mother found him, with his hand in the cookie jar! Many parents have also told me that they found their child on the kitchen or dining room table after their child figured out how to climb there from the chair.

Since your child will want to climb, it will be important to think about how to give her safe, appropriate climbing opportunities at home and in the community. You can use climbing equipment ("called climbers") for toddlers, with a ladder, a slide, and a swing. Sometimes they are called an activity gym, or playhouse gym. They even have inflatable gyms and bouncers. Your child may also like crawling through a tunnel. In the community, you can use toddler playgrounds or climbing facilities that are available at places such as Discovery Zone, Monkey Bizness, or McDonald's. Your child can participate in programs like My Gym or Gymboree.

Consider buying some climbing equipment, such as slides, available through Fisher Price, Little Tikes, Step 2, and other companies. Depending on the size of your home, you can keep it inside or outside. If you can keep it inside, you can set your child up to do climbing there. When choosing slides, begin with a slide that has 3-4 stairs. Make sure there is enough room at the top for your child to hold on and sit down safely before she slides down by herself.

## Guidelines

*Keep your child moving to the endpoint with momentum and consistency.* If you set her up from the beginning to always move to the endpoint, she will develop safe climbing habits. You want her to learn to keep climbing up or down the stairs until she reaches the landing at the top or the floor at the bottom. Help her to keep focused and avoid distractions, since they will cause her to fall.

*Remember that your role is to motivate her to climb up and down, help her move her hands, knees, or feet (if needed) so she is successful, and supervise her so she is safe.* Your child's role is to understand all of the components needed for climbing. First, she needs to learn the steps and then put together the sequence of steps. Second, she needs to develop the strength to execute the steps efficiently. Third, she needs to plan how to climb safely. Fourth, she needs to use judgment to climb safely. Since you want her to learn to climb independently, you only want to provide minimal strategic support when she needs it. If you provide too much support, she will learn to depend on you to keep her safe rather than learn to do it by herself.

*Use shorter flights of stairs, if possible.* If there are 6-7 stairs to the landing, this is easier to do than a flight of 12-13 stairs.

*If your child's legs are short, begin climbing off lower furniture so her feet reach the ground more quickly.* After she can climb off this furniture, you can challenge her with higher furniture. With her short legs, it will take longer for her feet to touch the ground when sliding off the furniture. This can be scary and would make climbing off furniture more difficult.

*Use carpeted stairs when she is learning to climb the stairs.* She will feel more comfortable with her knees on the carpet, and you can avoid little accidents, like bumping her head. If only wooden stairs are available, have her wear pants to pad her knees. Move her slowly and particularly watch her head so she does not bump it. As her climbing skills improve, she will anticipate how she needs to move her head and knees so she is safe and comfortable.

*If your house does not have any stairs, ask a friend or relative if your child can practice climbing the stairs at their house.* Climbing is a fun activity and an important skill to practice at this developmental stage. It improves arm, leg, and abdominal strength and also helps your child use coordinated movements between these parts. Any time you can arrange opportunities for climbing, your child will benefit from them.

## Temperament

If your child is an **observer,** she will climb up stairs when she is motivated. You will need to encourage her to keep moving because she will prefer to stop, sit, and play. She will generally be more attentive to being safe, but you still need to watch her—especially if she tries to sit on the stairs, rather than continue to climb. When she climbs off the sofa and down stairs, she will be fearful initially and will want to lower herself slowly and carefully. You will need to keep her moving and focused on reaching the bottom of the stairs.

If your child is **motor driven,** she will like to climb up and down stairs. She will like moving fast and will think it is fun. You will need to watch her because she may not pay attention to being safe. She will enjoy the feeling of sliding down as she is climbing off furniture. She will like sliding down the stairs when she is familiar with the movements.

## ACTIVITY #18: Climbing Up the Flight of Stairs

1. Place your child on the stairs with her hands on the #1 stair (from the top) and her feet on the #3 stair.
2. Place a toy on the landing so it is easy to see but out of reach.
3. Position yourself on your knees on the #4 stair.
4. See if she will try to move to the toy. She will need to do the following steps:
   a. Move each knee, one at a time onto the #2 stair.
   b. Then, while on the #2 stair, move one foot into the half kneel position and then move onto her other foot.
   c. Move each hand onto the landing, one at a time;
   d. Repeat steps a and b, on the #1 stair, until she climbs up on the landing.
5. Help her move her hands, knees, or feet if needed. After she places each knee or foot, support it to prevent sliding. Use your thumb to support behind her knee at the crease, and use your thumb and index finger web space to support behind her heel. If she tries to sit, help her keep moving forward and do not allow her to sit on the stair to take a break. Provide the least amount of support and supervise her so she is safe.
6. When she climbs up to the landing from the #3 stair, place her on the #4 stair. Gradually increase the number of stairs she climbs. Only practice the number of stairs that she is ready to do, and that she will cooperate with persevering to move all the way to the landing.
7. Work toward climbing up the entire flight of stairs.
8. Continue to practice climbing up the flight of stairs until it is automatic and she consistently climbs up safely.

## ACTIVITY #19: Climbing Off the Sofa

1. Place your child sitting on the sofa, with her back against the back cushion. This will give her adequate space to roll over before she slides down to the floor.
2. Place motivating toys on the floor, approximately 3 feet (.9 meters) in front of the sofa, so she can see them easily from where she is sitting. (If you place the toys too close to the sofa, she needs to move to the edge of the sofa to see them, which will encourage her to climb off head first.)

3. Sit on your heels on the floor in front of the sofa, next to the toys. This position allows you to help your child if needed but you are far enough away that she will not reach for you or lunge forward and expect you to catch her.

4. Say "down" and wait, watching to see her reaction. Wait for her to show that she wants to move down to the toys. If she does not show any interest, find other motivating toys.

5. When she chooses to climb down and starts to move, see whether she plans to move head first or rolls to her stomach to move down feet first. If she leans her trunk forward to come down head first, then give her the verbal cue "on your belly" or "turn over." See if she flips over onto her belly. If not, then flip her over quickly onto her belly.

6. After she is on her belly, watch her legs. See if she straightens them. If not, you straighten them, especially her hips.

7. Once she is on her belly, her hips are straight, and her trunk is resting on the surface, then give her the verbal cue "push."

8. She will push with her hands until her feet touch the floor. If she is timid or upset because her legs are dangling, then move her feet to the floor. Have her land on her feet, catch with her feet, and stop in standing. When she first practices the skill, you can guide her to land in standing quickly so she understands where she needs to go. Once familiar with the skill, you can let her legs dangle as she is climbing off, and she will need to keep pushing with her arms until her feet find the floor to land on. From standing, she will probably move to sitting on the floor to play with the toys.

9. Continue to practice this activity until she consistently and automatically climbs down safely, feet first.

10. When she chooses to climb down, if she moves from sitting to her side and props her hands to that side, support her trunk on that side (under her armpit) and wait to see if she moves her legs straight in preparation to move down feet first. Lessen your support when ready so she learns to do it by herself with control. When you do it with this kind of support, you are letting her choose her method and then providing support to shape her method into a safe method, by helping her learn the additional movements needed.

11. When she has mastered climbing off the sofa safely, have her practice climbing off other furniture—a bed, and a variety of chairs in the house.

## 🏃 ACTIVITY #20: Climbing Down Stairs

1. Place your child on her stomach on the stairs with her elbows on the #4 stair (from the bottom) and her knees on the #3 stair.
2. Place a toy on the floor at the bottom of the stairs.
3. Position yourself on your knees on the #2 stair.

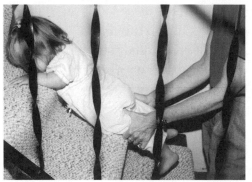

(fig. 5.49)

4. Hold her thighs near her buttocks (with your fingers on the front of her thighs, your palms on the side and back of her thighs, and your thumbs on her buttocks if needed to straighten her hips) and support her hips and knees straight (fig. 5.49). Gently lift her thighs and pull downward to cue her to move down the stairs.

5. Say "push" and wait for her to push with her hands, and then support her legs to slide down the stairs. Let her toes touch each stair so she feels stable. If needed, say "push" on each stair so she learns to continuously push on each stair until her feet touch the floor and she understands that she is at the bottom of the flight. Then let go and let her sit and play with the toy. Keep her focused on moving down the stairs and make it fun by varying the speed as you slide her down. Do not encourage her to play on the stairs or distract her.

6. When she is familiar with these movements, set her up on the #4 stair and see if she will climb down by herself. If not, strategically assist her as needed with as little support as possible.

7. When she can climb down from the #4 stair by herself, place her on the #5 stair. Gradually increase the number of stairs she climbs down.

8. Work toward climbing down the entire flight of stairs.

9. Continue to practice climbing down the flight of stairs until it is automatic and she climbs down safely.

10. The last component to develop is initiating climbing down the flight from sitting on the landing. See if she will move to her stomach and then start the prone slide method. If not, give her the verbal cue that you used to climb off the sofa, and see if she will move to her belly. If not, wait for her to show the intent to climb down and then move both hands to one side, and see if she will move to her stomach from this position. If not, move her to her stomach and then have her start climbing down.

# 🏃 ACTIVITY #21: Climbing on the Sofa and on Climbing Equipment

1. When she is standing in front of the equipment that she wants to climb on, wait for her to initiate climbing up. She will move her knee or foot, and then you can place it and stabilize it, or support it after she places it. Provide the least amount of support needed for her to be successful.
2. Watch her arms and guide her about where to hold on so she can grip and pull effectively.
3. Guide her and provide strategic support as needed so she learns to do it safely on her own.

# Plantigrade and Moving to Stand

During this stage, your child will discover and use the plantigrade position, which is being on her hands and feet (fig. 5.50), similar to the "downward dog" yoga pose. From hands and knees, she will lift her pelvis up so she is on hands and feet. She will first learn that she can move into this new position. She may also learn to use it for mobility by bear walking, and later, it will be very important to use to move up to standing. When she can move from plantigrade to

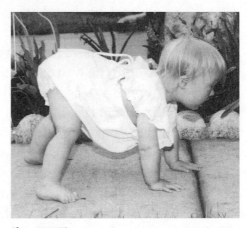

(fig. 5.50)

stand, she will be able to stand up anywhere in the house, and will no longer need to use furniture to pull to stand. Your child will need to learn this skill to be a functional and independent walker. If she needs to creep over to you or to furniture in order to stand up, she will choose to walk less because it will be more efficient to creep or bear walk where she wants to go.

## Components

The components to focus on are:
1. arm strength to push up and hold the plantigrade position, and to weight shift forward and back
2. abdominal strength to tuck the pelvis under, moving the pelvis into the rounded position rather than holding it in an arched position

3. leg strength to maintain the plantigrade position with knees bent, weight shift forward and back, and later to move upward from the squat position to stand
4. Strength, balance, and coordination to maintain the plantigrade position, and to be able to weight shift with control and move upward to standing
5. ability to weight shift backwards with fluidity in plantigrade and to find the precise point of balance, from which she will then use leg and trunk strength to move up to standing
6. ability to move her hands and feet close together while maintaining her balance in plantigrade
7. motivation to stand, and ability to maintain balance in standing

## Tendencies

The tendencies are:
1. to lock the knees and hold them stiff, and to stand with a wide base
2. to arch the back and pelvis and use the back muscles, without using the abdominal muscles
3. to have excessive flexibility in the hamstring muscles so she leans into the posture created in 1 and 2 (above) (without bending her knees or using her abdominals to tuck her pelvis)
4. to be stiff in the plantigrade position and hold herself with her pelvis over her feet, with her hands and feet too wide apart, or with her knees stiff and her pelvis behind her feet
5. to resist bending her knees
6. to resist weight shifting forward and backward
7. to learn to move to stand from plantigrade with her trunk and pelvis arched and stiff knees

---

### Steps in Learning the Plantigrade Position

Your child will progress through the following steps:
1. move into plantigrade;
2. move into modified plantigrade;
3. move from modified plantigrade to stand;
4. move from plantigrade to stand.

---

## Moving into Plantigrade

Watch your child to see when she starts initiating moving into the plantigrade position (fig. 5.51). She will be on the floor on her hands and knees and then straighten her knees and lift her buttocks up so she is propping on her hands and feet. She will experiment with moving in and out of the plantigrade position from hands and knees. She will also explore weight shifting forward, backward, and sideways. While in plantigrade, she will be intrigued, looking at the environment while upside down.

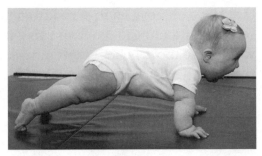

(fig. 5.51)

Your child's first experience of plantigrade occurred when she practiced climbing up stairs. When climbing up the stairs, she started on her hands and knees and then moved onto her feet, and at the moment she was in the plantigrade position. Now she will learn to use the position while on the floor. She will playfully use the position during this stage, and when she is taking independent steps, you can teach her that she can move to stand from this position.

The plantigrade position helps to build arm strength. To maintain the position, your child will need to prop on her hands and push upward with her arms to hold up her body weight while maintaining this inverted V position. She will also learn to weight shift with control, tolerating slight movements in all directions, while still maintaining the position. Playing around with weight shifting will help her later when she needs to find her point of balance so she can move up to standing.

The plantigrade position will also help her use her abdominals. When she first moves into the position, she will straighten her knees and move her pelvis upward. After she is familiar with the position, she will learn to use new movements. She will learn to bend her knees and move her pelvis backwards toward the squat position. She will combine knee bending and activating her abdominals, and you will see her tuck her pelvis under her trunk rather than hold her pelvis and back arched. When her trunk, pelvis, and legs learn these movements, she will weight shift easily through her legs and arms, which will prepare her for bear walking and moving to stand. You want to guide her to learn these movement transitions, and avoid having her learn to be stiff and rigid, particularly in her knees.

When she first moves into the plantigrade position, her feet and hands will be far apart. After she practices weight shifting in the position, bending her knees, and tucking her abdominals, she will move her hands and feet closer together with balance and control. She will need to be able to do this in order to move from plantigrade to stand.

When she initiates using the plantigrade position, encourage her to play with it and have fun in the position. Through her own play, she will develop the arm, trunk, and leg movements described above. Later you can teach her that she can move up to stand from plantigrade, and she can also lower herself from standing to the floor using it. On her own, she may learn to use bear walking to move in her environment, but this is an optional skill and not one that you need to teach her. If she bear walks, watch her knees so that she bends them as in figures 5.52 and 5.53.

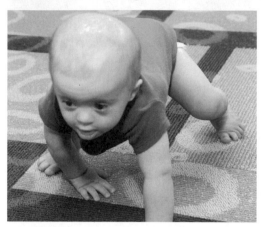

(fig. 5.52)

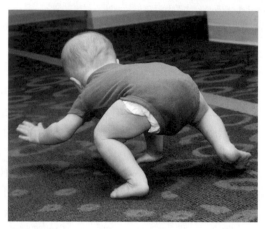

(fig. 5.53)

## Moving into Modified Plantigrade

When your child is ready to practice moving from plantigrade to stand, you will introduce her to the modified plantigrade position. In modified plantigrade, she will prop her hands on a sofa cushion (about 5 inches or 12.5 cm high), placed on the floor. When she props on this raised surface, her trunk will be horizontal. You can then encourage her to bend her knees, weight shift her pelvis backwards, and move her hands closer to her feet. Using this position will make it easier to learn where her pelvis needs to move to find that point of balance, before moving upward to standing. She will move into the position easily and feel stable in the position.

To set her up to move into the position, place a sofa cushion on the floor and place a toy on it. Place her sitting on the floor a few feet away. She will creep over to the cushion, and then place her hands on it and move to her feet. At this moment, you need to kneel behind her and move her pelvis back to rest against your thighs so she stays in the position. If you entertain her with the toy, she will play in this position. If you let her continue moving on her own, she will probably climb up on the sofa cushion rather than learn the new position of modified plantigrade.

## Moving from Modified Plantigrade to Stand

You will need to teach your child the connection between plantigrade and standing. On her own, she will just keep using plantigrade playfully and may bear walk, but she will not discover that it is a transition position from which she can move to standing. To see that she can move to standing, she needs to learn to move from plantigrade to almost a squat position. When playing in plantigrade, she will probably keep her weight shifted forward onto her arms and look downward rather than experimenting with weight shifting her pelvis back over her legs toward the squatting position. Once she explores moving back to the squat position, then she can look upward and discover that she can move up to standing.

To show her how easy it is to transition to standing, it is best to start her in the modified plantigrade position. You can set her up to move into the modified plantigrade position, as described in the section above. She will move into the position more easily if she does it by herself rather than you placing her in the position. Once she is in the position, then you will kneel behind her, and help her to stand, positioning your thighs in the exact position where you want her pelvis to move back to. You will set her up to discover where her point of balance is—where her pelvis needs to weight shift back to—so her pelvis is behind her heels. From this position, you can help her to move to stand as described in Activity #22 (figs. 5.54–5.58).

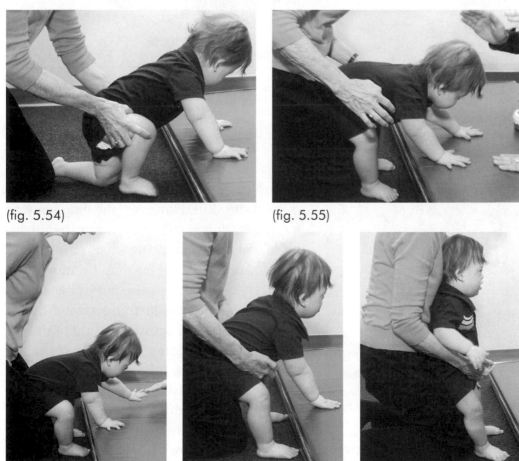

(fig. 5.54)  (fig. 5.55)

(fig. 5.56)  (fig. 5.57)  (fig. 5.58)

To practice all of the uses of the plantigrade position, after she moves to stand, you can add falling down (to modified plantigrade) and catching with her hands. You will give the verbal cues "stand UP" and "fall DOWN." By practicing falling down and catching with her hands, she will learn how to fall to the ground effectively and safely, and these are called protective reactions. They will be needed after she begins walking. To have reliable protective reactions, she will need to move her arms quickly so she props in time to catch herself, and her arms will need to be strong enough to stop the fall and prevent her head from bumping into the ground.

## Moving from Plantigrade to Stand

Once your child can move from modified plantigrade to stand, you can start practicing moving from plantigrade to stand (figs. 5.59–5.61). You want to time your practice to coincide with when this skill is functional for her. It will be most useful to her after she can take independent steps, and this

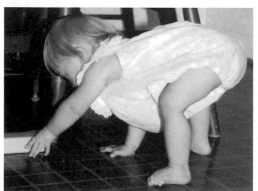

(fig. 5.59)

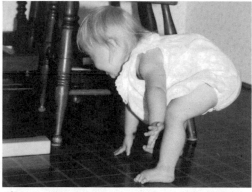

(fig. 5.60)

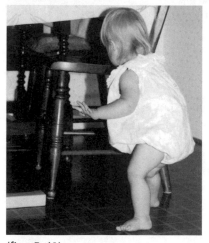

(fig. 5.61)

will be the critical time that you want her to learn the skill. However, she may want to practice it sooner, so if she is interested in doing it and likes balancing in standing, then you can practice it. She may be motivated to do it because you praise her or because it is a fun game to her. Just understand that if she learns the skill before it is functional for her, she may stop doing it and then resume it when she needs it to move to stand and walk.

The prerequisite skills are to be able to balance in standing for 5-10 seconds and to like standing. The focus will be to understand the connection between plantigrade, standing, and walking so that she learns to move from plantigrade to stand, and then take independent steps.

To move from plantigrade to stand, your child will need to learn to move from plantigrade to the squat position (steps 1-4 below), and then from the squat position to standing (step 5). The steps are:

1. to move into plantigrade from quadruped, by first placing one foot in the half kneel position, and then placing the other foot firmly on the floor so she has a stable base
2. to maintain the plantigrade position with knees bent and trunk horizontal
3. to balance in plantigrade and be able to weight shift the pelvis behind the heels and move her hands back closer to her feet (approximately 4-6 inches or 10-15 cm from toes to wrists)
4. to shift her weight back to her point of balance, knowing precisely where to place her pelvis behind her heels, and then pause and balance herself in this position until she is ready to move to standing (fig. 5.60).
5. to simultaneously balance herself and use her leg and trunk strength to lift herself upward to standing
6. to balance in standing for a few seconds, frequently using foot balance reactions, and when ready, initiate the waddle and take a step

Each step builds on the previous step and each step needs to be done perfectly for her to move up to stand independently. For the first step, if she does not plant each foot firmly on the floor, she will not have a stable base. If she does not move her hands and feet close together, she will not be able to weight shift her pelvis behind her heels. If she does not weight shift her pelvis back far enough to her point of balance and tries to move to stand too early, then she will fall forward. When she first learns to stand up, she will move slowly through these steps (figs. 5.62, 5.63). With practice, she will be fast and the steps will be precise, efficient, and automatic.

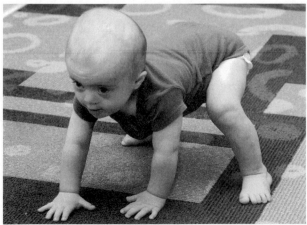

(fig. 5.62)

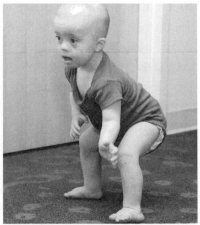

(fig. 5.63)

To learn to move from squatting to standing, your child will need to use leg, foot, and trunk strength while moving forward and upward. To prepare her, practice Activity #23—moving from sitting on a bench to standing. In stages 3 & 4, she practiced moving from sitting on the bench to standing so she is familiar with this activity. The difference now is that she will do it without hand support. She will need to move to stand and then prop on the supporting surface after she is in standing.

With her first practices of moving from squatting to standing on her own, she will probably fall back to sitting. She will either weight shift her pelvis too far back, or she will try to move to stand but not be able to simultaneously balance herself and use leg and trunk strength to move upward to stand. If you see her try to move from squatting to stand, you can kneel behind her and provide support behind her pelvis so she is successful. She may be creative and figure out that she can position her pelvis against the sofa or the wall, and then move to stand. She may also do this in the crib or playpen, and position her pelvis against the crib rails or net of the playpen. Some children first move from plantigrade to stand on a large bed or on a mini-trampoline. Once your child knows the steps, observe how she practices them and where she is most comfortable.

Your child may learn to move from plantigrade to stand before she takes independent steps, or she may take a few independent steps and then need to learn to move from plantigrade to stand. You can help your child learn the steps to move from plantigrade to stand, but she will only do it spontaneously when she is ready—when *she* wants to stand up. She will choose standing when she knows she can stand well, is comfortable in standing, and is motivated to stand. After she stands up, see what she is motivated to do. She may want to stand a few seconds and then fall to sitting, or she may want to dance, or she may want to clap and play "so big." If she can take independent steps, you can show her that she can take a step from this position. At first, you can do it with one-hand support and later, you can sign and say "walk" and then she can shift her weight sideways on her own (waddle) and take a step.

## Guidelines

*Wait for your child to initiate moving into plantigrade, or set her up to move into the modified plantigrade position.* I don't recommend trying to put her in the plantigrade position because it will feel awkward, and she will probably resist it. Your job is to watch her and notice when she starts using this position, and then you can build on it.

*Expect your child to keep her feet wide apart when she first learns to move from plantigrade to stand independently.* By positioning her feet wider than her hips, she can more easily balance herself as she moves from plantigrade to stand. With practice, her strength, balance, and efficiency will improve and she will spontaneously narrow her base. When she uses a wide base, it will be difficult to take a step, so you may need to narrow her base to set her up to be successful with stepping.

*As your child is practicing plantigrade, modified plantigrade, and moving to stand, make sure she learns to bend her knees and to activate her abdominals to tuck her pelvis under her trunk.* These are critical movements to develop in order for her to succeed with the final goal of moving from plantigrade to standing, and initiating stepping.

*Set your child up to move to stand by labeling the game and sitting on the floor with her.* Say and sign "stand" to let her know the game you want to play. If you stand over her when she is sitting on the floor, and you say "stand up," she will reach out to hold your hands so you can help her pull to stand while she is looking upward at you. It is better if you sit on the floor and say it. When you are at the same level as she is, she will more easily move from sitting (facing you) to plantigrade (facing downward), and then up to standing (at eye level to you).

## Temperament

If your child is an **observer,** she will probably learn to move from plantigrade to stand before she takes independent steps. She will approach walking carefully and will want to develop moving to stand and standing balance before she tries to take steps. She may move from plantigrade to stand and then stand for 10 seconds or more, or she may move to stand and then sit down again. She will surprise you the first time she does it, and she will be proud of herself!

If your child is **motor driven,** she will probably take independent steps first. Later, she will be willing to learn to move from plantigrade to stand when it is functional for her. She will learn standing balance as she is learning to step longer distances. When she wants to walk 5- to 15-foot distances, she will be motivated to learn to move to stand from plantigrade. If you help her learn how to do it at this point, she will learn quickly so she can move to stand and walk.

 ## ACTIVITY #22: Moving from Modified Plantigrade to Stand

1. Place a sofa cushion on the floor and place a motivating toy on it.
2. Place your child sitting on the floor a few feet away from the cushion.
3. She will creep, crawl, or bear walk to the sofa cushion.
4. Anticipate that she will move to the cushion and as soon as she places her hands on the cushion with her feet on the floor, quickly kneel behind her, positioning your thighs in the exact position that you

want her pelvis to move back to (where her point of balance is, with her pelvis behind her heels). Then immediately place your fingers on the front of her thighs where her pelvis and thighs meet. Move her pelvis back so it is stabilized and rests against your thighs. You need to move quickly because once her hands touch the sofa cushion, she will start climbing up on the cushion, and you need to guide her to move to stand rather than do her habit of climbing.

5. When her hands are propping on the sofa cushion and her pelvis is resting against your thighs, her trunk should be horizontal, her knees bent, and her pelvis tucked and rounded. If her knees are straight, and her trunk and pelvis are arched, then tickle her belly to see if you can activate her abdominals so she bends her trunk, pelvis, and knees.

6. Tell her "stand up" and sign "stand" and see if she lifts her trunk to move to standing. If not, then place your hand on her upper abdomen and do intermittent tapping with lifting movements to cue her to move her trunk up straight. Once she moves her trunk up to standing, then kneel up tall behind her so she stands with your support. Then praise her and clap for her to celebrate! (It is important to label the game by saying "stand up" so later you can just give the verbal cue and she will know what to do.)

7. From standing, add the new game of falling down to plantigrade and catching with her hands. Say "down" and assist her with moving her trunk and hands down to the cushion. You can play this game with a sibling doing the same movements, kneeling in front of her on the other side of the cushion. You can also set her up to do these movements by playing a game. For example, she can bend down to pick up a ball and then stand and shoot a basket with a low hoop. She can also bend down to pick up a shape and then stand up and put the shape in the shape sorter container.

8. Once she knows how to move from modified plantigrade to stand, with you providing support behind her pelvis, then you can experiment using these methods with less support:

    a. Lie on the floor on your back and have your child prop on your chest or abdomen and then move to stand.

    b. Sit on your heels on the floor and have your child prop on your thighs and then move up to stand. If she needs a little support, she can prop her hand against your chest to move up to stand. Or, you can offer your finger, and she can hold it to help her move to stand.

    c. When she stands, clap for her and praise her.

d. When she uses these methods, if she does not bend her knees and move her pelvis behind her heels, then go back to providing the support described in steps 1-6.

## ACTIVITY #23: Moving from Sitting on a Bench to Standing

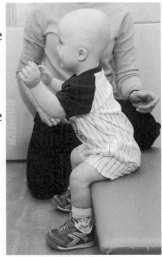

1. Seat your child on a bench, with her feet firmly stabilized on the floor (fig. 5.64). The height of the bench should be 1 inch (2.5 cm) more than the measurement from the back of her knee to the bottom of her foot. With this height bench, her buttocks will be higher than her knees, which will make it easier for her to move up to standing.

2. Place a high (21-24 inches or 53 to 61 cm) soft surface in front of her that she will move toward. (Examples of surfaces to use: very large ball, play kitchen set, mat placed vertically against the wall, sofa with two cushions on the seat.)

(fig. 5.64)

3. Start by placing the bench and the surface 15 inches (38 cm) apart.

4. Place a motivating toy on the surface and say/sign "stand up."

5. See if she stretches her arms forward to reach toward the surface, leans her trunk forward, and then straightens her legs to move upward to standing (fig. 5.65). Once in standing, she can prop her hands on the surface and then take 1-2 steps to the surface (figs. 5.66-5.67).

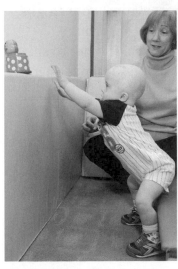

(fig. 5.65)

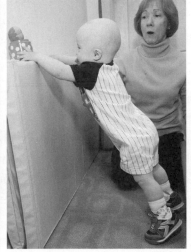

(fig. 5.66)

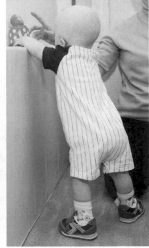

(fig. 5.67)

  a. If she can touch the surface while she is sitting on the bench, place the bench and surface 16 inches (40.5 cm) apart.

  b. If she moves from sitting on the bench to sitting on the floor, start with the surfaces closer together so she learns the game of standing up, even if she touches the surface. When she is familiar with the game, then move the surfaces back to 15 inches (38 cm) apart.

6. When she is standing at the surface, clap for her and praise her.

7. When she is comfortable with this game, and she is able to take 2-3 independent steps, then place the bench and surface 16-18 inches (40.5-46 cm) apart. Say and sign "stand up and walk." The goal will be to move to stand, balance in standing, and then take 1-2 steps to the surface.

## ACTIVITY #24: Moving from Plantigrade to Stand

This activity can be done after your child can move from modified plantigrade to stand.

1. When your child is on hands and knees, kneel behind her. Say "stand up." See if you can get her to move into the plantigrade position by placing one leg in the half kneel position (with her foot on the floor) and then placing her other foot on the floor. Provide assistance if needed to place both feet firmly on the floor.

2. Position your knees so your thighs are at the precise place that her pelvis needs to move back to, her point of balance.

3. See if she moves her pelvis back to your thighs. If not, place your index fingers at her upper thighs, the crease where her pelvis and thighs meet, and move her pelvis back to rest against your thighs.

4. Say and sign "stand up" and see if she will move her trunk and legs to rise up to standing. Then kneel tall behind her so she can balance against you in standing. Praise her and clap for her to show your excitement.

5. Practice steps 1-4, frequently lessening your support, until she can do it by herself.

6. If she can take independent steps, then combine moving to stand with taking a couple of independent steps. After she moves to stand, then say and sign "walk" and encourage her to take an independent step. When she is ready, increase the distance she walks after she moves to stand.

# Standing

During this stage your child will learn to balance herself in standing without holding onto a support. The goal will be to stand 5-10 seconds without support. Until she is ready to stand alone, standing with one-hand support will be the main position she will use to practice standing balance. In Stage 4, she learned how to stand with an optimal posture with a narrow base, knees and feet pointing straight ahead, knees unlocked, and abdominals tucked. With this posture, she was active with bouncing in standing, and rising up on tiptoes. She also started working on balance by learning to stand with one-hand support. In this stage, her leg, foot, and abdominal strength will improve, and she will learn to use foot balance reactions. The combination of these components will help her stand on her own.

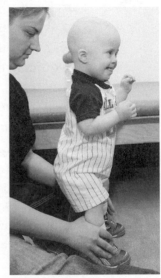

(fig. 5.68)

In addition to learning these components, she will need to gain the confidence to practice this skill. You will need to wait for the right time for her to be willing to practice the skill. Frequently, this skill is scary, so you do not want to force it before she is ready to do it. She will show you when she is ready, and then she will be motivated to figure out how to balance herself when you practice it. Some children like playing standing balance games. You hold them in standing and then let go, and they balance briefly and then fall toward you so you catch them (fig. 5.68). Other children wait and learn standing balance when it is functional for them, when they are learning to take independent steps. She will learn to balance herself when she takes two or more steps. Once she has the confidence and motivation to work on maintaining her balance, and she has the strength and balance strategies to use, she will persevere with practicing this skill.

## *Components*

The components to focus on are:
1. standing posture with trunk vertical and abdominals tucked, heels in line with hips, knees and feet pointing straight, and knees unlocked
2. the ability to activate the feet and use foot balance reactions when weight shifting to maintain balance
3. the ability to tolerate mild weight shifting in all directions, and to maintain balance

4. coordination of movements between the trunk, legs, and feet to maintain balance, and recover balance when her weight is shifted off balance
5. fluidity of movement and the ability to control small gradations of movement to maintain and recover balance
6. motivation to challenge herself to balance in standing without support, and hold the position for a few seconds

## Tendencies

The tendencies are:
1. to stand stiffly with the trunk and pelvis arched, the knees locked, and the buttocks behind the heels
2. to position the feet wide apart, turned outward with collapsed arches and with the toes flexed (grasping the surface)
3. to avoid weight shifting and use the trunk, leg, and foot posture described in 1 and 2 to hold the body stiff and balanced
4. to quickly move to the floor, probably to the plantigrade position, if she feels off balance, rather than try to recover her balance in the standing position
5. to resist standing without support

---

### Steps in Learning to Stand

Your child will learn to stand:
1. propping her hands against a vertical surface;
2. propping on one hand, and reaching to the side, behind, or down with her other hand;
3. without support.

---

## Propping Hands against a Vertical Surface

Your child is already familiar with maintaining her balance with one or both hands propped on top of a surface. With this setup, her arms can help her maintain her balance by pressing into the surface. The next challenge is to balance with her hands propped against a vertical surface, such as the refrigerator or mirror (fig. 5.69). When she stands with this support, her hands help her hold her trunk vertical, but she needs to use her trunk, legs, and feet to balance herself.

Since this is a stressful position, you need to see if she tries to stabilize herself by using the compensatory pattern of standing with a wide base and toeing-out. You will need to teach her to balance herself with her heels in line with her hips, and her feet pointing straight. With her feet in this position, she will learn to weight shift through her feet, activate her muscles to move in all directions, and use the subtle movements needed for foot balance reactions. If she places her feet wide apart and turned outward, this position will block movements in her feet, and she will not learn foot balance reactions.

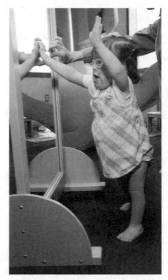 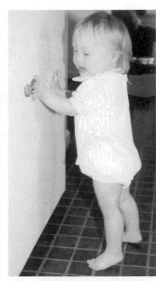

(fig. 5.69)          (fig. 5.70)

When she is comfortable with this new standing position, she can practice propping on one hand and reaching forward and playing with a toy with her other hand. For example, she can prop on one hand and play with a refrigerator magnet with her other hand (fig. 5.70). She can also turn to you at her side and reach for the magnet. When she practices turning her trunk to the side with her feet positioned facing forward, she will weight shift sideways through her feet, onto the outer border of one foot and onto the inner border of her other foot. You can also place the magnet up high on the refrigerator, and then she will need to rise up on tiptoes to reach it. If you place the magnet at the level of her knees, then she will bend her knees and weight shift through her feet toward her heels. By practicing weight shifting in all directions (sideways onto the inner and outer borders of the feet, forward onto tiptoes, and backward onto heels), she will develop strength in these movements and be able to use them as needed for balance.

## Propping on One Hand, and Reaching with her Other Hand

You can continue to challenge your child's balance by placing the toy behind her, further to the side, or down on the floor (fig. 5.71). She can be standing at the coffee table and prop on one hand, and when she reaches for the toy, she will need to rotate her trunk to reach behind, or side bend her trunk to reach to the side. To reach downward to the floor, she will need to bend her knees and move to a squat. If her feet are placed in line with her hips and pointing

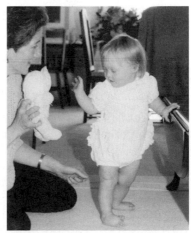

(fig. 5.71)

straight, when she moves her trunk, she will weight shift through her feet. By practicing reaching, she will strengthen her trunk, leg, and foot muscles, and this will prepare her for all of the movements needed to balance in standing.

## Standing without Support

After practicing the standing skills described above, your child will develop the movement components and strength needed for the ideal standing posture—trunk erect, abdominal muscles activated, knees unlocked, feet in line with hips and pointing straight, and foot movements in all directions—

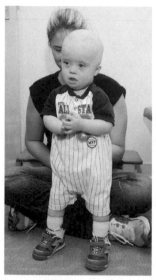

(fig. 5.72)

and for accessing balance reactions (fig. 5.72). Once she has these prerequisite skills, she will probably surprise you (and herself) the first time she balances in standing on her own. She may be playing at a table and suddenly let go of the surface briefly to play with a toy. Once your child realizes that she is standing alone, she may quickly prop again or sit down. If you praise her and clap for her, she will learn you are proud of her, and then she will want to practice this new game with you.

You can playfully test when your child will tolerate standing without support, as described in Activity #27A. If she is not interested in playing the standing balance game in Activity #27A, then she will learn to balance in standing when she is practicing independent steps.

If she is setup to move from sitting on the bench to standing (Activity #23, step 7), she may balance in standing before taking a step. Or, if you are practicing taking two or more independent steps (Activity #13 & 14), she may pause when doing the waddle and balance herself momentarily. If you watch your child and read her cues, you will know the best way to practice this skill. If she is comfortable balancing herself in standing, but taking steps is still challenging for her, she may choose to stand rather than take a step.

With practice, she will learn to stand without support for ten seconds or more. She will choose standing when she knows she can do it, and is comfortable and motivated to stand. When she has this level of standing readiness, then she will be successful with the skill of moving from plantigrade to stand.

## Guidelines

*Make sure your child uses the proper standing posture when practicing each position.* To stand properly, her feet need to be in line with her hips and pointing straight ahead, her knees unlocked, her trunk up straight with abdominals tucked and not leaning against the surface, and her hands propping on or against the surface. With this posture, when she sways off balance, she can use her trunk, legs, or feet to regain her balance back to the centered position. This posture will also help her strengthen her feet as she moves up on tiptoes, back onto her heels, and over the inside and outside borders of her feet. By developing strength in these foot movements, her foot balance reactions will be more effective.

*Have your child practice while barefoot, if possible.* To use foot balance reactions, your child needs to be barefoot and to have her feet in the optimal posture. If she is wearing shoes, she will hold her feet rigid within the shoes. If her feet are wider than her hips and turned outward, she will learn to balance herself by using this stiff posture in her hips, knees, and feet. This leg and foot posture will block access to using smooth and controlled balance strategies.

*Determine whether your child needs foot support with shoes to stand.* If your child needs to use foot support with shoes (described in Stage 4), the ankle stability she feels from the support will free her up to use the desired standing posture of the trunk, hips, and knees. She will learn to weight shift through her feet, but within a limited range, to move up on her toes, sideways, and back onto her heels.

When she is ready to work on balancing in standing, you can test to see if it is easier to do it with or without the foot support. When she is first practicing moving from plantigrade to standing, she may be more successful doing it barefoot so she can access foot balance reactions. These instances of standing without foot support will be temporary, just to help her learn to do the skills in the beginning. Once the skills are established, then she can learn to do them with the foot support and shoes. The ultimate goal is to have the foot strength to be dynamic using the foot support and shoes, rather than be rigidly held within this support.

*Make sure the height of the table or surface is around nipple level.* If the height is too low, your child will lean her trunk over the surface in order to prop on her hands. If the height is high, she will stand with her head and trunk up straight when propping on her hands. With this setup, she will learn the movements needed to balance in standing.

*Choose motivators depending on the standing skills your child is practicing, and place them in a strategic spot.* When she stands with her hands propping against a surface such as a sliding glass door or refrigerator, you can use colorforms or magnets.

When she can stand with one-hand support, have her play with lightweight toys with her other hand. Some examples include: maracas, rings to place on a ring stack, blocks to place in a sort box, small balls to put in the gumball toy, push button toys or books, playing a xylophone, popping bubbles, turning pages in a book, and pointing to pictures in a book.

When she is standing with support behind her back or standing alone, it is best if you sit on the floor so that you are at eye level to her. When she looks at you, her head and trunk will be up straight, which will help her balance herself. If you are higher, when she looks up at you, she will lose her balance. You can entertain her by talking to her, whistling, singing favorite songs or singing gesture songs like "Itsy Bitsy Spider," "Wheels on the Bus," "If You're Happy and You Know It," and "Pat-a-Cake." Her hands are free to clap or play games like "So Big." She also might like it if you count and show your fingers. This is your chance to be a creative entertainer so she focuses on you rather than thinking about what she is doing. She may stand because she is preoccupied by what you are doing. With practice, she will know the standing game and be comfortable playing it with you.

She can also practice standing facing favorite toys placed on a 21- to 24-inch high (53- to 61-cm) soft surface (a large ball, kitchen set, or a 24-inch (61 cm) mat placed vertically against the wall). The toy placed on the surface will motivate her and she will either watch it or want to move to it. She will stand longer if you use a toy that she can watch, like watching a musical video, music box, or musical playhouse.

*Provide verbal cues and label the standing game.* It is important to say "stand" every time you practice it so she learns what standing is, and anticipates playing the standing game with you.

*Move at your child's pace when developing standing balance.* If you force her to stand, she will quickly develop strategies to avoid standing. Test her readiness by doing it for brief periods, providing the best entertainment and motivators. You need to realize this position may be scary to her. She will be ready to challenge herself when she feels secure in the position, and the motivator is worth standing for.

*She will not need to be able to stand alone before practicing independent steps.* She can practice her first independent steps through lunging steps. With the setup to walk to a vertical surface, she will learn to hold her head and trunk up straight, and this will guide her posture toward the balanced standing position.

## Temperament

If your child is an **observer,** she will need to be tricked into practicing the standing game. Even though she tends to be cautious and careful, she might be willing to do this risky game with you if you make it playful and she trusts you! Once she is enrolled and knows the game, she will learn how to do it with control.

Her initial preference will be to stand with hand support since she will feel stable and secure. She will probably first balance in standing when she lets go of the support, not knowing she is standing on her own. With practice, she will learn to balance herself very well, and may choose to keep standing rather than take a step.

If your child is **motor driven,** she will not want to stand still, so it will be hard to motivate her to stand and balance herself for a few seconds. She will develop balance through standing with one-hand support. When you test her to see if she can balance in standing, she will probably try to step to you or will move down to the floor. She will learn standing balance through stepping activities.

## ACTIVITY #25: Supported Standing with Hands Propped against a Surface

1. Place your child standing with her hands propped against the refrigerator, sliding glass door, or kitchen cabinet.
2. Position her legs with her feet in line with her hips and pointing straight ahead. Position her trunk up tall and discourage leaning her trunk against the surface.
3. Look at her side view and make sure her trunk is straight, she is activating her abdominals, and her knees are unlocked.
4. Entertain her with pictures or magnets at eye level (in front of her) and have her balance herself in the standing position. You can also play music and have her dance in this position. If she leans in any direction, see if she can move herself back to the centered and balanced position. If not, help her.
5. When she is ready, encourage her to let go with one hand and use it to play, while maintaining her balance. Begin by having her hold a magnet or Colorform picture placed in front of her. With practice, she will be able to maintain standing with one-hand support for a few seconds or more.
6. When she can keep her balance with one-hand support while reaching for toys in front of her, encourage her to reach for a toy placed at the side of her trunk. Hold the toy at her side, at the level of her middle trunk, and have her twist (rotate) her trunk to reach for it. Watch her feet and see if she weight shifts sideways onto the outer border of one foot and the inner border of the other foot. Also practice placing the toy to the opposite side and watch her weight shift through her feet in that direction.
7. Practice reaching up so she rises on tiptoes.

8. Practice reaching down for a toy placed at the level of her knees, and watch her bend her knees and weight shift toward her heels.

9. When she is reaching to the side, up, and down, reposition her feet in line with her hips (narrow base). Place them straight if she widens her base or turns her feet outward.

## ACTIVITY #26: Reaching in Supported Standing

1. Place your child standing at a sofa, chair, or coffee table with her hands propped on top of the surface. The height of the surface should be at nipple level or up to 3 inches (7.5 cm) below.

2. Position her legs with her feet in line with her hips and pointing straight ahead. Position her trunk up tall and discourage leaning against the surface.

3. Place a lightweight toy at the side of her trunk, at the level of her chest, so she needs to rotate her head and trunk to look at it and reach for it. After she does this easily, then hold the toy behind her so she has to rotate her head and trunk in a larger range. Look at her feet to see if she is weight shifting onto the outer border of one foot and the inner border of the other foot. Also watch her knees to see if they are unlocked. Practice reaching in each direction.

4. Practice reaching to each side, with her elbow straight, at the level of her shoulder. After she can do this, place the toy 1-2 inches (2.5-5 cm) further and see if she will stretch for it, while maintaining her balance. To make the game easy, have her pop a bubble. You can blow a bubble and catch it on the wand, and have her reach to pop it. Watch her feet to see if she moves onto the outer and inner borders. Practice in each direction.

5. Practice reaching down to the side, to a toy placed on a step stool. After she can do this, place the toy on the floor. She will need to bend her knees and move toward the squat position to reach it. Practice to each side.

6. When she is reaching to the side, behind her, and down, reposition her feet in line with her hips (narrow base) and place them straight if she widens her base or turns her feet outward. If she locks her knees, touch the back of her knees (at the crease) with your thumb and index finger to cue her to unlock them.

# ACTIVITY #27: Standing Alone

## A. *Playing the Standing Game*

1. Sit on the floor and place your child standing in front of you. You will be at eye level to her. Talk to her and set her up to play the game. Label the game and make it exciting!

2. Hold her trunk and pelvis and balance her, then let go. You may want to count so she anticipates when you are going to let go. (Say "1, 2, 3, stand up!")

3. Hold your hands out, and see if she will balance for a second or two, and then fall toward you. Clap and praise her while she is standing. With practice, she will stand for longer periods.

4. If she can stand for longer periods, you can sing gesture songs (like "Itsy Bitsy Spider" or "Wheels on the Bus") to entertain her (and distract her).

## B. *Balancing in Standing While Practicing Stepping*

1. Sit her on a bench, with her feet firmly stabilized on the floor. The height of the bench should be 1 inch (2.5 cm) more than the distance from the back of her knee to the bottom of her foot. With this height bench, her buttocks will be higher than her knees when sitting, which will make it easier for her to move up to standing.

2. Place a high soft surface (21-24 inches or 53-61 cm) ) in front of her, which she will take a step toward. (Examples of surfaces: very large ball, mat placed vertically against the wall, parent sitting on her heels and leaning her chest forward so her child can prop against it, play kitchen set.)

3. Place the surface about 18 inches (46 cm) away from the bench, so when she is standing, she cannot touch the surface or prop on it.

4. Place a motivating toy (musical toy is helpful) on the surface and sign/say "stand up."

5. When you child rises to stand, she will need to balance herself since she cannot prop on a surface. Her lower legs will feel stable against the support of the bench. When she is standing, you can entertain her (for example, playing music) and she may balance in standing for a couple of seconds. (If relaxed enough, she may dance.) From this position, she will either try to take a step or sit down.

6. If she is willing to take a step, sign/say "walk" and encourage her to take a step to you or the surface with the toy. Since the surface is high, she will hold her head and trunk up straight so she can look at the toy. This setup will help her balance in standing as she initi-

ates the waddle to step. (If she looks downward, then her head and trunk will lean forward, and she will move down to the floor.)

7. When she balances in standing, praise her and clap for her, play games (like "so big"), or sing songs, so she is happy and proud of what she has done.

8. As she continues to practice taking independent steps, she will constantly work to maintain her balance, and recover it when she briefly loses it, in order to persevere to keep stepping to the endpoint.

## ☆ MOTOR MILESTONE CHECKLIST

### Cruising

- ☐ She cruises 1-2 steps
- ☐ She cruises 3-4 steps
- ☐ She cruises from one end of the sofa to the other, in each direction
- ☐ She cruises around the corner of a table
- ☐ She cruises from one piece of furniture to another, with the surfaces next to each other
- ☐ She cruises from one piece of furniture to another, with the surfaces parallel to each other
- ☐ She cruises with her hands against a surface

### Walking

- ☐ She walks with trunk support for 10 feet (3 meters)
- ☐ She walks with two-hand support for 10 feet (3 meters)
- ☐ She walks with two-hand support for 100 feet (30 meters) or more
- ☐ She walks with a push toy or posterior walker with support for 10 feet (3 meters)
- ☐ She walks with a push toy or posterior walker for 100 feet (30 meters)
- ☐ She pulls to stand at the push toy or posterior walker if it is stabilized
- ☐ She pulls to stand at the push toy or posterior walker, and then walks with it
- ☐ She steers the push toy or posterior walker around furniture and obstacles
- ☐ She lunges to the sofa, props her hands, and then takes 1-2 steps
- ☐ She walks with one-hand support, using the waddle pattern, for 10 feet (3 meters) with:
  - ☐ you standing behind her and providing maximal support
  - ☐ three points of support
  - ☐ two points of support
  - ☐ index finger support
- ☐ She walks with one-hand support for 100 feet (30 meters) or more
- ☐ She takes 1-2 independent steps to a high surface, and props her hands against it
- ☐ She consistently takes 3 independent steps
- ☐ She walks a distance of 2-3 feet (60-90 cm)
- ☐ She walks a distance of 3-5 feet (.9-1.5 meters)

(continued on next page)

❏ She walks a distance of 5-7 feet (1.5-2.1 meters)
❏ She walks a distance of 7-10 feet (2.1-3 meters)
❏ She walks a distance of 10-15 feet (3-4.5 meters)
❏ She walks a distance of 15 feet (4.5 meters) consistently
❏ She walks long distances in the house (level surfaces)
❏ She walks all of the time in the house (level surfaces)

### Climbing

❏ She climbs up 5-6 stairs
❏ She climbs up a flight of stairs
❏ She climbs off the sofa with verbal cues
❏ She climbs off the sofa by herself
❏ She climbs down the bottom 4 stairs
❏ She climbs down half the flight of stairs
❏ She climbs down the flight of stairs
❏ She climbs up a small slide and slides down

### Plantigrade

❏ She moves into the plantigrade (hands and feet) position on the floor
❏ She bear walks to move around a room (optional)
❏ She moves into the modified plantigrade position
❏ She moves from the modified plantigrade position to standing with knees bent and support behind her pelvis
❏ She moves from the modified plantigrade position to standing without support
❏ She moves from sitting on a bench, through squatting, to standing
❏ She moves from plantigrade to standing with knees bent and support behind her pelvis
❏ She moves from plantigrade to standing without support
❏ She moves from plantigrade to standing, and then takes independent steps

### Standing

❏ She stands 3-5 minutes with two hands **propping against** a surface
❏ She stands 3-5 minutes with one hand **propping against** a surface
❏ While standing with one hand **propping against** a surface, she balances herself while reaching for a toy placed at her side, up high so she is on tiptoes, and down at the level of her knees

(continued on next page)

❑ While standing with one hand **propping on top of** a surface, she plays with a toy placed at her side, behind her, and on the floor
❑ She stands without support for 2-5 seconds
❑ She stands without support for 10 seconds
❑ She balances in standing after moving from plantigrade to stand

# PART TWO:
## Post Walking Skills

# 6

# Introduction to Post Walking Skills

Congratulations! If you are reading this section of the book, your child has learned to walk, and he is now ready for a whole new period of exploration and gross motor skill development. It is time for him to be independent, have fun, gain confidence, and be proud of what he can do. Part Two of this book is about the Post Walking period of development, and *the goal of this period of development is to refine your child's walking pattern.* This will be accomplished by practicing targeted gross motor skills, the post walking skills, and by providing customized foot support. This chapter is divided into three sections: *post walking skills, foot management,* and *guidelines* for this new period of development.

In Stage 5, your child learned to walk using the new walker pattern. Since walking independently is such a difficult gross motor skill to do, he figured out a method that was stable for his body, with his degree of hypotonia, ligamentous laxity, and strength. The *new walker pattern* of a child with Down syndrome (fig. 5.27) is similar to that of a one-year-old (fig. 6.1). Components include:

1. a wide base, with heels wider than hips
2. feet turned outward or toeing-out
3. weight bearing on the inside borders of his feet (with flat arches if barefoot)
4. full sole weight bearing when stepping, like taking marching steps
5. trunk vertical, trunk and pelvis moving as a unit, with no pelvic rotation
6. short step length
7. stiff knees
8. arms in the high guard position

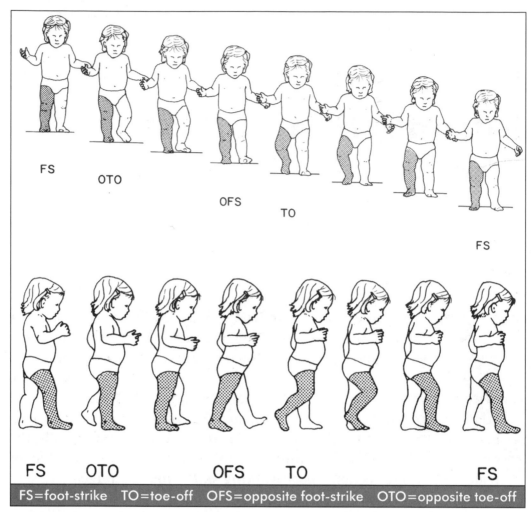

FS=foot-strike   TO=toe-off   OFS=opposite foot-strike   OTO=opposite toe-off

Fig. 6.1—Gait cycle of one-year-old. Used with permission from: D.H. Sutherland, R. A. Olshen, E.N. Biden, and M.P. Wyatt, *Clinics in Developmental Medicine No. 104/105: The Development of Mature Walking* (London, England: Mac Keith Press, 1988), p. 129.

Your child's walking pattern may not have all of these components, but these are the areas to monitor. Through using this stable pattern, your child gained confidence in walking and learned to walk all of the time. Now that he is motivated to walk, and this is his established method of mobility, he will be comfortable with being challenged to refine his walking pattern.

The components that need to be developed for the ***refined walking pattern*** (see p. xi) are:

1. a narrow base with heels in line with hips
2. feet and knees pointing straight ahead
3. feet in optimal alignment (heels vertical) so weight bearing is through the center of the foot

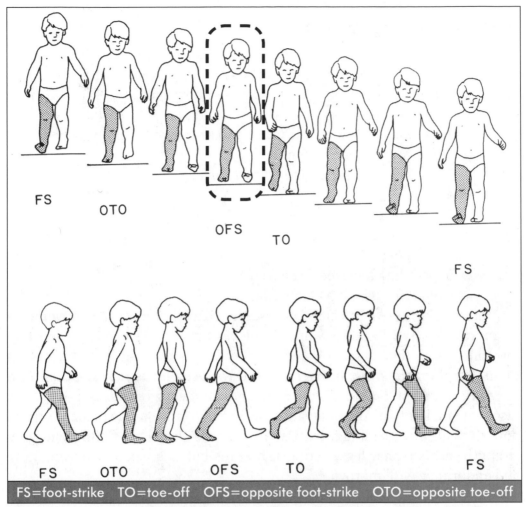

FS=foot-strike   TO=toe-off   OFS=opposite foot-strike   OTO=opposite toe-off

Fig. 6.2—Gait cycle of two-and-a-half-year-old. Used with permission from: D.H. Sutherland, R. A. Olshen, E.N. Biden, and M.P. Wyatt, *Clinics in Developmental Medicine No. 104/105: The Development of Mature Walking* (London, England: Mac Keith Press, 1988), p. 135.

4. weight shifting from the heel to the ball of the foot, progressing to toe push-off when stepping
5. trunk leaning forward and pelvis rotating on the trunk
6. longer step length
7. knees unlocked and moving smoothly between bending and straightening
8. hip hyperextension (side view: thigh moving behind the hip joint; see circled area, fig. 6.2) in combination with toe push-off for propulsion and efficiency
9. legs in vertical alignment without tilting at knees or ankles
10. arms at sides and reciprocal arm swing
11. increased speed and endurance

# Post Walking Skills

These new components for the refined walking pattern will be developed through practicing the following post walking skills and using proper foot support. (Foot support will be discussed on pages 299-311.) The post walking skills are:

1. walking on uneven surfaces, and around or over obstacles
2. fast stepping and running
3. walking up and down inclined surfaces
4. kicking a ball
5. walking up and down curbs
6. walking up and down stairs
7. jumping
8. pedaling and steering a tricycle
9. walking across a balance beam

These skills were selected because they contribute specific movements to improve walking, and they are also necessary skills for independence in the community and at school, and for playtime with siblings and peers. ***In the beginning, the most important skill to focus on is fast stepping and running.*** In chapters 7 to 15, the components of each of these skills will be discussed in detail so you understand the specific movements to focus on and how they improve walking. By practicing these skills, your child will gain strength in his trunk, legs, and feet, and his balance, speed, coordination, and endurance will improve.

In this period, you will have a new set of questions:

- My child walks with his feet wide apart; when will he walk with his feet closer together like other kids?
- He wants to run and tries to go fast, but when will he learn to run really fast rather than use a jogging pace?
- He prefers to climb up and down the stairs rather than walk; when will he safely walk up and down the flight of stairs by himself?
- He says "jump," and he wants to jump, but he can't get both of his feet off the ground simultaneously. When will he learn to jump?

Your child can learn to do all of these skills with proficiency, and the following chapters will teach you the strategies to use. The ages for these skills are approximately 2 to 6 years. Your child will be ready to start practicing these skills when he can walk in the house all of the time, is motivated to walk, and is confident and competent with walking on level surfaces.

How you practice gross motor skills in the Post Walking period of development will be different from how you practiced skills in the Birth to Walking period. In the birth to walking period, you focused on the skills of the stage the child was in, and he achieved the goals of each stage within a few months. In the post walking period, you will introduce all of the skills and practice what he is interested in at any given time. So he will be working on learning many skills at the same time. I advise you to read all of the post walking chapters, focusing on his level in learning each skill.

It will take awhile for him to achieve the goals in each skill area, and in the meantime, he will be working on each step in the process toward the goal. By focusing on the steps toward the goal, you will be able to measure his progress in that skill. You will appreciate his progress by looking at the improvements in the components that he uses, refinements in executing the skill, and the subtle changes that ultimately will result in achieving the goal. For some skills, such as curbs, stairs, and the tricycle, he will need to grow. For other skills, such as learning to generate lift-off for jumping, he will need to be confident and adventuresome. According to the data I have collected, *the average ages to achieve the gross motor goals of the post walking period* are:

| *Average ages to achieve the gross motor goals of the post walking period:* | |
|---|---|
| Walk down a 4-inch (10-cm) curb, without support | 35 months |
| Walk up a 4-inch (10-cm) curb, without support | 36 months |
| Fast step 100 feet (30 meters) in 25 seconds | 37 months |
| Walk across 7.5-inch (19-cm) wide balance beam | 38 months |
| Walk up stairs, two feet per stair, with one hand holding the rail | 39 months |
| Walk down stairs, two feet per stair, with one hand holding the rail | 40 months |
| Jump on floor with both feet together | 47 months |
| Walk down 8-inch (20-cm) curb, without support | 47 months |
| Walk up 8-inch (20-cm) curb, without support | 49 months |
| Run 100 feet (30 meters) in 15 seconds | 52 months |
| Walk up stairs, one foot per stair, with one hand holding the rail | 56 months |
| Pedal tricycle 15 feet (4.5 meters) | 61 months |
| *The following skills have a wide range of variability:* | |
| Walk across 4.5-inch (11-cm) wide balance beam | 64 months |
| Walk down stairs, one foot per stair, with one hand holding the rail | 6-8 years |

# Factors That Affect the Development of Post Walking Skills

A number of factors will influence your child's ability to master the nine skill areas of the Post Walking period of development. These factors fall into four categories:

1. Physical problems: including hypotonia, decreased strength, increased joint flexibility due to lax ligaments, short arms and legs, and difficulty with balance;
2. Temperament;
3. Attention;
4. Readiness and motivation to do a skill.

## Physical Problems

The physical problems observed in children with Down syndrome are covered at the beginning of the book on pages xii-xv. Now that your child is older, his **hypotonia** has decreased and you probably will not notice it when he is doing an established skill that he executes efficiently. However, when he is learning a new skill such as running or jumping, you will notice it in the area of coordination. You will also notice it in his abdomen when he stands still in a relaxed position. When he is at rest, his abdomen may protrude due to hypotonia. However, if you watch his abdomen when he is active, you will see that he has strong abdominal muscles when he activates them.

Your child's **strength** will improve with repetition and practice. The key is to find the activities that he likes to do, and then he will naturally do them often and for long periods. As he practices, watch his movements and help him do the skills properly so he develops strength in the right muscles, and in the optimal way.

**Increased joint flexibility** will be present and the primary areas to focus on are his feet, knees, and neck. Your child will have his own unique degree of laxity. The goal is to be proactive to protect his joints so he does not stretch his ligaments further. He may have ligamentous laxity in his ankles and knees, and need foot support to walk with a refined pattern and for improved gross motor skill performance. The next section of this chapter will address foot management. Also watch his sitting posture on the floor. If he makes a habit of w-sitting, encourage him to sit instead on a child's chair or a bench (90/90 sitting), or to sit with legs crossed (criss-cross position). When a child uses the w-sit position, he excessively stretches the medial knee ligaments and this adds to the knee tilt (valgus) when standing and walking.

People with Down syndrome are also at risk for **atlantoaxial instability,** due to ligamentous laxity at the first two bones of the neck. In this condition, one of the topmost vertebrae in the neck slips forward on the next vertebra and compresses the spinal cord. (See page 313.)

The **length of your child's arms and legs** will be short relative to the length of his trunk. This will affect the following skills: walking up and down stairs and curbs and pedaling a tricycle. Sometimes you will need to wait for his legs to grow before he can achieve the next goal in these skill areas.

Children with Down syndrome have difficulty with **balance skills** and need practice to gain competence in this area. They may need foot support to be successful (see "Foot Management," below). They also need to be motivated to persevere with practicing it, so the setup needs to be fun for them. For example, a child may not want to stand on one foot for several seconds in the clinic setting, but he may want to do the tree pose in yoga class or the passé pose in dance class. He will also learn balance by practicing skills such as kicking a ball, walking up and down curbs (without hand support), and walking across a balance beam (without hand support).

## Temperament

Whether your child is motor driven or an observer, he will be active during the Post Walking period of development. It is still important to observe which temperament your child tends to have as he learns each new skill and be sensitive to his learning style in your approach to teaching the post walking skills.

If he is **motor driven,** he will prefer vigorous gross motor activities such as running, climbing, walking up and down inclined surfaces, kicking the ball, and jumping. When practicing skills, he will enjoy it if you move fast. He will not want to move slowly and pay attention, for example with balance beam skills. He will tend to be risky and do activities without paying attention to how to do them safely. He will need to be supervised closely to see what he is up to and to make sure he is safe. As he practices the skills, he will learn how to do them safely, and he will learn to pay attention.

If your child is an **observer,** he will pay attention to each skill and try to do it with control. He will like walking on a balance beam and walking up and down stairs with support. He will tolerate practicing all of the post walking skills with support, so he can learn how to do each skill. Once he is comfortable with doing the skill, he will do it on his own. He will enjoy running fast with support and will need encouragement to learn to run fast on his own. He will tend to be careful, so will feel safer practicing skills that he knows how to do.

## Attention

Certain post walking skills will require your child to move slower and pay attention. When your child walks on uneven surfaces, around obstacles, and from one surface to another, he will need to look down at the ground to plan how he can walk and avoid falling. When he walks across the balance beam, he will need to watch his feet and step within the boundary. When walking up and down a 2-inch (5-cm) curb, he will need to be aware of it and plan how to step up and down with control. By practicing these skills, he will learn to slow down and pay attention to what he is doing so he can be successful.

If your child is an observer, he will pay attention to the details of what he sees and feels, and will react with a plan of how to move safely. If your child is motor driven, he will tend to take the trial-and-error approach and react in the moment. If you give verbal and visual cues to elicit his attention, then he will begin to notice the details that he needs to attend to for each skill. He will learn to pay attention by practicing the skills that require it.

When needed, help your child focus his attention by giving visual, verbal, or tactile cues. Set the equipment up in such a way that he sees different surfaces, or he watches a sibling model the skill so he can imitate how his sibling did it. Give him verbal cues like "up" and "down" so he notices that he needs to step up and down the mat surface. He will experience the tactile cues as he practices the skill. For example, if you practice balance beam skills by walking across a 7.5-inch (19-cm) wide piece of wood placed on the floor, your child will notice when he steps out of the boundary. This setup will get his attention better than walking between two pieces of tape or a painted stripe on the floor. With each skill, there are ways to help your child pay attention in order to learn how to do it. You will learn to be creative in finding ways to help him focus his attention.

## *Readiness and Motivation to Do the Skill*

Let your child choose the skills he wants to practice since he will naturally show you what he is motivated to do. If he likes a skill, he will automatically challenge himself to the next level, and he will initiate practicing it for many repetitions. To broaden what he chooses to practice, encourage siblings and peers to practice certain skills with him. If he sees that they like to do the skill, then he will want to do it with them. Practicing with his siblings and peers will give him models to imitate but even more importantly, he will be motivated to do the skill because they are doing it. If your child is not showing an interest in a particular skill, practice it briefly in a fun way to keep it familiar while you wait for him to show the desire to do it. When he is ready and motivated to do a skill, he will figure out what he needs to do to be successful.

# Foot Management
## *What Causes Flat Feet in Children with Down Syndrome?*

As discussed in Chapter 4, children with Down syndrome are at risk for foot alignment problems, primarily due to ligamentous laxity. The ligaments that hold the bones of the feet together have more stretch, so they do not hold the bones together tightly for optimal alignment and function. The joints of the foot have excessive flexibility, which causes instability and inefficient mechanics when standing and walking, and doing post walking skills.

The foot has 26 bones and can be divided into 3 sections: the **hindfoot** (the heel bone and the talus, which sits on top of the heel bone), the **midfoot** (5 small bones in close contact with the bones of the hindfoot), and the **forefoot** (5 long bones of the foot, and the 14 bones of the toes). In children with Down syndrome, ligamentous laxity can cause the following alignment problems in these areas of the foot:

1. **Hindfoot:** The top of the heel bone tilts inward (rather than being held vertically), which causes the talus to slide downward and toward the inside border of the foot, resulting in a flat arch. (See figs. 6.4-6.5.) You can observe this heel tilt by standing behind your child and watching his heels as he stands and walks barefoot.

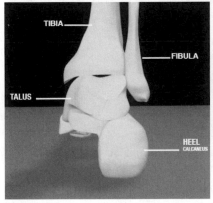 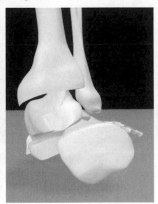 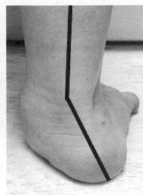

(fig. 6.3) Optimal alignment, heel vertical   (fig. 6.4) Heel tilt   (fig. 6.5)

2. **Midfoot:** Depending on the degree of laxity, the bones of the midfoot may be pulled inward by the sloping talus, and then the arch is flattened further. (See figs. 6.7-6.8.) You can observe the flatness of the arch and the length of the flatness by looking at your child's arch from the side view.

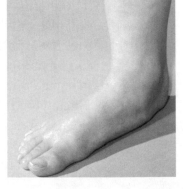

(fig. 6.8)

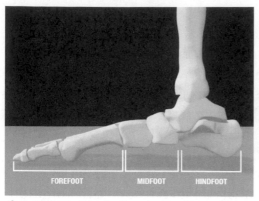
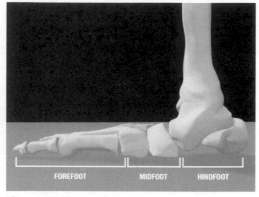

(fig. 6.6) Optimal alignment with arch        (fig. 6.7) Flat arch

**3. Forefoot:** After you have observed your child's hindfoot and midfoot, stand in front of him and observe whether his feet point straight ahead or turn outward (called toeing-out). With the heel tilt and the collapse and stretch of the medial arch, the long bones of the foot and the toes may turn outward. (See figs. 6.10-6.11.)

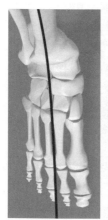
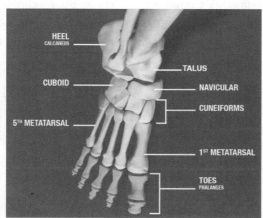
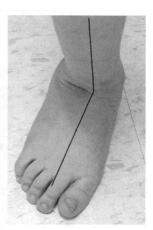

*left* (fig. 6.9) Optimal alignment, foot pointing straight; *center* (fig 6.10); *right* (fig. 6.11) Toeing out

4. If the heel tilts and the entire inside border of the foot is collapsed, you may also see that the **big toe** turns and bends (toward the second toe) or tilts sideways toward the second toe (fig. 6.12).

5. If your child has toeing-out (3 and/or 4) as described above, he will also have excessive weight bearing on the **ball of his big toe.** Eventually, this can cause callous formation, and walking can be painful, especially when he is older and bigger.

6. In some children, you see the opposite position of the big toe. The big toe tilts inward, and it is caused by an overactive muscle, the abductor hallucis longus (fig. 6.13). The degree of the toeing-in may just involve the big toe, or it may cause the forefoot to turn inward.

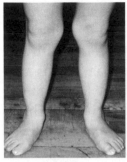

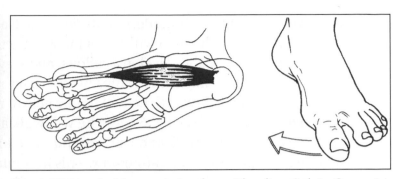

(fig. 6.12)

(fig. 6.13) Used with permission from: Blandine Calais-Germain, *Anatomy of Movement* (Seattle, WA: Eastland Press, 2007), 284.

## *Why Is Flat Footedness a Problem?*

If your child has any of the alignment problems described above, there will be functional consequences in all gross motor skills involving standing. Not only does it affect the foot and ankle movements, but also the movements of the joints above—in particular, the knees and hips. The individual joint movements do not occur properly, and then you have the added effect of several joints moving improperly. A simple comparison is to see how a door swings on its hinges. It glides when it is working properly but scrapes, impinges, and stops moving when it is not hung right, and it takes more power to move. If your child has faulty foot alignment, he cannot use his strength effectively because the muscles are not aligned for efficient activation. Since his strength does not generate efficient power, he uses more energy to do the skill and fatigues more quickly.

Since walking is vital for your child's mobility for his entire lifetime, it is very important to be proactive in promoting optimal alignment and function, beginning when he learns to walk. The consequences of faulty mechanics range from impaired performance to pain, which can result in limitations in walking.

Examples of **common alignment problems and their consequences** are:

1. If your child's heels tilt an he has flat arches and walks bearing weight on the inside borders of his feet, he will walk with a wider base, with his heels wider than his hips. If you look at his knees, they will probably tilt inward. When you look at his legs and feet, they will not be in the optimal vertical alignment but instead will have varying degrees of tilting at each joint (fig. 6.14). When he walks and runs using toe push-off, he will take excessive

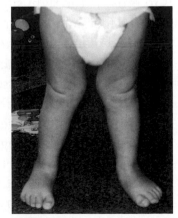

(fig. 6.14)

weight on the inside borders of his feet, especially under the ball of his big toe. This area will take a lot of impact and shearing forces and will probably develop a callous, and may become painful.

2. If your child walks with his hips in external rotation (thighs and knees turned outward), he will not be able to move his hips into hyperextension (see fig. 6.2), so he will walk and run with shorter steps. He will walk and run with hips and knees bent, like a jogging pattern. If he cannot move his hips into hyperextension, he will not be able to use toe push-off for efficient propulsion. (In order to move the hip into hyperextension, the hip needs to be in neutral rotation.)

3. If he uses the walking and running patterns described above, he will learn to do these skills using faulty mechanics, and will not learn to do them efficiently or progress to his optimal performance level. As his growth increases over time, his ligaments will be further stretched in this pattern. The long-term effect will be muscle tightness, and his feet will become rigid in the position. However, if you provide foot support, his feet will remain flexible enough to accommodate the support and he will have flexible flat feet (that can be supported in the optimal position) rather than rigid flat feet.

## What Can Be Done?

Your child will need to be evaluated to see *if* foot support is needed. If it is needed, then it is important to determine **when** the best time is to start using foot support. The vast majority of children with Down syndrome will need support to provide stability. Some children begin using foot support when they are learning to walk with support, and others use foot support after walking is mastered, in order to refine their walking pattern. The goal is to provide the right support for two purposes: 1) optimal alignment of the legs and feet, and 2) improved function. Your child needs to be able to use the support dynamically for efficient walking and running, so he can walk and run with speed for long distances.

The best time to first evaluate whether your child needs foot support is after he pulls to stand (from sitting on the floor) by himself and is motivated to play in standing (Stage 4). When he can pull to stand, he is ready to practice cruising and stepping with your assistance (Stage 5). The foot support is only beneficial when he is in standing, so the best time to begin using it (if needed) is when he is at this skill level. Therefore, when a child pulls to stand and wants to stand much of the time, I evaluate his standing posture to determine whether foot support is needed. (See box on pages 184-85.)

If your child did not need foot support when first evaluated, then continue to watch his foot posture as he spends more time in standing and practicing stepping with support. When he practices walking with support several times daily for long distances, his foot posture may change and foot support may be needed. If he does not need foot support when he is learning to walk, then evaluate his feet after he is walking independently, all of the time. At this time, evaluate whether foot support is needed to refine his walking pattern.

To evaluate your child's foot posture to determine whether he needs foot support, you need the best setup. Watch his feet while he is walking barefooted to observe his best performance and the variations he tends to use.

Here are recommended guidelines to follow:

1. Have him walk *quickly and directly* to a specific endpoint about 30-50 feet away. If possible, use a long hallway so he is not distracted. He needs to walk a long distance so he is motivated to use an efficient pattern. If he walks slowly, turns his head to look at something, deviates to the right or left, or is distracted, you will see changes in his foot posture. Practice in this space for several repetitions to observe his best performance.

2. Observe his walking pattern from these 3 views:

    **A. Standing behind him**:
    - Look at the width of his base by observing how close together his heels are. See if he walks with a wide base (heels wider than hips) or a narrow base (heels in line with his hips).
    - Look at his heels and see if they are vertical or if they tilt while he is walking. Watch one foot at a time if you need to so you can really study how it moves as he walks the long distance.
    - Look at his knees and see if his thighs and lower legs are vertical or if his knees tilt inward.

    **B. Standing in front of him**:
    - Watch his feet and see if they point straight ahead or if they turn outward.
    - Observe his knees to see if they tilt inward or if his legs are straight.

    **C. Standing at his side**, on the right and on the left
    - Look at the arch area of each foot and see if it is flat or if he activates his muscles to lift the arch a little.

3. The optimal walking posture is with a narrow base, his knees and heels vertical, and his feet pointing straight ahead.

4. If he does tilt the top of his heel bones inward, has flat arches, and his feet turn out, check the flexibility in his feet while he is standing. (His feet will need to be flexible to accommodate the support.) Sit on the floor in front of him and position his heels in line with his hips (narrow base) with his feet pointing straight. If needed, place your feet on the outsides of his feet to maintain them in this position. Then hold his heels and move them to the vertical position and see if you can move his feet so he has a lifted arch. If he does not tolerate the heel support, then cross your hands (palms up) and use your fingertips to lift his arches. Feel if he has the foot mobility to be supported in this position. When you are moving his feet to test the flexibility, let him hold onto a support if he feels unstable.

5. Do not evaluate his foot posture when standing and playing because he will automatically use a wider base and turn his feet out for stability. With a wider base and toeing-out, his heels will tilt and his arches will naturally be flat.

## What Types of Foot Support Are Recommended?

If your child needs foot support, a variety of types are available depending on his age, needs, size and weight, and what he will tolerate. His leg and foot posture will need to be evaluated along with his activity preferences and motor performance. What is needed for a 3-year-old is different than what is needed for a 13-year-old. The foot support will be a tool to improve his walking posture and gross motor skill performance. The goal of the foot support is to improve his function by providing support for optimal alignment so he can use his strength, balance, and coordination more efficiently. By improving his function, he will be motivated to be active, his endurance will increase, and his overall activity level will increase.

The type of support for each child needs to be determined on a case-by-case basis, and depends on the factors listed above. A critical factor is whether your child will tolerate the support, because it will not help him if he will not wear it. To determine the type of support needed, it is best to have a team approach, and the team needs to be experienced with the best types of foot support for children with Down syndrome and the goal of the support. The team can include the PT, orthotist, parents, pediatrician, and orthopedist. The recommended foot support will need to be tested for effectiveness and modified until the desired results are achieved.

In my experience, children with Down syndrome generally tolerate flexible supports better than rigid supports. Rigid supports tend to reduce the foot's ability to move naturally through the gait cycle. Many types of support are available, including a wrap-around support, also referred to as an SMO (supra-malleolar orthosis, above the ankle support), shoe inserts, and arch supports. The supports range from providing maximal support to minimal support.

I recommend that the support be used when the child is physically active, because that is when it will provide the most benefit. I focus on providing more support (SMO) when the child is a new walker and during the early years of walking in order to refine the walking pattern from the beginning. This strategy also is proactive in preventing further stretching of the ligaments. If this is achieved within the first 3 to 5 years of walking, while he is mastering the post walking skills, then I decrease the support to using shoe inserts in athletic shoes. The type of shoes used with the support is critical and is addressed in the next section. If your child is provided with support in the early years, then when he is an adolescent or adult, he may only need athletic shoes with good arch supports (already in them) or with inserts added.

If a child is learning to walk or is a new walker, the most direct way to align the foot is to support and stabilize the heel bone toward the vertical position. If the heel bone is held vertical, the surrounding bones move with it toward the desired position. (You can see this for yourself: If you hold your child's heel bone and move it vertically, you will notice that the inside border of his foot moves into an arch.) However, this support also needs to be dynamic and allow movement from side to side and from the heel to the ball of the foot. One brand that offers foot support that fulfills these criteria is the **SureStep**SM **Dynamic Stabilizing System.** (See fig. 6.15; website www.surestep.net.) This foot support has the following patented features in its design:

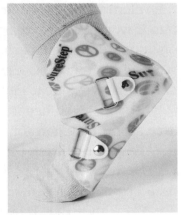

1. Thin, lightweight, flexible plastic: allows for more natural movement of the foot and ankle, assists the muscles to work efficiently, and maintains proper alignment when standing, walking, and running

2. Compression fit: the plastic stabilizes the foot and ankle by compressing them into alignment, and the foot can remain dynamic while stabilized (this allows for the development of much more natural movement patterns)

(fig. 6.15)

3. Trim lines: leave the toes free for squatting, running, jumping, and walking up and down inclines, curbs, and stairs.

In my experience, children tolerate the SureStep system well once they are accustomed to it (fig. 6.16). If they are learning to walk, they feel the sup-

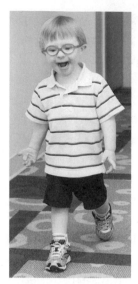

(fig. 6.16)

port and stability of standing and stepping with optimal alignment, and the skills become easier for them and require less energy. When a child uses this type of support after he has mastered walking, he learns how to use it dynamically, particularly when fast stepping and running. When weight shifting from the heel to ball of the foot, he develops the strength and movements needed to break them in (like a new shoe) and flex the plastic. With strategic practice designed to teach your child how to use these supports dynamically, he will develop an efficient walking pattern with toe push-off and improved performance and endurance in gross motor skills.

The SureStep system can be ordered by an ABC or BOC certified orthotist. (An orthotist is a professional who measures, designs, fabricates, fits, or services orthoses. An orthosis is a broad term to describe a device that will support or correct the positioning of a body part and is synonymous with the term "brace.") The orthotist needs to have training on measuring for the SureStep system and have experience with fitting and servicing it. If you need a referral for an experienced orthotist in your area, call 877-462-0711 or contact SureStep through their website. The SureStep system is covered by most health insurance policies, but discuss your insurance coverage with the orthotist who measures your child.

The SureStep system will be effective if it is put on properly, the circumference and length fit properly, the straps are tightened for a compression fit, the Velcro straps have adequate shear strength (gripping power), and the system is worn with the right type of shoe. Refer to the website for instructions on donning, tightening the straps, proper fit and trimlines, and replacing the straps. If your child is having problems, contact your orthotist right away to determine what is causing the problem and how to fix it.

If your child needs less support, you can investigate shoe inserts and arch supports. When you use these types of support, you are indirectly aligning the foot by lifting the bones of the arch to assist the heel alignment toward a more vertical position. Orthotists can provide a custom-made insert or fit an off-the-shelf model. Some examples of inserts are:

1. Cascade Dafo HotDog® inserts (fig. 6.17; www.cascadedafo.com) can be purchased through this company in Ferndale, Washington. These inserts have two layers of dense foam, a partial heel cup (concave space for the heel), a medial longitudinal arch (with optional foam arch filling), and a flexible toe lever. The arch area is long and wide to fully support the length and width of the child's arch. (I recommend adding the foam arch filling.)

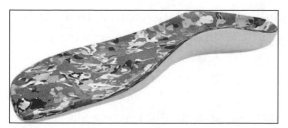

(fig. 6.17)

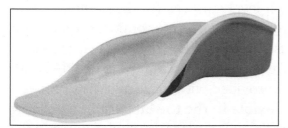

(fig. 6.18)

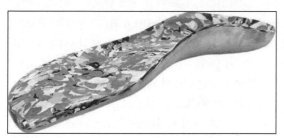

(fig. 6.19)

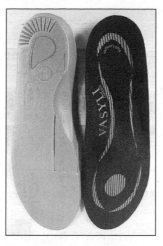

(fig. 6.20)

The flexible toe lever of the insert supports the foot from the ball of the foot to the toes, and makes toe push-off easier. Athletic shoes (lace-up) with good support provide vertical support to the heel, and hold the foot over the support of the insert base. When using these inserts, you will need to remove the original insole from the shoe and place the HotDog insert in the shoe.

Depending on the support your child needs, there are other products available from CascadeDafo, including the Chipmunk® (fig. 6.18) and PattiBob® (fig. 6.19). The PattiBob is similar to the HotDog, but has one layer of foam and one layer of plastic. The Chipmunk provides more support and has a plastic base, full heel cup, and full support to the medial side of the foot.

2. SUPERfeet® insoles (www.superfeet.com) can also be used. Colors vary depending on the support that is needed and what the insoles are used for. Many dealers sell this product, so they are available locally.

3. Vasyli® custom orthotics (fig. 6.20; www.vasylimedical.com) are another option. Check the website to see the products available. In my experience, the medium density (blue) full length custom orthotics for athletic footwear work well in athletic shoes.

4. You can also visit running shoe stores or sporting goods stores to see what types of shoes and support are available for "pronators."

5. For some children and adults, good athletic shoes with a good fit, base, and arch support insole will provide the stability and comfort needed when physically active.

## What Shoes Are Best?

Whether your child uses foot support or not, the type of shoes worn when he is physically active is critical. If he is a new walker and working on the goal of walking all of the time on level surfaces (in the home), he will probably walk longer distances if barefoot. When he is a confident walker and walks all of the time on level surfaces, then he will be ready to learn the new skill of walking with shoes. It will take time for him to adjust to walking with shoes, and he will learn most easily if provided with the ideal type of shoes.

It is best if the **shoes are very flexible in the toe box area**, so bending the soles of the shoes is easy. To test for flexibility, place your index finger in the shoe where the ball of the foot will be positioned. Then place your thumb and fingers on the outside edges of the soles. Place the shoe on a firm surface and feel the force needed to bend the sole of the shoe where the ball of the foot will be. If there is significant resistance, then see if you can flex the shoe in this area to "break" it in. If it does not bend easily, then your child will not be able to bend it, and he will limit his foot and ankle movements due to the stiffness of the sole of the shoe. He will feel the stiffness of the soles and will not have the strength or initiative to push against it in order to break them in. If these shoes are used, he will learn to walk with a marching pattern (full-sole weight bearing) and will not progress to walking with a heel-toe pattern (weight shifting from the heels to the balls of his feet), ultimately using toe push-off.

If your child is not setup with ideal shoes, his performance and leg and foot posture will be compromised. He may totally resist wearing shoes, he may walk with knee stiffness, slap his feet, or use a heavy-footed pattern when stepping.

When selecting shoes for daily use, lightweight, supportive **athletic shoes** with flexible soles are the best type. Since styles change, you will need to experiment with different brands of athletic shoes to determine what is best for your child. Ideally, the base of the shoe will support the bottom of the foot, and the sides and heel of the shoe will hold the foot up over the base. Therefore, you need to examine the base, medial counter, and heel of the shoe.

It is best if the shoe has a **narrow fit** so the heel and the arch area can be supported effectively. If it is a wide fit, his heel and arch will have a big space to move within the shoe, and the heel will tilt and the arch will be flat. The **medial counter needs to be firm and supportive** to lift the long arch of the foot. If it is flimsy, it will tilt inward to take the shape of the child's flat-footed posture. The **heel counter needs to be firm and raised,** since its purpose is to hold the heel vertically.

**Lace-up closures** are better than Velcro closures to hold the foot over the support of the base. With Velcro, it is difficult to close the shoe tightly, and the loose fit allows the foot to tilt into the flat-footed posture. Even if the Velcro can be fastened tightly, over time the shear strength of the Velcro wears out. You can also use the **Yankz! Sure Lace System** (www.yankz.com) to avoid having to tie the laces.

The **rubber nonslip soles** of the athletic shoes will prevent sliding on slippery surfaces and provide traction so your child will feel more stable. Also look at the side view of the shoe to see if the **toe box** is flat on the floor or if it **curves upward** at the end of the shoe. It is best if it curves upward because if it is flat, your child will trip more easily. High top shoes are not recommended because they will limit ankle mobility. When the laces are tightened, it will be difficult for your child to bend his lower leg forward over his foot so this will limit his performance when learning running, walking up and down curbs, stairs, and inclines, bouncing, and jumping.

After you have found the perfect shoes, your child will need time and practice to learn how to walk with them. He may resist them in the beginning and want to take them off. Or, his stepping pattern may change as he learns how to walk in them, and he may start by using a wider base, stiff knees, and toeing out. He may also trip often, which may frustrate him.

To help your child become familiar with shoes, set him up to be successful. Start with using the shoes for brief periods when he is at his physical best. Practice with hand support, either holding your hand or pushing a grocery cart or push-toy. Also practice fast stepping with two-hand support because this will help him break in the shoes and learn to step quickly in them. If he can step quickly, he will be able to avoid tripping. When he is more comfortable wearing the shoes, then gradually increase the time he wears them. His leg and foot strength and coordination will improve with practice. When he is ready, you can focus on refining his walking pattern in the shoes so he uses them dynamically to walk with a narrow base, feet pointing straight, with hip hyperextension and toe push-off.

If your child uses foot support inside the shoes, additional details need to be checked when selecting shoes to use with them. **If he uses the SureStep system**, the shoe needs to have extra room over the front opening to expand to fit over the SureStep. The shoe also needs to lace down far enough (toward the toes) so the shoe can be opened up wide enough to place the SureStep and foot into the shoe. A broad, rounded toe box design tends to work best. The adjustability of the lace closure is needed, since the Velcro strap will probably be too short to fit over the extra width of the SureStep in the shoe. I am currently recommending the Cohesion model of Saucony shoes (www.saucony.com) for children with Down syndrome. There is also a SureStep athletic shoe that is flexible and is specifically designed to accommodate any type of foot support with a wider, deeper heel, toe box, and instep.

**If he uses inserts such as HotDogs,** the shoe needs to provide support to hold his foot up over the support, and lace closures are best. If your child uses the orthoses or inserts, the insole in the bottom of the shoe needs to be removed. With the insole removed, he will have more room for a comfortable fit in the toe box area, and his foot will fit more deeply in the shoe so the shoe can provide stability and support.

After your child is comfortable and familiar with walking with shoes and the foot support in the shoes, his walking pattern will likely improve by using this foot management and practicing post-walking skills. However, if his walking pattern does not improve, it may be due to the shoes used. If the shoe is too long, too wide, or feels heavy, cumbersome, or stiff to him, he may walk with a clumsy or awkward pattern. If this happens, experiment with different brands and styles of athletic shoes to see which shoes promote the best walking pattern in your child.

Try to find a child-friendly shoe store where the employees are willing to remove the insoles of shoes so your child can try them out with his type of foot support (orthoses or inserts). Parents in a local Down syndrome support group may be able to direct you to an accommodating store.

## Once My Child Has the Right Foot Support and Shoes, Then What?

When your child has the ideal foot support and shoes, he needs to practice post-walking skills to learn to use them dynamically. With structured practice, he will gain the strength and coordination to bend the support and shoes to move efficiently for each of the post walking skills. It is critical for your child to learn to weight shift through his feet from the heels to the toes, and to use toe push-off. Fast stepping and running will be the best skills to practice to achieve this. Using the foot support and shoes will improve the alignment of his feet and improve his mechanics for walking and running. He will fully benefit from them if he learns to use them dynamically for each skill.

When he can move efficiently with his foot support and shoes, you will notice that he is light on his feet. He will use his leg and foot strength and achieve the final components for a refined walking pattern. He will hold his trunk erect and lean it forward, use hip hyperextension and toe push-off, and have a longer step length. The foot support and shoes will improve his alignment and he will be able to use his strength, coordination, and balance more effectively. His endurance will improve and he will be motivated to be active since his movements will be more energy efficient.

Now you have seen the benefits of using proper foot support and shoes. It will be important to watch your child's foot and leg posture over his lifetime and provide the right foot support and shoes when he is physically active. Exercise will be an important part of his life. It will be critical to give him the foot support and shoes that will give him access to an active lifestyle.

# Guidelines

*Provide an environment* **with equipment that is safe and offers a variety of activities to do.** Now that your child can walk, he will want to be independent and explore more than ever before. To encourage his independence, you will need to select or setup environments where he can play with minimal intervention from you. You can setup a room in your home or your backyard, or go to the park, especially one with a toddler playground. He can go to Discovery Zone, Monkey Bizness, or to community toddler programs, such as Gymboree, My Gym, The Little Gym, or the YMCA. He will love playing with the other children in these programs, using the equipment, and having fun. You can take long walks around the neighborhood, at the zoo, or at the mall. With these environments, he can choose where he wants to walk and what he wants to do. You can let him be the leader and supervise him so he is safe.

*Introduce all of the skills* **and see what he is interested in doing.** Let him focus on the skills he likes so they become familiar and he learns the routines for practicing those skills. With practice, he will love to do them on his own, and will do several repetitions. He will enjoy the independence and the freedom to be in control. Gradually add in other skills as tolerated. Over time, he will be motivated to practice all of them.

*Let your child choose the order of activities* **he wants to do.** After you have selected or setup an environment, let him move from one activity to another in the order he chooses. Let him repeat each activity as long as he is interested. You can help him practice activities that are hard for him to do by himself.

**Alternate** *easier* **and** *harder* **skills.** Watch your child and see which skills he finds easy and which are hard. Look for a pattern and see if he prefers vigorous activities, like running and jumping, or slower moving and attentive activities, like walking across a balance beam or walking up/down curbs. Once you figure out which skills are easier for him, guide him to try a challenging skill after he has gained confidence from practicing the easier skill. If he will practice the challenging skill, make it fun by doing it with his sibling, and make sure he is successful. Give extra support if needed. Let him practice it as long as he wants to and then let him do his preferred skills again.

In the beginning of the post walking period, he will want to explore, so the easier skills to practice will be walking on uneven surfaces, walking up and down inclined surfaces, fast stepping, and kicking a ball. The intermediate level skills will be walking up and down curbs and stairs, running, jumping, and walking across balance beams. The advanced level skills will be walking across a 4-inch (10-cm) wide balance beam and riding a tricycle.

*Follow the sequence of steps* **within each skill area.** Each skill area will have goals, and there will be a list of steps to practice to achieve the goals. You will determine what your child can do and what is next for him to learn to do. Begin at his level, and, when he is ready, help him practice what is next.

*Motivate* **your child to practice the skills.** Your child will love practicing skills with other children. He will practice longer and the repetitions will improve his performance. He will watch the other children and imitate what he sees them doing. He will also take turns with them, which will give him a few seconds to recover in between practices.

**Provide** *visual* **cues and simple** *verbal* **cues.** Your child will learn best by *watching* other children and *hearing key words* to label the game they are playing. If there is a special way to do the skill, have his friend demonstrate it or exaggerate the movement, and then your child will imitate him. For example, when walking up and down the 2-inch (5-cm) mat, the playmate can march and say "march, march, march" as he walks on the floor, and then say "up" and "down" when walking up and down the mat. If you show your child and name what he is doing, he will learn the routine and be ready to practice the skill.

**Do activities for short periods, or** *for as long as he wants to.* Your child will show you how long he is motivated or physically able to practice an activity. If he no longer wants to practice a skill, it is best to stop at that time, and he may choose to go back to it later. He will perform the skill better when he chooses to do it.

*Be prepared* **for toddler experiences.** Your child will use his newly developed skills wherever he is. He may use his new running skills to run away from you when you are in the grocery store or department store. He may use his climbing skills to get something you never imagined he could reach. For example, Elizabeth was in her bedroom, which had been "child proofed." She figured out that if she moved the hamper over to the dresser, she could climb on the hamper and up on her dresser to get the Balmex cream. She did this and had a few seconds of fun putting Balmex on her face and on the mirror before her mother found her!

**Test whether your child can do a** *new* **skill better when using shoes (with/without support) or when barefoot.** When he is first learning a skill, his success may depend on what he has on his feet. Once he has the strength to do the skill, he will be able to do it barefoot or with shoes (with/without support).

Children with Down Syndrome are at increased risk for Atlanto-axial Instability (AAI) and Occipital-Atlantal Instability (OAI). It is important to know about these conditions so they can be quickly diagnosed, managed, and treated if present. These conditions occur due to instability at the joints of the first two vertebrae (bones) of the neck (AAI) or the joint between the skull and the first bone of the neck (OAI). In Down syndrome, a combination of bony abnormalities, lax ligaments, and hypotonia can contribute to instability in these joints. The instability, if symptomatic, can cause impingement with one of the vertebrae pressing on the spinal cord.

If there is spinal cord impingement, you may suddenly see any of the signs listed in the box about atlantoaxial instability below. If you see any of these changes, your child needs medical attention immediately, as detailed on the flyer.

Since children with Down syndrome are at risk for these conditions, you want to avoid movements or activities that put excessive stress on the neck.

---

### Atlantoaxial Instability

Children with Down syndrome are at increased risk of developing compression of the spinal cord due to a condition called atlantoaxial instability. This problem is caused by a combination of low tone, loose ligaments, and bony changes. The spinal cord can be pressed by the bones and cause nerve damage. Symptoms of nerve damage can occur at any time and there is no test or x-ray that can tell who is at risk.

Parents should watch their child for any changes in how they walk or use their arms or hands, a head tilt, complaints of pain in the neck, change in bowel or bladder function, change in general function, or new onset weakness.

> **Contact physician immediately for an x-ray of the neck in neutral position if your child has:**
>
> - Change in how he or she walks
> - Change in how he or she uses arms/hands
> - Change in bowel or bladder control
> - Head stays tilted
> - Neck Pain
> - New onset weakness
> - Decreased activity level or function
>
> If the x-ray is abnormal or symptoms persist, the child should be referred as soon as possible to a pediatric neurosurgeon or pediatric orthopedic surgeon experienced in managing atlantoaxial instability.

*Used with permission of the Down Syndrome Program at Riley Hospital for Children at Indiana University Health*

You want to prevent wild or sudden movements of the head, either forward or backward. Restrict participation in contact sports or physical activities that place the neck at risk for trauma.

For more information, refer to *Babies with Down Syndrome: A New Parents' Guide* (Woodbine House, 2008, pages 83-84); the article by Marilyn Bull in the References; or the Down Syndrome: Health Issues website (www.ds-health.com).

**Avoid the w-sitting position when sitting on the floor to play.** If you notice that your child uses this position in his pre-school program or when sitting and playing on the floor, you need to be proactive to limit it. You can teach him the new position of crossing his legs (criss-cross or ring sit position), and you can encourage sitting in a child's chair (90/90 sitting) when playing at a table or watching TV. If he uses this w-sit position regularly, it will put stress on the medial aspects of his knees, and stretch these ligaments. Your child may already have increased laxity in these ligaments, and he may stand with his knees tilting in (in combination with his flat footed posture). Since the goal is to encourage vertical alignment in his legs when standing, it is best to avoid the w-sit position.

**While practicing post walking skills, his** *abdominal strength will improve*. Toddlers typically walk with the low back arched and the belly protruding. Through practicing post walking skills, your child will learn to activate his abdominal muscles when standing and walking, and his strength will improve. Don't judge his abdominal strength by looking at his belly when relaxed in standing. (Just as you would not look at your belly when relaxed!) To see him contract his abdominals, take his shirt off and look at his belly when he is fast stepping and running, kicking a ball, walking on uneven surfaces (like sand), walking up and down inclined surfaces, stepping up and down curbs and stairs, bouncing and jumping, and walking across balance beams. He will also improve his abdominal strength through climbing, squatting, carrying large objects, pushing a weighted cart, and reaching up to open and close doors or pushing heavy doors open.

Through activating his abdominal muscles in standing, he will balance the strength between his back and abdominal muscles, and his trunk posture will be erect and easily move between arching and tucking. At this age, it is best to strengthen abdominal muscles through doing a variety of gross motor activities that he is naturally motivated to do.

# How to Use Chapters 7 through 15

Each of the chapters will focus on one of the nine skill areas of the Post Walking period of development. There will be a goal or goals for each skill area. The steps needed to achieve each goal will be explained, along with instructions on how to practice the steps properly. Tips or guidelines will be provided to let you know how to practice the skills most effectively.

Each chapter ends with a checklist of motor milestones. Using it, you can keep track of what your child can do in each skill area. Since you will be practicing many of the skill areas at once, the checklist will help you keep track of what has been accomplished and what to focus on next.

With practice in the post walking skills and with proper foot support, your child will develop a refined walking pattern, achieve the skills he needs to play with peers, and gain the skills for independence in his home, school, and community. He will learn to run, jump, walk up and down curbs and stairs, and ride a tricycle. He will build the foundation needed for exercise and fitness for life. Once this foundation is established, then he can practice what he is motivated to do in order to further develop strength, coordination, speed, balance, and endurance.

# 7

# Walking on Uneven Surfaces

## Introduction

Your child has mastered walking on level surfaces and is confident and motivated to walk. The next skill for her to learn is walking on all types of surfaces, for example, on a mat or other squishy surface, grass, sand, sidewalk, wood chips, and gravel. You can practice on any surface your geographic location has to offer, including snow. The goals will be to walk on all types of surfaces, to walk smoothly from one type of surface to another, and to walk over or around obstacles on the floor.

To learn to walk, your child figured out the most stable and reliable method that worked best for her body. This is now her automatic habit for walking, and she will use it consistently when walking on level surfaces. Her walking pattern is typical for a "new walker": a wide base, stiffness in her knees, feet turned out, and full sole weight bearing. She may also slap her feet or use a heavy-footed pattern. *To change this pattern, you need to change the surface she walks on.* By changing the surface, you will challenge her to find a new way to move her body and balance herself with each step.

When she takes a step on the new surface, her foot will be in an unfamiliar position due to the uneven nature of the surface, and she will need to learn how to move her foot, leg, and trunk to keep her balance and take another step without falling. Initially, she will meet the challenge by stiffening her knees and continuing to use a wide base. With practice and lots of repetitions, she will learn new strategies such as weight shifting through her feet, bending her knees, narrowing her base, and activating her abdominals. Her balance and strength will need to improve to effectively walk on these surfaces.

---

## Steps in Learning to Walk on Uneven Surfaces

Your child will learn to achieve the goals in this skill area using the following steps:

1. Walking on a variety of surfaces:
   a. walking on a firm or squishy mat (or some other kind of soft, squishy surface like a mattress, a sofa bed mattress, a futon, a float, or a water bed)
   b. walking on grass
   c. walking on sand
   d. walking on a sidewalk with cracked, uneven pavement
   e. walking on wood chips and gravel
2. Walking from one surface to another (same height)
3. Walking around or over obstacles on the floor

---

## Components

The components to develop are:

1. weight shifting in her feet in all directions, onto her heels, from her heels to the balls of her feet, and sideways
2. strength in her feet to balance in all directions, and toe push-off to propel herself forward
3. weight shifting the trunk and pelvis forward over her foot, which also causes her lower leg to move forward over her foot
4. bending her knees and using her abdominals for balance as needed
5. willingness to challenge herself by walking on these new surfaces, and to quickly regain her balance
6. looking down at the surface to notice obstacles on the floor or the new surface she is approaching

## Tendencies

The tendencies are:

1. to have inactive feet and continue to step with full sole weight bearing and foot slap
2. to march, stepping with her trunk and pelvis vertical over her feet
3. to stiffen her knees and widen her base for balance
4. to be afraid and freeze on the new surface, or to move to the ground and creep or bear walk
5. to look forward and not pay attention to the surface or obstacles in her path

## Setup for Learning

When your child is beginning to practice walking on a new surface, think about how it feels to her as she takes each step. As you step with her, feel what the surface is like and how your feet and body move on it. This will be hard for you since your body already knows how to walk on this surface. To appreciate how it feels to your child, imagine stepping onto a surface that is challenging to you; for example, stepping on ice. You might take one or two steps and fall. Then you would know to pay attention to the new surface. You would move your body differently than how you ordinarily walk. You would be conscious of each step and would constantly work to maintain your balance. You would learn how big a step to take and how fast to move. Initially, you would move stiffly, but with practice, would move more freely. Your child will go through this learning experience with each surface she walks on.

Below is the typical sequence in which children learn to walk on surfaces, from easier to harder. Each surface requires different movements and strategies for balance. When practicing walking on these surfaces for the first time, your child will need hand support while becoming familiar with how the surface feels and figuring how to step on the surface. With practice, she will develop the strength needed to walk on the surface. When she is ready to walk on the surface without hand support, she will work on the balance strategies needed for that surface.

## Sequence of Surfaces

### Mat

When your child first steps on a squishy mat, her feet will feel the surface moving, and she will feel off balance (fig. 7.1). Keeping her balance will be her first priority, and her reaction will be to put out her hands and activate her abdominals to balance herself. She may also widen her base, take smaller steps, and move stiffly. Her feet will sink into the surface, so she will need to activate her calf muscles to use toe push-off to take a step. The softer the surface, the more she will sink in. It will be easier if you begin with a firmer surface and then gradually try softer surfaces when she is ready.

It is best to use a surface large enough so she practices for several steps before she reaches the edge. For example, use a sofa bed mattress rather than a sofa cushion because

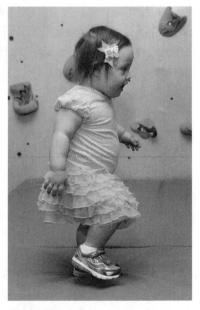

(fig. 7.1)

she would only take a few steps on the cushion and then be done. At home, you can practice walking on crib and bed mattresses. If you go to a gym, recreation center, or toddler gym program, you will have an assortment of mats to walk on, from a 1- to 2-inch (2.5- to 5-cm) high firm mat to a 4-inch (10-cm) high squishy mat. You can also be creative and see what you have around the house, like a pool float or interlocking foam squares.

### Grass

Walking on the grass is challenging because the unevenness of the surface is unpredictable. Your child constantly needs to pay attention and make adjustments. When first walking on this surface by herself, she will fall often. You need to watch her reaction to falling and provide support if she becomes frustrated. If she is fine with falling and quickly moves back to standing, then she does not need support. Using her hands to catch herself when she falls will help her gain the arm strength and speed needed for effective protective reactions. She will practice this skill until she can walk across the grass without falling and can move at the same speed as she does on level surfaces.

Many children are also affected by the texture of the surface and do not want to touch it with their hands or feet. When your child is walking on the grass, experiment with walking barefoot. If she cannot tolerate the texture on her bare feet, have her wear shoes. If she does not mind walking barefoot, have her practice with and without shoes.

### Sand

Walking on sand is similar to walking on a mat, but much more difficult. Your child's foot will sink deeper into the sand and she will need more strength to take steps. At first, she may use the method of marching to walk on the sand. With practice, she will learn to weight shift through her feet from her heels to the balls of her feet. After she can do this movement, she will develop strength to generate propulsion for toe push-off to take steps. To be most effective walking on sand, she will also need to lean her trunk and pelvis forward over her toes, and move her lower leg forward over her feet. She can practice walking on wet and dry sand, and figure out what adjustments to make. When she is comfortable walking on sand, the next challenges will be to walk longer distances and faster on this surface.

### Sidewalk

Walking on a sidewalk is dangerous since your child could injure herself if she falls. It is best to wait until she is an experienced walker and ready to walk on this surface. She will need to have fast and effective protective reactions, be able to walk well on uneven surfaces, and be able to pay attention to the surface and obstacles on the ground. She will need shoes to protect her feet, so she needs to be used to wearing shoes, and they need to be broken in. It is easy for her toes or the rubber edge of the shoe to catch, causing her to trip and fall.

You need to help avoid falls by watching the surface. If it slopes or the pavement is cracked or uneven, provide hand support for your child's safety. Initially, you will need to point out the changes in the surface; later, she will notice them herself.

### Wood Chips and Gravel

To walk on wood chips and gravel, your child needs to learn to walk on a variety of irregularly shaped, hard, uneven surfaces. As she places her foot on the surface, her foot position will dramatically change. Her ankle will be torqued and she will need to move her leg and body to balance over her foot in this new position. With each step, she will make new, quick, unique adjustments due to the inconsistency of the surfaces.

### Other Surfaces

Depending on where you live and where your child plays, you may have additional types of surfaces to walk on. At the park, you may have a "swinging bridge" to walk across (fig. 7.2). She can practice walking across it, balancing on it while moving it, or walking on it while someone else is moving it. She can also practice walking inside inflatable gyms and bouncers. If you have access to nature trails, she can learn to go on hikes with you. If you have snow, she can learn to walk on it. First let her practice walking in her boots on level surfaces, and then add the surface of the snow. Be on the lookout for all kinds

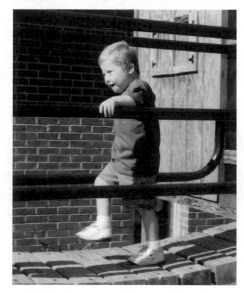

(fig. 7.2)

of surfaces in your area. Encourage your child to walk on each type of surface, because each surface will teach her new ways to move her body and to balance herself while walking.

### Walking from One Surface to Another (Same Height)

When your child is comfortable walking on a variety of surfaces, you can challenge her to walk from one surface to another. In the house, she can walk from the hardwood floor onto the area rug, or she can walk from one room to another over the threshold strip. Outside, she can walk from the sidewalk to the grass, or walk from the grass to the sand to the wood chips at the park. When she first does this, if she pays attention to the change in the surfaces, she will probably choose to use a climbing method to transition from one surface to the other. She will walk to the edge of one surface, move to plantigrade and bear walk onto the new surface, and then stand up and resume walking on the new surface.

If you provide hand support and say/sign "walk," you can teach your child that she can walk from one surface to the other using her usual stepping pattern. If she does not pay attention to the change in surface, she will probably trip as she moves onto the new surface. To teach her to pay attention to surfaces, point out the new surface as she approaches it. It will also help her if you give her verbal cues like "walk" or "march." With practice, she will pay attention to the change in surfaces and know how to walk from one surface to another.

### Walking Over or Around Obstacles

As your child is practicing walking on different surfaces, she is learning to look downward and pay attention to the floor. This will help her notice obstacles on the floor so she can plan to step over them or maneuver around them, rather than tripping on them. To help her pay attention, you can deliberately place obstacles in her path to see what she will do. At first, pick obstacles that are easy to step over, and are noticeable because they are colorful or make sounds. For example, stepping over a long ribbon or scarf, jump rope, or tissue paper. (Make sure it is stable and does not slide if she steps on it.) When she is successful with these easy obstacles and is paying attention to the floor, you can pick less observable items and see if she notices them.

When she consistently notices obstacles on the floor, you can challenge her ability to step over or around the obstacles, and maintain her balance. You can start with a broom handle, a hula-hoop, rings, pom pom, 9-inch (23-cm) diameter spot markers (assorted shapes), and alphabet foam squares, and then progress to toys on the floor, Beanie Babies, Koosh balls, bean bags, or a swimming noodle. Depending on the size of the obstacle, she will need to figure out the best method, whether to move over it or around it.

## *Guidelines*

*Practice within your child's tolerance.* She will need to adapt to walking on uneven surfaces. See how she responds and help her be successful, with her temperament. When she begins walking on the new surfaces without hand support, she may fall a lot and may get tired of falling. The falls may have a cumulative effect, and she may get upset and frustrated. To minimize the stress, alternate walking with support and without support. If she is too tired to practice, stop the activity. If she wants to keep doing the activity, then provide hand support for success.

*Motivate your child to walk on the new surface by having her walk to someone or something she wants.* She will practice walking on the new surface best if she has an endpoint with a favorite motivator. For example, at the park, she will walk on the wood chips to get to the swing or slide. At the beach, she will walk on the sand to move to the water. She will walk across the mat to get the ball.

*Begin with hand support, and then let go when she is familiar with the new surface.* She needs the hand support to feel the new surface, figure out how to walk on it, and then gain the strength to walk on it for longer distances. Once she can do these components, let go. She will then need to figure out the final component, which is balancing herself.

To provide hand support, have her hold your index finger (placed horizontally) and control her own balance while holding your finger. If you hold your child's hand and balance her, she will rely on your support and not learn to do it by herself. It is also important to place your index finger in front of her, at the level of her shoulder or chest. If you place your finger high, above her shoulder, then you are providing too much support.

*Choose relatively flat surfaces, rather than inclined surfaces.* If a surface is uneven and inclined, you will be challenging your child to do two hard gross motor skills at once. She will need to practice each skill area separately—walking on uneven surfaces and walking up and down inclines (Chapter 9). She can practice walking on uneven surfaces that are flat, and, at the same time, she can practice walking on even surfaces that are inclined. When she is familiar with both, you can combine them and have her walk up an uneven surface that is also inclined, like a sand dune or a grassy hill.

*Prepare for falls by practicing falling.* Your child will fall when she is learning to walk on uneven surfaces without your support. She will use her hands to "catch" herself and prevent falling forward and bumping her head. By practicing falling and learning to use effective protective reactions, she will become experienced with falling, develop strategies to fall safely, and no longer be upset by falls. Give her lots of practice falling on soft surfaces so she masters falling before practicing walking on hard surfaces like concrete or gravel.

*Use different footwear for different surfaces.* Since her primary long distance walking will be on level surfaces, she will use the foot support and shoes that are best for her walking pattern. When she is walking on uneven surfaces, she can experiment with the footwear she uses. If she wants to fully feel the surface—like the soft surfaces or grass—she can be barefoot. On the hard surfaces, like the sidewalk, gravel, and wood chips, she will wear shoes with flexible soles. If your child is walking in the snow with boots, she will first need to learn to walk using boots, and then she will need to learn how to walk in snow.

### *Temperament*

If your child is an **observer,** she will be very detail-oriented and will notice the new surface and step slower. She will tolerate it when holding your hand and you will need to be responsive to the pace she chooses. When it is time for her to walk by herself, she may stand still or sit down, if she does not want to walk on a particular surface. She will not want to fall, and so may refuse to walk on a surface if she feels too challenged. When she walks from one surface to another, she will take her time and try to do it without falling. With practice, she will learn how to walk on each surface and from one surface to another.

If your child is **motor driven,** she will walk on the uneven surface at full speed and then fall. She may tolerate holding your hand, or she may let go because she wants to do it by herself. She will learn how to walk on the new surface through trial and error and falling. She will learn she has to slow down in order to walk without falling. When she is familiar with the surface, she will learn to walk on it using her regular "fast" speed. When she walks from one surface to another, she will initially trip and fall. Later, she will learn to move her legs quickly to stagger and recover her balance.

 ### ACTIVITY #1: Walking on Uneven Surfaces

1. Pick one surface at a time. If you are walking on grass, pick an area that is level.
2. If the surface is soft, have your child walk on it barefoot. If not, have her wear flexible-sole shoes that she is comfortable walking in.
3. Have your child hold your index finger and balance herself while walking on the surface, for approximately 10 feet. Continue to practice this distance until she is familiar and comfortable with walking on this surface.
4. When she can walk on the surface comfortably with hand support, let go and begin practicing walking for short distances without hand support. If needed, position yourself squatting or kneeling five feet in front of her. Encourage her to walk to you without support.
5. Continue to increase the distance she walks by herself when she is ready.
6. As she practices walking on the surface by herself, she will figure out how to catch herself effectively when she falls.

7. Repeat steps 1-6 on all types of surfaces until she can walk on them confidently and comfortably.

## ACTIVITY #2: Walking from One Surface to Another

1. Pick two adjacent surfaces; for example, the sidewalk and grass. Make sure your child is comfortable walking on each surface.
2. Position your child on the sidewalk, standing with her feet perpendicular to the edge of the sidewalk.
3. Stand next to her or kneel on the grass in front of her and let her hold your index finger.
4. Sign and say "walk" and encourage her to walk from the sidewalk to the grass.
5. When she is familiar with walking from the sidewalk to the grass with hand support, try doing it without hand support. Kneel in front of her on the grass and encourage her to walk to you. When she does that well, let her spontaneously walk from the sidewalk to the grass while playing—for example, when chasing a ball.
6. When she walks from the sidewalk to the grass by herself consistently, begin practicing walking from the grass to the sidewalk.
7. Practice on all types of adjacent surfaces. Practice moving in one direction until your child masters it and then begin moving in the opposite direction.
8. When your child pays attention to the floor, place obstacles on it so she needs to figure out how to move around them or step over them. Use one obstacle at a time. See if she notices the obstacle, and if she does not, point it out to her. Start with easy obstacles like a ribbon, scarf, or jump rope. Progress to larger obstacles like a broom handle, hula hoop, rings, foam squares, toys, or a swim noodle. Encourage her to walk around the room, paying attention to the floor, and figuring out how to step over or around the obstacles safely. Later, you can progress to hiking on trails.

# MOTOR MILESTONE CHECKLIST

### Walking on Uneven Surfaces

❑ She walks on a mat or other squishy surface, holding your index finger

❑ She walks by herself on a mat or other squishy surface

*She walks on the following surfaces, holding your index finger:*

| 10 feet (3 meters) | 50 feet (15 meters) |
|---|---|
| ❑ grass | ❑ |
| ❑ sand | ❑ |
| ❑ sidewalk (with cracks) | ❑ |
| ❑ wood chips | ❑ |
| ❑ gravel or rocks | ❑ |
| ❑ other: _____ | ❑ |

*She walks without hand support on the following surfaces:*

| 10 feet (3 meters) | 100 feet (30 meters) |
|---|---|
| ❑ grass | ❑ |
| ❑ sand | ❑ |
| ❑ sidewalk (with cracks) | ❑ |
| ❑ wood chips | ❑ |
| ❑ gravel or rocks | ❑ |
| ❑ other: _____ | ❑ |

❑ She walks on all types of surfaces by herself without falling

### Walking from One Surface to Another

*She walks from one surface to another, holding your index finger:*

❑ sidewalk to grass
❑ grass to sidewalk
❑ grass to gravel
❑ gravel to grass
❑ other: _____

(continued on next page)

*She walks from one surface to another without hand support:*
- ☐ sidewalk to grass
- ☐ grass to sidewalk
- ☐ grass to gravel
- ☐ gravel to grass
- ☐ other: _____

☐ She walks from one surface to another by herself, using all types of surfaces

## Walking on Obstacles

- ☐ When walking, she consistently looks at the floor, and notices obstacles
- ☐ She walks around obstacles
- ☐ She walks over obstacles
- ☐ While walking, she consistently pays attention to obstacles on the floor, and figures out how to step over them or walk around them without falling

# 8

# Fast Stepping and Running

## Introduction

When your child is able to walk all of the time on level surfaces, he is ready to practice fast stepping with hand and trunk support. *This is the most important skill for a new walker to practice because it will transform his "new walker" walking pattern into a refined walking pattern.* Just as you needed to guide your child to learn the leg stepping pattern and waddle when you were teaching him to walk, now you will need to guide him to learn the refined walking pattern. Otherwise, he will continue the walking habit he knows. Through practicing fast stepping and running, you will teach him the components needed for an efficient walking pattern. So, there are really two goals to be achieved in this skill area:

      1. walking with a refined pattern;
      2. fast stepping and running skills.

As a new walker, your child will move his trunk and pelvis together as one unit, which will cause him to take short, wide steps. With short steps, he will use a marching pattern and weight bear on the full sole of each foot. Since walking is a new skill, he will turn his knees and feet outward for extra stability. If barefoot, the wide base and toeing-out posture will cause the inside borders (arches) of his feet to collapse into the ground.

Practicing fast stepping with hand and trunk support (method described later in that section) will introduce him to a whole new way to move his trunk, legs, and feet. *Through this experience, he will learn to rotate his pelvis on his trunk, enabling him to take longer steps and narrow his base.* He will also lean his trunk forward and feel weight shifting through his feet from the heels to the balls of his feet, eventually learning to propel himself with toe push-off. When he swings his legs forward quickly, this will cause his knees and feet to point straight ahead. With lots of practice, his walking speed and endurance will spontaneously improve. His leg coordination will also improve and tripping will diminish because he will be able to step quickly enough to avoid tripping.

Your child will need to practice for several repetitions, on a level surface, for 50-100 foot distances in order to assimilate the new movements. Your child will love the feeling of the speed and will smile while practicing. He will probably say or sign "more" spontaneously when you stop. As you practice the steps toward running speed, you will need to constantly train him to the next level of speed so he learns there is "faster to go."

## Steps in Learning Fast Stepping and Running

To achieve the goal of this skill area, your child will need to practice the following steps:

1. Fast stepping with two-hand and trunk support on level surfaces
2. Fast stepping down an incline with hand support, then without hand support
3. Fast stepping with one-hand and trunk support
4. Fast stepping swinging one or both arms for momentum
5. Fast stepping for 100 feet (30 meters) in 25 seconds
6. Running 100 feet (30 meters) in 15 seconds with reciprocal arm swing

## Components

The components to focus on are:

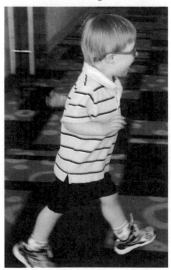

(fig. 8.1)

1. rotation of the pelvis on the trunk ("diaper/buttock wiggle"), seen when walking behind your child
2. longer steps (stride length), seen from the side view (fig. 8.1)
3. heels in line with hips so he has a narrower base, seen when walking behind him
4. knees and feet pointing straight ahead, seen from standing in front of him
5. increased leg speed, and coordinated leg movements with the increased speed
6. leg movements that match, and are uniform from side to side, if you compare both sides
7. the ability to practice for several repetitions and increase endurance

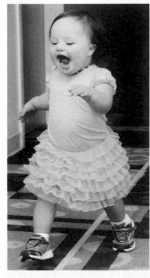 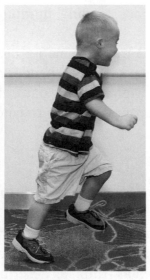 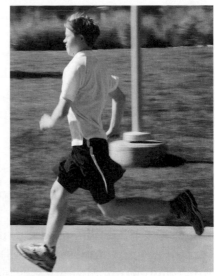

(fig. 8.2)          (fig. 8.3)          (fig. 8.4)

8. weight shifting from the heels to the balls of the feet, progressing to running on toes, and later using toe push-off (fig. 8.2)

9. trunk and pelvis leaning forward, and lower legs moving forward over feet (fig. 8.3)

10. eyes looking forward at the endpoint and watching where he is going, for safety

11. coordinated arm swing, progressing to reciprocal arm swing (fig. 8.4)

12. running with the leg and foot strength to use hip hyperextension and toe push-off (p. xix)

## Tendencies

The tendencies are:

1. to resist hand support so your child does not practice this skill and learn the new movement of pelvic rotation

2. to try to do it on his own (without support) so he moves his legs faster but keeps his trunk and pelvis moving together as a unit, taking short steps, with his heels wider than his hips (wide base), and his knees and feet turned outward

3. to be cautious and move slower to feel in control

4. to move each leg differently, with one leg wider and turned out, and perhaps moving slower with that leg

5. to do a couple of practices and then want to stop

6. to fast step with his trunk vertical and maybe progress to jogging on toes, but without leaning his trunk and pelvis forward over his toes

7. to look down when fast stepping, bumping into obstacles and falling

8. to use uncoordinated arm movements, or to focus on swinging arms with elbows bent so his leg speed is at a slower pace

9. to never learn an efficient running pattern with hip hyper-extension and toe push-off because the movement pattern was never taught

## Setup for Learning

### Fast Stepping with Two-Hand & Trunk Support on Level Surfaces

Your child will need maximal support to learn this new movement pattern of pelvic rotation (fig. 8.5). Two adults are needed, one on each side of him, supporting his hands as well as trunk, as described in Activity #1. This

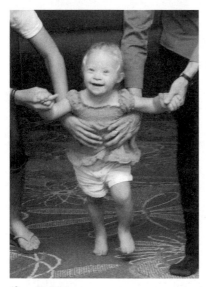

hand and trunk support is needed to guide his trunk to lean forward, to help your child feel balanced, and to catch him (with his trunk) if he falls, trips, or lifts his legs. If you just provided hand support and he fell or lifted his legs, you would be supporting him just by his arms. This is too unsafe and risky with the lax ligaments in his shoulders.

Once he is strategically supported, he is ready to practice fast stepping. You will position his hands in front of his chest, at the level of his shoulders, and you will lean his trunk forward. The primary support is at his trunk, and the hand support is for balance. With this posture, you will fast step down a long hall-

(fig. 8.5)

way (50-100 feet or 15-30 meters) on a level surface, like carpet. You want to step faster than his usual pace, but not so fast that he is out of control or lifts his legs up. He will need to move his legs fast to keep up. By leaning his trunk forward and positioning his hands at shoulder height, he will take full weight on his feet, and this will drive the forward and backward pelvic movements. If you hold his hands above shoulder level, you will be lifting him upward, and he will not use pelvic rotation. When he uses pelvic rotation with the increased speed, he will take longer steps, his base will narrow, and his knees and feet will point straight ahead. With the longer steps and narrower base, he will weight shift through the centers of his feet, from his heels to his toes. With both sides of his body supported, he will move each leg with an optimal pattern. As you increase the speed, he will learn to

step faster, and his leg coordination will improve.

When your child first practices fast stepping, he will be
shocked by the experience of
moving so fast. He will quickly
respond by moving his legs to
keep up with you. He will be challenged and will enjoy it too. After
you practice the increased speed
for a few repetitions, let go and
see if he will try to imitate moving
faster without your support. He may also practice fast stepping holding the
handle of a push toy or ride-on toy, or the Little Tikes grocery cart (fig. 8.6).
You can encourage fast stepping by playing chase games with you or siblings.

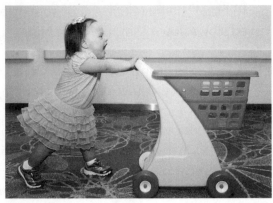

(fig. 8.6)

### Fast Stepping Down an Incline

When your child is familiar with fast stepping on level surfaces and can
move his legs fast, try inclined surfaces. The incline will help him step faster
than his usual speed. To use inclines, he will need to already be familiar with
walking up and down them with hand support (Chapter 9). By practicing fast
stepping down the incline, you are encouraging him to be risky and a little
out of control. You can start with two-hand support (an adult on each side
of him), and progress to one-hand support. He can practice with you using
small, medium, and large inclines. He can also practice on his own, holding
onto the handle of a push toy or Little Tikes grocery cart, down a small incline
of a driveway or sidewalk.

### Fast Stepping with One-Hand & Trunk Support

Practice fast stepping with one-hand and trunk support if you notice
that one of your child's legs lags behind the other when walking, or that his
walking pattern is less coordinated on one side. You may notice that the base
is wider on that side, or the knee and foot turn outward to a greater degree
when compared to the other side. To practice fast stepping with one-hand and
trunk support, you will provide support on the side having difficulty. With
practice, your child will learn to move both legs with equal coordination.

You can also practice one-handed fast stepping when your child is experienced with two-handed fast stepping and you want to challenge him by providing less support. When you choose to do this activity, I recommend alternating
which hand you support so each side receives practice. When only one hand is
supported, the unsupported side needs to work harder to keep up with the sup-

ported side. If you notice the unsupported side hanging back or if your child's speed slows down a lot, then it is better to practice with two-hand support.

### Fast Stepping Swinging One or Both Arms for Momentum

As you keep practicing fast stepping with hand support, you will notice your child spontaneously stepping faster when he walks and plays. He will step fast to move to his sister, to chase the dog, to run to something he wants, and to run away. He will be motivated to move faster and will experiment with his body to see how to move faster. You will notice he will lean his trunk forward, take longer steps, be on his toes, and begin to swing one or both arms for momentum (fig. 8.7).

Usually, he will swing one arm first. He will position his arm with his hand at his side and his elbow fairly straight. He will swing it forward and back quickly as he is fast stepping. He will generally hold his other arm stable, either straight at his side, or with his elbow bent. He will prefer swinging one arm, and later, he will swing both. When you notice him swinging his arm for momentum, then you know that he wants to move fast, and that is the time to help him increase his speed, and maintain the faster speed over longer distances.

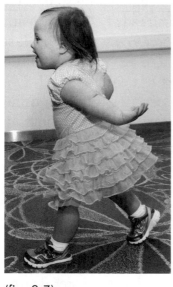 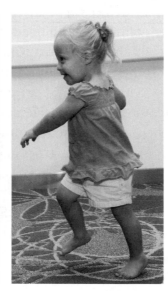 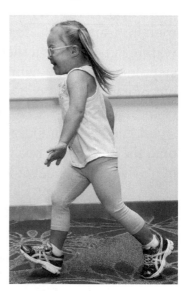

(fig. 8.7)          (fig. 8.8)          (fig. 8.9)

### Fast Stepping for 100 Feet (30 Meters) in 25 Seconds

At this point, your child has developed the components needed to fast step, and he is ready to work on the goal of fast stepping 100 feet (30 meters) in 25 seconds. To move at this speed, he will lean his trunk slightly forward, use moderate pelvic rotation, step quickly at a jogging pace, weight shift onto his toes, and have the endurance and motivation to keep going fast for the whole distance (fig. 8.8).

This goal will take time to achieve. He will need to keep practicing with hand support to *develop the speed* and confidence to use this fast speed when unsupported. He may automatically step faster when he has hand support because he feels more stable and balanced. He may fast step more slowly on his own because he feels more in control with that pace and stepping faster feels too risky. He also will need the motivation to *move this long distance.* He may prefer to fast step for 50-foot (15-meter) distances and then lose interest. He also needs to *want to move faster,* to challenge himself to race someone to the finish line. All of these factors need to be focused on for him to achieve this goal.

As you practice fast stepping, play chase games and have races with siblings so he practices trying to move faster. You can generate excitement by saying "Ready, set, go" or "1, 2, 3, go." He will try to move faster to keep up with you or his siblings, or maybe even to chase the dog.

### Running 100 Feet (30 meters) in 15 Seconds with Reciprocal Arm Swing

To move 100 feet (30 meters) in 15 seconds, your child will need to change his movements from the fast stepping pattern to the running pattern (fig. 8.9). He will need to lean his trunk more forward, move his legs into hip hyperextension (as described in the "Components" for Chapter 6), use toe push-off for propulsion, and take longer steps. To run, he will need to use these movements with the strength necessary to propel his body forward, and he will need to have speed and endurance to achieve the goal of 100 feet in 15 seconds. To develop this pattern, he will need lots of practice with hand support.

After he develops the speed to achieve this goal, he will learn to swing his arms with coordination. With continued practice and increased speed, he will learn to use reciprocal arm swing, which is the ultimate goal. Reciprocal arm swing occurs when the opposite arm and leg move simultaneously together, and it is indicative of a refined running pattern. You cannot teach reciprocal arm swing through imitation or modeling. It emerges with very fast leg speed, when the whole body is working together to move as fast as possible.

Once your child achieves this running goal, he can continue to practice, increasing his speed and distance, even using it for exercise. Running will improve his leg and abdominal strength, and his overall level of fitness. He will enjoy running while playing chase or tag, participating in sports, and having races with friends and siblings.

## Guidelines

*Use level surfaces and open spaces.* At first, your child will need a level surface so he can focus on moving fast. You can use a long hallway or a school gym. It is best if the area is free of distractions, and he can see the endpoint that he is moving to.

If the surface is uneven, like grass, he will trip and fall more easily, and he will not increase his speed because he will feel unstable. Once he can fast step or run and does it spontaneously, then he can practice on uneven surfaces, but he will not use his fastest speed on these surfaces. Examples are: your backyard, parks, playgrounds, golf courses, or football fields.

***Ensure that he looks forward at the endpoint.*** It is urgent to setup the game for him to look forward, because the tendency for many children is to look downward. He can look forward at the person at the endpoint, or he can race his sibling, with the sibling a little ahead of him, so he looks at her while running to the endpoint.

***Alternate using hand support and providing no support, and place his arm parallel to the ground.*** When your child is learning to fast step, he will need hand and trunk support to learn the new movements and to practice moving fast. By having him also practice without support, you can observe what he has learned. After he can do fast stepping, he will need support to increase his speed and distance and learn the movements for running. Continue alternating hand support and no support until he is using the running pattern with reciprocal arm swing.

When you support his arms, you will need to position them to provide the appropriate "pull." You want him to feel a gentle *forward pull* rather than an *upward pull*. To give him the forward pull, position his arms in front of his chest, at shoulder level. With the forward pull, he will learn the action of leaning his trunk forward, pelvic rotation, weight shifting onto the balls of his feet, and stepping fast with his legs. If you hold his arms up with his hands above his shoulders, you will be providing an *upward pull*, which will support his trunk vertically and will not achieve the desired movements. Depending on your height and your child's, you may need to bend down to provide the forward pull.

***Motivate your child to fast step and run.*** Many games can be used to motivate your child to step quickly or run. The best motivator will be his brother, sister, or friend. If they run, your child will probably try to run to keep up with them. They can run while playing together or when playing games such as chase, tag, and races. When you want to challenge your child's speed and distance, a race will motivate him to do his best. Later, a variety of sports can be used that combine running and ball skills.

***Provide verbal cues.*** You will use a wide assortment of verbal cues depending on what you want your child to do. To cue him to go, you can say "ready, set, go," or "1, 2, 3, go." To cue him to move faster, you can say "go, go, go" or "faster, faster, faster." These cues help him focus on what he needs to do now. Keep them simple and clear and say them when you want him to do the action.

*Use fast stepping and running for breaks between other activities.* Your child will love to practice fast stepping and running after he has been sitting for awhile or has been doing something hard, requiring concentration. Taking a running break will release any stored up energy or frustration and help him feel alert, awake, and energized. Your child may even initiate running to get away from something he does not want to do!

*Build speed, distance, and endurance.* As he is practicing fast stepping and running activities, make sure you also work on maintaining the speed for long distances. Many children can use the fast stepping speed but have not trained to do the 100-foot distance. If you practice speed and long distances for many repetitions, his endurance will improve.

*Be prepared for your child to spontaneously use fast stepping and running.* Your child will go through four stages in learning to move fast. First, he will experience moving fast with your support, and he will enjoy the feeling. Second, he will gain the strength and movement patterns to move fast. Third, he will see how to move fast when playing games like chase or races. Fourth, he will spontaneously move fast when he is motivated. At this point, he will realize what he can use fast stepping or running in his own life! An early sign is running away from you in a store, particularly when you are in the check-out line. He also will use running to get something he wants but probably is not allowed to have. Now you will be challenged to keep up with him!

*Wear appropriate footwear.* Your child needs to wear sneakers with flexible soles to practice fast stepping and running outside. Since he will need to lean his trunk forward and weight shift onto the balls of his feet, he needs shoes that bend easily to allow that foot motion. If your child has new shoes that are not broken in, you need to flex them in the toe box area to break them in for him. High top sneakers are not recommended because they will limit bending at the ankle, specifically moving the lower leg forward over the foot. If your child wears SureStep orthoses (described in Chapter 6), he will need to develop the strength to flex the plastic in order to dynamically use toe push-off, while benefitting from the stability and alignment provided by the orthosis.

*Don't try to teach your child how to swing his arms.* When he fast steps on his own, let him use whatever arm swing he uses spontaneously. If you focus on arm swing and have him imitate you, then his leg speed will slow down. His arm swing will become more coordinated once his leg speed is established, after he is able to run fast.

## Temperament

If your child is an **observer,** he might prefer to start practicing fast stepping at a slower speed. However, after he is familiar with it, he will smile when you do it, showing you he likes it because it is so much fun. He will like practicing fast stepping and running with hand support because it will feel safer to him. When you hold his hand, he may initiate moving at his fastest speed, because he will feel balanced holding onto your hand. He will also be willing to fast step and run down inclines with hand support. On his own, he will move at a slower pace to feel in control. With practice, he will learn to move faster and faster on his own.

If your child is **motor driven,** he will love fast stepping and running from the very beginning. Since he will love to move fast, he may spontaneously initiate it after you show him, or he may say or sign "more" so you can help him do it again. He will practice fast walking on his own and will like to do it with hand support or down inclined surfaces in order to move faster. He will be motivated to increase his speed, even if he feels out of control. When he is out of control, he will try to regain his balance by stepping faster.

Your motor driven child will practice fast stepping and running until he is fatigued. He will not necessarily need a game in order to practice. He will be self-motivated to move fast and run and will easily tolerate increasing his distance and speed.

 ## ACTIVITY #1: Fast Stepping with Support

1. Use a flat, level surface with a distance of 50 feet (15 meters) or more. It is best if it is straight rather than curved. A long carpeted hallway is ideal.
2. If practical, remove your child's shirt so you can support his trunk firmly without slippage.
3. Have one adult stand sideways on each side of your child. The child's right hand holds the right index finger of the adult on the child's right side; the child's left hand holds the left index finger of the adult on the child's left side. Then the adult holds the child's wrist. The adult's other palm rests against the child's abdomen, thumb down.
4. Position your child's hands in front of his chest, at shoulder level, and lean his trunk forward. The primary support is at his trunk, and the hand support is for balance. (You do not want to pull his trunk forward with his hands. Instead, he will lean his trunk forward against your hand on his abdomen.)
5. Give the verbal cue "ready, set, go" or "1, 2, 3, go." With this strategic support, step quickly down the hallway (50-100 feet; 15-30 meters). You want to step faster than his usual pace but not so fast that he is out of control or lifts his legs up. He will need to move his legs fast to keep up. If he trips, falls, or lifts his legs, catch him using

your hand on his trunk. (Do not catch him by pulling him up with his arms, due to the lax ligaments in his shoulders.)

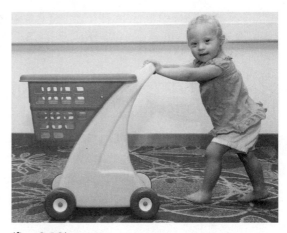

6. Watch his pelvis and legs, looking for pelvic rotation, longer steps, feet pointing straight, and a narrower base.

7. Increase the speed as tolerated, continuing to watch the movements of

(fig. 8.10)

the pelvis and legs. With the increased speed and longer steps, he will also weight shift through his feet, from his heels to his toes.

8. After you practice the increased speed for a few repetitions, let go and see if he will try to imitate moving faster without your support.

9. He can also practice fast stepping holding the handle of a push toy or ride-on toy, or the Little Tikes grocery cart (fig. 8.10). You can encourage fast stepping by playing chase games with you or siblings.

10. When he is ready, increase the distance to 100 feet (30 meters).

11. When he is experienced with fast stepping with hand and trunk support, then just provide hand support (fig. 8.11). He will hold on for balance and initiate moving faster with this support. Since you are not providing trunk support, you need to move at a slower pace in case he trips or falls.

12. When he is familiar with inclines (Chapter 9) and fast stepping, begin practicing fast stepping down small and medium inclines. Provide two-hand support initially and then decrease your support to one hand. When he is ready, try it without support.

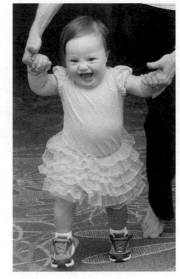

(fig. 8.11)

13. When he is experienced with fast stepping and moving fast with two-hand support, try providing only one-hand support. Stand beside him, have him hold your hand, and position his arm in the proper position. Then fast step together and have him balance himself by holding your hand. Alternate hand support so each side re-

ceives practice. If one leg is less coordinated, practice fast stepping while supporting the arm and trunk on that side.

## ACTIVITY #2: Fast Stepping and Running 100-Foot Distances

1. Use a flat, level surface with a distance of 100 feet (30 meters).
2. Make sure your child is focused on the endpoint and not distracted so that he will move at his fastest speed. Either you or a sibling stand beside your child, and have someone standing at the endpoint to motivate him.
3. Motivate your child to fast step or run as fast as he can by setting up a race.
4. Say "1, 2, 3, go."
5. Encourage him to go fast for a distance of 50-100 feet (15-30 meters) without stopping.
6. To help him increase his speed, setup some races with hand support (either two-hand or one-hand) so he experiences the faster speed and later tries to imitate it when running without support.
7. Practice increasing his speed and distance until he achieves the fast stepping speed of 100 feet (30 meters) in 25 seconds.
8. When he is ready to train for running, you will need to teach him the new posture he will need to use by initially providing support to lean his trunk more forward. When he leans his trunk forward, he will learn to use hip hyperextension and toe push-off, and eventually gain the leg and foot strength to propel himself with these movements and take longer steps. Alternate practicing with and without hand and trunk support as you work with him on increasing his speed and running the distance. Continue to practice until he achieves the goal of running 100 feet (30 meters) in 15 seconds.
9. Practice races and running in motivating ways so that you cultivate your child's desire to move faster and faster. As his speed increases, observe his arm swing. Continue to practice increasing his leg speed until you see him use reciprocal arm swing.
10. Use running for fun, and this is the perfect exercise. Combine running and kicking a ball to improve coordination and timing of leg movements with speed.

## 🏃 MOTOR MILESTONE CHECKLIST

❑ He fast steps for 50 feet (15 meters) with two-hand and trunk support

❑ He fast steps for 100 feet (30 meters) with two-hand and trunk support

❑ He fast steps down a medium incline with hand support

❑ He fast steps down a medium incline without hand support

❑ He fast steps for 100 feet (30 meters) with one-hand and trunk support

❑ He fast steps for 50 feet (15 meters), swinging one or both arms for momentum

❑ He fast steps for 100 feet (30 meters), swinging one or both arms for momentum

❑ He fast steps 100 feet (30 meters) in 25 seconds

❑ He runs 100 feet (30 meters) in 15 seconds

❑ He runs fast, with reciprocal arm swing

❑ He runs with hip hyperextension, toe push-off, and reciprocal arm swing

# 9

# Walking Up and Down Inclined Surfaces

## Introduction

Walking up and down inclined surfaces is another important skill for children with Down syndrome. First, it can improve your child's walking pattern and help her be independent when walking in the community. Second, it is the best skill to practice if your child walks with her knees stiff and straight because she will need to unlock her knees to walk up and down with balance and control. Third, if your child slaps her feet when stepping with full sole weight bearing, this skill will teach her to weight shift through her feet and strengthen her feet, which will lessen this habit by teaching her more advanced foot movements.

Examples of inclined surfaces are: inclined sidewalks or driveways; ramps; sloped areas in yards, playgrounds, parks, and malls; school or church hallways; and nature trails. You will need to look around and see what is available in your community. You will need to find small (2-4 degrees), medium (5-10 degrees), and large (15-25 degrees) inclines for your child to practice on. The goal will be for your child to walk up and down all types of inclined surfaces by herself.

Your child's early walking pattern on level surfaces will be with her trunk vertical, her knees straight, and with full-sole weight bearing. Some children also slap their feet against the surface, making a sound, and it becomes a habit if we let it. When your child walks up or down an inclined surface, her whole body position will change, and she will learn to balance herself in forward and backward directions while using strength to step up and down the inclined surface with control.

When walking up, her ankles will tilt with her toes upward, and then she will need to lean her head, trunk, pelvis, hips, and knees forward to keep

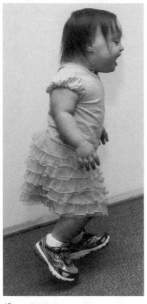

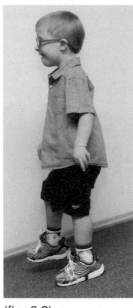

(fig. 9.1)                    (fig. 9.2)

her balance (fig. 9.1). She will activate her abdominal muscles and bend her hips and knees to lean her trunk and legs forward for balance. From this posture, she will need to use strength and power to straighten her hips and knees, and use toe push-off in her ankles to walk up the incline. When she does it well, she will use hip hyperextension and toe push-off with her knees and feet pointing straight ahead.

When walking down, your child's ankles will tilt with her toes downward, and then she will need to lean her head, trunk, and pelvis backward, keeping her hips and knees mildly bent, to maintain her balance (fig. 9.2). She will step down the incline by holding her hips and knees in this bent position, activating her abdominals, and taking small steps. She will need strength to decelerate her movements, to move slowly with control.

---

### Steps in Learning to Walk on Inclined Surfaces

To achieve the goal of this skill area, your child will practice these steps in the following order:

1. Walk up and down small (2-4 degrees) inclines with support, then without support
2. Walk up and down medium (5-10 degrees) inclines with support, then without support
3. Walk up and down large (15-25 degrees) inclines with support, then without support

---

## Components

The components to focus on are:

1. strategies for moving the head, trunk, pelvis, hips, knees, and feet to the effective position for balance when walking up and down
2. strength needed in the hips, knees, and ankles to walk up/down the incline when she initially places each leg, takes

weight on it and moves her body forward, and then swings her leg to step forward

3. hips in neutral rotation so knees and feet point straight ahead
4. strength in ankle muscles to *dorsiflex* (lift toes above the level of the heel) and *plantarflex* (toe push off with the toes below the level of the heel)
5. the ability to walk down using *eccentric actions,* so she moves slowly with control. ("Eccentric actions" means that the contracting muscle lengthens, acting as a "brake" to slow down and control the movement taking place. They are also used when walking down curbs and stairs.)

## Tendencies

The tendencies are:

1. to lose her balance when she is walking up and down, because she does not effectively move her head, trunk, pelvis, hips, knees, and feet for the length of the incline
2. to have difficulty walking up and down due to muscle weakness in the hips, knees, and feet
3. to use hip external rotation and turn the knees and feet outward
4. to march with her feet and take small steps due to weakness or because she has not learned to weight shift through her feet (heels to toes)
5. to walk down the incline too fast and without control because she has not learned to use eccentric actions

## Set Up for Learning

When your child first tries walking up or down a small inclined surface, she will feel the tilt, feel off balance, and not know what to do. She may freeze, try to step and fall, or move to hands and knees to climb. She will need hand support to become familiar with her new orientation on the surface, to figure out how to balance herself, and to develop the strength needed to walk up and down. You can start with two-hand support and then decrease your support to one hand when she is ready. When you provide hand support, if you hold her hand and guide her, she will become dependent on your support. It is best if *you* **have her hold your index finger**, placed at her shoulder level, and then let her control her own balance as she walks up or down the incline.

Your child will adjust to walking up inclined surfaces holding your index finger easily. Walking up will be easier than walking down. The real challenge will be for her to do it without hand support. She will be wobbly at first and will waver forward and back until she figures out how to

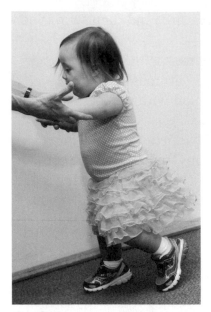

(fig. 9.3)

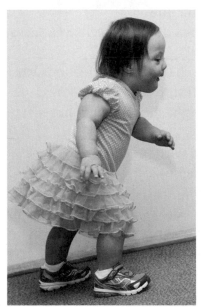

(fig. 9.4)

position her body for balance. You will need to be close enough to give her support when needed. With practice, she will learn to automatically move to her point of balance when she feels an inclined surface.

Walking down a small inclined surface will require a different strategy than walking up, and the biggest challenge will be controlling her speed (fig. 9.3). Your child will need hand support while she learns how to balance herself, how to take small steps, and how to use her muscles to control the descent. When she can walk down the incline holding your index finger, you will let go so she can learn how to do it by herself. At first, she will not be able to control her speed. You will need to be close to help slow her down. An alternative way to practice is to play the "crashing" game described in the activity below. By practicing stepping fast and falling, your child will overcome her fear of the skill, and eventually learn to slow herself down using a speed that she is comfortable with. Her temperament will influence her preferred speed.

With practice, she will learn to position her body and use her strength to walk up and down inclined surfaces, for the entire length of the inclined surface (fig. 9.4). She will need to maintain her posture and movements and pay attention, or she will lose her balance. She will also need to learn to transition from walking on the incline to walking on the adjacent level surface, and change her movements with precision at the right time.

When your child is able to walk up and down small inclines without support, you will progress to medium and then large inclines. The same principles of learning to walk up and down will apply, but the balance and strength required will be more dramatic. Continue to practice this skill area until she can walk up and down all grades and lengths of inclines automatically without hand support.

## Guidelines

*Vary the angle of the incline and the length.* It may be helpful to measure the angle of the incline so you know which size incline you are using. To measure the incline you can use a tool called an angle finder or protractor. It is easily available at a hardware store.

You will probably tend to overestimate the angle of an incline. You will see a 25-degree incline and you will think that it is 45 degrees. For the really small inclines, you may not even notice the slope, but your child will notice it, and you will observe how it challenges her balance. When you measure the inclines you and your child use in your community, you will see that small ones are 2-4 degrees, medium ones are 5-10 degrees, and large ones are 15-25 degrees. You will begin with small inclines and gradually progress to medium and large inclines when your child is ready.

It is also important to pay attention to the length of inclines. The shorter the length, the easier it will be to walk up and down. To help your child develop the strength and balance needed to walk up and down inclines, you can start with inclines that are 5-10 feet (1.5-3 meters) long and progress to inclines that are 40 feet (12 meters) or longer. As your child learns to walk up and down each grade, the next challenge is to increase the length. For example, when your child can walk up and down a 5-10 foot (1.5-3 meter) medium incline, try a 20-foot (6-meter) medium incline; when she can do that, try a 40-50 foot (12-15 meter) medium incline. Continue to practice on medium inclines until she is ready to try large inclines. You can also challenge your child by having her transition from inclines to level surfaces.

*Walking up is generally easier than walking down.* Walking up an incline is easier because the pace is slower and the ground is closer to prop on for support if needed. Your child will feel more in control, and, if she does lose her balance and fall, she can easily catch herself with her hands or choose to climb up rather than walk. When she walks down an incline, the tendency is to move faster and feel out of control, so she may become fearful. It is also harder for her to catch herself with her hands and stop herself effectively because the ground is so low. As your child walks up and down, watch her reaction so you can practice this skill in the best way to accommodate her temperament and learning style.

*Use surfaces that are familiar and safe to your child.* Familiarize her with walking on a particular type of surface before you add walking up and down an incline on that surface. For example, after she is familiar with walking on the grass, then she can practice walking up and down a grassy incline. If she is not ready to walk on uneven surfaces such as grass, use a level surface such as a carpeted or tile floor. You may be able to find small inclines with carpet or tile surfaces in churches, schools, or malls. Concrete driveways can be used with close supervision to avoid falls. Later, when your child is ready for medium and large inclines on uneven surfaces, you can practice walking on hiking trails.

***Begin with hand support and then let go.*** You child will need hand support until she learns how to move her legs on the inclined surface, balance herself, and use her strength to walk up and down. When providing hand support, have your child hold your index finger (placed horizontally) and learn to balance herself with this type of support. After she holds your finger, place her hand in front of her chest, at the level of her shoulder or chest. If you hold her hand and place her hand above shoulder level, you will be controlling her, and she will become dependent on your support rather than learning to do it by herself.

When walking up or down inclines, you will begin with two-hand support, progress to one-hand support, and work toward no support. When walking up the incline with two-hand support, you can walk behind her. If two people are available, you will walk on each side of the child, stepping sideways. (Your child's right hand will hold the right index finger of the person on her right, and your child's left hand will hold the left index finger of the person on her left.) When she is ready for one-hand support, you will walk at her side, stepping sideways, with the hand support already described. When walking down the incline with two-hand support, you will be in front of your child, stepping backwards. When she is ready to try walking up without hand support, you can walk behind her and provide intermittent support as needed to help her be successful. When she is ready to walk down without support, it is best if you are in front of her so she can prop against you if needed for balance, or you can assist her balance or give hand support when needed.

Walking up and down requires your child to use her strength in different ways. Once she has the strength to walk up and down with one-hand support, then practice without hand support so she learns how to balance herself.

***Encourage her to walk up and down the incline rather than climb.*** Your child will naturally feel safer if she climbs rather than walks, particularly with the medium and large inclines. To move up the incline, she will use the plantigrade position or creep on hands and knees. To move down, she will slide down on her belly, try to sit and scoot, or slide down in sitting as she would move down a slide. She can use these climbing methods when she is playing by herself or when you do not give her hand support and she does not feel ready to walk. When you are practicing the inclines with her, encourage her to walk up and down by giving her one hand support until she will do it by herself.

***Provide verbal and visual cues.*** As she is walking up or down the incline, pick an appropriate verbal cue to say. You can say (and sign) "walk," "up," or "down." To keep her focused, you can repeat the word with each step she takes. She will also pay attention to visual cues, such as watching another child walk up and down the incline ahead of her, and they can follow each other or take turns doing it. To make it more exciting, you can think of different ways to walk up and down. For example, you can march up and run down and say "whee" (fig. 9.5). You can also roll a ball up the incline, and then she can follow it; when she reaches the top of the incline, then she can push it down the incline and follow it. If it looks like fun, she will participate.

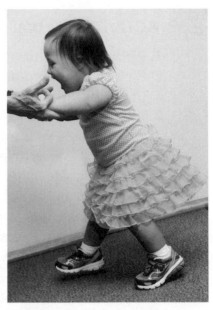

(fig. 9.5)

***Wear appropriate footwear.*** Since many of the inclined surfaces are going to be outside, she will wear shoes suitable for the environment. She will need to weight shift through her feet, from the heels to the balls of her feet, so the soles of her shoes need to be flexible and broken in, especially in the toe box area. She will also need to be able to move her lower legs forward over her feet, so the shoes cannot restrict this movement. This is why high-top shoes are not recommended. If your child wears SureStep orthoses, she will develop the strength in her ankles and feet to dynamically use toe push-off with optimal alignment of the knees and feet.

## Temperament

If your child is an **observer,** she will feel the change in the surface and become alert and cautious. She will want to move slowly so she feels in control. She will prefer hand support until she feels comfortable doing it by herself. When she first does it without support, she may sit or stop walking if she feels she will fall. With practice, she will become confident and walk up and down, maintaining a careful speed.

If your child is **motor driven,** she may not notice the incline, or if she does, it will not stop her. With her adventuresome nature, she will continue to walk at her regular speed, whether she falls or not. She will need hand support, particularly when walking down the incline, to slow down her speed. With practice and when she is motivated, she will learn to walk up and down maintaining her balance, while moving at her normal fast speed.

## ACTIVITY #1: Walking Up and Down Inclines

1. Pick a small incline (2-4 degrees) to walk up and down. Make sure the surface is familiar and your child is comfortable walking on that surface.

2. To walk up with two-hand support, stand behind your child and have her hold your index fingers, placed horizontally in front of her chest, at the level of her shoulders or lower. (Or, one person could be on each side of her, and she could hold the right index finger of the person on her right, and the left index finger of the person on her left. Each person would walk up the incline sideways.) Your child will feel stable with the hand support, and she will figure out how to move her body to walk up the incline. She will also need to manage her balance. Have her hold on when you reach the top of the incline so she adjusts herself to the transition of walking from the incline to walking on the level surface.

3. To walk down with two-hand support, stand in front of your child, facing her, and walk backwards down the incline. Place your thumbs horizontally in front of her chest, at the level of her shoulders or lower. (Or, this could be done with one person on each side of her, with her holding your index fingers as noted in step 2, stepping sideways down the incline.) She will figure out how to step down the incline and control her speed. If she moves too quickly, you can help her to move slowly with control. Have her hold on when you reach the bottom of the incline to help her transition to walking on the level surface.

4. To walk up or down with one-hand support, position yourself at her side, stepping sideways. She will hold your index finger (either your right index finger with her right hand or your left index finger with her left hand), and then position her hand in front of her chest at shoulder level or lower.

5. When she is familiar with walking up the incline with one-hand support, see if she will do it by herself. You walk behind her to provide intermittent support when needed so she is successful.

6. When she is familiar with walking down the incline with one-hand support, you can play a "crashing" game for fun to help her work on controlling her speed. Place 2 or 3 stacked beanbag chairs in front of her, about 3 feet (90 cm) from the top of the incline. You can give her one-hand support to help her learn the game. She will hold your index finger and step quickly to the beanbags and then "crash" into them, propping on and falling into the

soft surface. When she is familiar with the game, she can do it by herself. When she is ready, you can place the beanbags further away so she has to maintain her control stepping down the incline before crashing into the soft support.

7. With practice, your child will learn how to walk down the incline without support, and how to control her speed. When she is ready to practice doing it without hand support, stand in front of her, facing her, and walk down backwards so you can give intermittent support, as needed. She can also prop against you if needed to control her balance.

8. Provide verbal and visual cues when walking up and down.

9. Clap and praise her when she reaches the top or bottom of the incline.

10. When she can walk up a small incline on one type of surface, try it on a variety of surfaces.

11. When she can walk up and down small inclines for 5-to-10-foot (1.5-to-3-meter) distances, try longer inclines.

12. Follow the steps above using medium and large inclines when she is ready.

13. When she is competent and confident with doing inclines and 10-inch (25-cm) wide balance beams (as discussed in Chapter 15), you can teach her to walk up an incline with neutral hip rotation (knees and feet pointing straight ahead) by using a 10-inch (25-cm) wide balance beam (2 x 10 board) and placing it on a stair or other firm surface (fig. 9.6). You can create the angle you want, depending on the height of the surface you use. It is very important that the setup is stable because if she feels any wobble, she will be setup to fail.

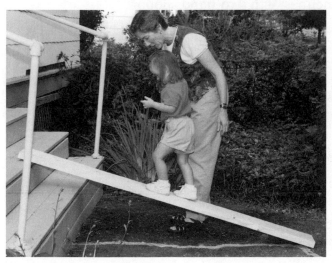

(fig. 9.6)

## 🏃 MOTOR MILESTONE CHECKLIST

❑ She walks up small inclines with two-hand support

❑ She walks down small inclines with two-hand support

❑ She walks up small inclines with one-hand support

❑ She walks down small inclines with one-hand support

❑ She walks up small inclines without support

❑ She walks down small inclines without support

❑ She walks up medium inclines with two-hand support

❑ She walks down medium inclines with two-hand support

❑ She walks up medium inclines with one-hand support

❑ She walks down medium inclines with one-hand support

❑ She walks up medium inclines without support

❑ She walks down medium inclines without support

❑ She walks up large inclines with two-hand support

❑ She walks down large inclines with two-hand support

❑ She walks up large inclines with one-hand support

❑ She walks down large inclines with one-hand support

❑ She walks up large inclines without support

❑ She walks down large inclines without support

❑ She walks up and down all types of inclined surfaces by herself

# 10

# Kicking a Ball

## Introduction

Learning to kick a ball will teach your child to balance on one foot, and the components that he will learn from this skill will improve his walking pattern. First, he will need to learn the action of kicking the ball with hand support, and then he will need to learn how to balance himself on one foot and kick a ball. He may have learned the action of kicking a ball with hand support when you were motivating him to walk longer distances. He also may be familiar with this skill from watching his siblings play soccer. It will be a fun and dynamic activity for practicing balancing on one foot. The goal will be to kick the ball 10 to 20 feet (3 to 6 meters). When he is able to fast step and kick a ball, he can combine these skills and learn to run and kick the ball.

Learning to kick the ball will be a two-step process. First, your child will need to learn how to stand on one leg, by weight shifting over it and maintaining the position with strength and balance. Second, he will need to maintain his balance while lifting and swinging his other leg to kick the ball. Learning this skill will improve his foot posture, standing balance, and leg and foot strength. These components will improve his walking pattern by teaching him to use a narrower base, with his feet pointing straight ahead.

The first challenge will be teaching your child how to balance on one foot. His typical standing position will be with his feet wider than his hips, his knees and feet turned outward, and his weight on the inside borders of his feet. To balance on one foot, his knee and foot will need to be pointing straight ahead, and he will need to weight shift over his foot, from the inside border to the outside border. He will need to find his point of balance and then use his leg and foot strength to maintain the position. If his foot is turned outward, it will block weight shifting over it. Learning to place his foot pointing straight ahead will be critical in learning to balance on one foot.

---

### Steps in Learning to Kick a Ball

Your child will learn to achieve the goal in this skill area using the following steps:

1. Kicking a ball when provided with two-hand support and assistance to swing his leg (if needed)
2. Kicking a ball with one-hand support
3. Kicking a ball without support
4. Kicking a ball 10 to 20 feet (3 to 6 meters) by swinging his leg and straightening his knee when his foot hits the ball.
5. Running and kicking the ball with coordination and timing

---

## Components

The components to focus on are:

1. positioning the hip in neutral rotation with the knee and foot pointing straight ahead
2. standing with the feet in line with the hips (narrow base)
3. the ability to weight shift the pelvis over the leg and foot, so he weight shifts from the inside border to the outside border of his foot
4. strength in the abdominals, leg, and foot to hold the posture and maintain balance on one foot
5. the ability to find the point of balance and maintain it while swinging the other leg to kick the ball (fig 10.1)
6. eye-foot coordination and timing to kick the ball effectively

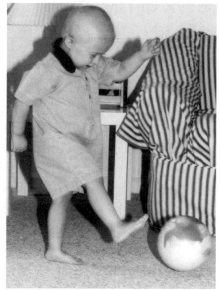

(fig. 10.1)

## Tendencies

The tendencies are:

1. to stand with hip external rotation with the knees and feet pointing outward
2. to stand with the feet wider than the hips (wide base) and to weight bear on the inside borders of the feet

3. to be unable to weight shift the pelvis over the leg and foot because weight shifting is blocked by the wide base and toeing-out posture
4. to try to balance while standing in this posture (combination of 1, 2, and 3)
5. to trip over the ball when he tries to kick it
6. to resist this new activity and persist with the familiar game of throwing the ball

## *Setup for Learning*

Your first job is to introduce your child to the game of kicking a ball. You will show him the object of the game is to move his foot to hit the ball. When he does this, the ball will move. You will say "kick" as his foot touches the ball so he begins to label the game. When he kicks the ball, praise him and clap for him. Since he is familiar with rolling or throwing the ball, his tendency will be to bend over and pick up the ball rather than kick it. You will need to provide two-hand support to teach the new game, make it easy to practice, and structure kicking the ball rather than throwing it.

When you give two-hand support, you will stand behind him and have him hold your index fingers in front of his chest, at the level of his shoulders. You will place the ball in front of his foot so it is easy to kick. At first, you may need to hold his hands and swing his leg to demonstrate the kicking motion. When he understands the game, he will know to move his foot to kick the ball. His initial method of kicking will be to lift his leg with his hip and knee bent. With the ball placed in front of his foot, this leg movement will make his foot hit the ball and the ball will move forward two or three feet.

When your child easily and consistently kicks the ball with two-hand support, then give him one-hand support. You will stand at his side, and he will hold your index finger, placed in front of his chest at the level of his shoulder. You will support the hand opposite the kicking leg to guide him to weight shift over the standing leg. Have him hold your finger and balance himself rather than you holding onto his hand and wrist and controlling his balance. With one-hand support, his kicking pattern will improve, and he will start swinging his leg and kick the ball farther. With one-hand support, he will learn how to position the standing leg, with the knee and foot pointing straight, and how to weight shift over it, onto the outer border of his foot. With practice, his strength will improve in his abdominals, legs, and feet, and he will feel confident with kicking the ball.

When your child is ready, test whether he will kick the ball without holding your finger. Place the ball in front of his foot and say "kick." Praise any motion he makes toward kicking the ball. Kicking the ball without hand support will be a challenge because he will need to figure out how to balance

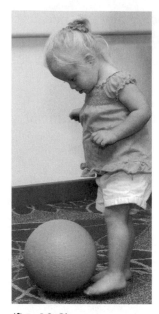

(fig. 10.2)

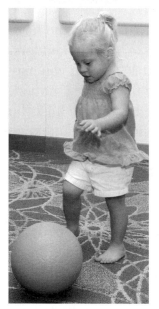

(fig. 10.3)

himself without any support. With practice, he will learn how to use the strength he developed through kicking with one-hand support and combine it with balancing himself. You will need to stand beside him as he practices kicking the ball to help him be successful. A common mistake is to trip and fall because his foot gets stuck on the ball after he swings it.

Learning to kick the ball is a combination of using the right leg posture, weight shifting, strength, and balance. Your child will need to combine balancing on one foot and dynamically swinging the other leg to kick the ball. He will first learn to do it with the ideal setup—standing with the ball placed in front of his kicking foot (fig. 10.2). When he has mastered the components with this ideal setup, then he can be challenged to walk to the ball and stop to kick it. With this setup, he will need to figure out where to stop in front of the ball and position himself to kick it with his preferred foot, rather than step too far or too close to it and trip over it, or have the wrong foot in front of it.

The next goals will be to walk and kick the ball (without stopping) (fig. 10.3), and then to run and kick the ball. Your child will first learn these skills with hand support because he will have new components to figure out. He will need to develop coordinated leg movements to kick the ball with either leg, to time when to kick the ball as he is moving, and to use eye-foot coordination to kick effectively. Even though running and kicking the ball will be the ultimate challenge for him, he will love moving fast and kicking the ball and playing this game with siblings. When I practice this skill with children in PT sessions, I use a carpeted hallway 100 feet (30 meters) long. This is the ideal setting, since it is a level surface without distractions. The children focus on the ball and are attentive to the game for the length of the hallway, and they want to practice for several repetitions.

As your child has more experience kicking the ball, he will learn the most efficient method of swinging his leg to kick. He will swing his leg and extend his knee as he contacts the ball. He will be able to kick the ball harder and farther using this method. It will require more balance because he will need to balance on one foot longer and maintain his balance while he swings his kicking leg with momentum and speed. Using this method, he will be able to kick the ball 10 to 20 feet (3 to 6 meters).

## Guidelines

*Choose a ball with the appropriate size and weight.* In the beginning, use a ball that is 8-10 inches (20-25 cm) in diameter, soft, and lightweight. You can use a beach ball, foam ball, Gertie ball, or inflated plastic ball from the toy store. My favorite ball is the Gopher Softball™, 8.25-inch diameter (www.gophersport.com). It is a low-density coated foam ball, which is soft and lightweight. When your child is familiar with kicking and likes to kick, he can use any size. When he kicks well, you can vary the weight and use heavier balls, such as a soccer ball, which will further challenge his strength and balance.

*Practice kicking the ball when your child is motivated.* Your child may want to throw the ball or play catch rather than kick the ball. If he is not interested in kicking the ball, try again another time. It will help if he watches his brother or sister do it, and they play the game together. For example, when Blaine watched his brother play soccer with his friends in the backyard, he became motivated to kick the ball too. Your child will have the desire to learn to kick the ball, so you want to look for his readiness and give him role models to imitate and play with.

*Let your child kick with the leg he chooses.* When your child practices kicking the ball with hand support, place the ball in front of each foot to see if he kicks the ball better with one foot or if he prefers to use one leg more than the other. If he does prefer one leg over the other, let him practice kicking with that leg. He will learn to have a dominant leg, just as he develops a dominant hand. He will show you which leg is easier to kick with, and, in many cases, it will be with his dominant leg.

*Provide verbal, visual, and tactile cues.* Give verbal cues by saying "kick" to identify the game to him, and to structure the ball game you are going to play. Say it every time the ball is to be kicked, and this will help him focus his attention on kicking the ball.

Give him visual cues and models to imitate. He will watch you or a sibling kick the ball, and then he will be motivated to imitate you. When you do the kicking motion, exaggerate it with a big movement, and say "kick" so he pays attention. When he imitates you, he will do a smaller scale version of what he saw.

Provide tactile cues to help him feel the motion or action you want him to do. For example, when you give him two-hand support and help him kick, move his leg in a big range, with a fast speed, and hit the ball with impact. If you move his leg slowly and gently touch the ball with his foot, he will barely notice what he needs to do to kick. By moving his leg with a big movement, fast, and with impact, the action will get his attention, and he will feel what he needs to imitate. When he is ready to learn to kick the ball by straightening his knee, you will also give him that tactile cue and kick the ball with momentum and force.

*Choose the right surface and space to practice kicking.* When your child is first learning to kick, it will be easier for him to weight shift and balance on a firm, level surface inside the house (tile, hardwood, and carpeted floors). When he is familiar with kicking and is motivated to kick, you can use uneven surfaces like the grass. When kicking is a fun game for him and he likes to chase the ball and kick it again, or he wants to run and kick the ball, you will need to use a large area like a gym or long hallway for level surfaces. Later you can practice on uneven surfaces like the backyard, parks, or playground areas.

*Use appropriate footwear when practicing kicking.* When your child is first learning the game of kicking the ball in the house, he will need to learn to move his foot to hit the ball so he can be barefoot. When he is ready to work on the components needed to balance on one foot, then the type of footwear used will be important. He will need to position his hip in neutral rotation with his knee and foot pointing straight, and to weight shift from the inside to outside border of his foot, so will need to use the footwear that will assist (facilitate) these components. If he wears SureStep orthoses or inserts in his shoes, or is wearing shoes, he will need shoes with flexible soles. When he kicks a heavier ball, he will need to wear shoes to support and protect his foot as it hits the ball.

## Temperament

If your child is an **observer,** he will prefer hand support to feel secure when learning to kick the ball or run and kick the ball. When you let go, he will be careful to control his balance and will kick gently. When he is learning to walk to the ball and kick it, he will be upset if he trips over the ball. You will need to be proactive to help him be successful and prevent falls. If he becomes frustrated, he may temporarily stop kicking the ball and choose to squat and hit the ball with his hand. When he is comfortable kicking the ball, he will play kickball until he is tired or bored with it.

If your child is **motor driven,** he will progress to kicking the ball without hand support more easily. He will trip when kicking the ball without support because he will be too close to the ball, moving too quickly, or not paying attention. The tripping will not bother him, and eventually he will plan how to kick the ball without tripping. He will be motivated to practice the game of kicking the ball even if he trips. He will enjoy kicking the ball and will love the combination of running and kicking the ball.

## ACTIVITY #1: Kicking the Ball with Support

1. Place your child standing on a flat, level surface. Position his feet in line with his hips (narrow base), with his knees and feet pointing straight ahead.

2. Place an 8- to 9-inch (20- to 23-cm) diameter ball (soft foam, lightweight) in front of his foot. As you practice, check to see if he prefers to kick with a particular foot, and then continue practicing with that foot as he is learning the skill.

3. Position yourself standing behind him. Place your index fingers horizontally in front of his chest at the level of his shoulders. Have him hold onto your fingers and balance himself with this support.

4. With this setup and support, say "kick" and see if he will move his leg so his foot hits the ball. If he does not initiate any leg movement, then hold both of his hands in one of your hands, and use your other hand to move his leg to kick the ball. Swing his leg in an exaggerated way so he feels a big movement and experiences the action of kicking the ball. Say "kick" as you do it. Then see if he will kick the ball on his own when you give him the verbal cue.

5. If his foot contacts the ball in any way and the ball moves, praise him and clap for him so he feels successful and learns the game.

6. Practice with siblings or friends so he can watch them kick the ball, and then imitate them.

7. Practice kicking for several repetitions so this is a familiar game, and he develops the strength to kick the ball easily and consistently with two-hand support.

8. When he is ready, begin practicing kicking the ball with one-hand support. Make sure he is standing with the right leg position and the ball is placed in front of his foot. Stand at his side, on the opposite side of his kicking leg. Have him hold your index finger, placed horizontally in front of his chest at the level of his shoulder, and balance himself with this support. Say "kick" and praise him when he kicks the ball. Practice until he can kick the ball easily and consistently with one hand support.

9. When he is ready, practice kicking the ball on a variety of surfaces, like grass.

**ACTIVITY #2: Kicking the Ball without Support**

1. Place your child standing on a flat, level surface. Position his feet in line with his hips (narrow base), with his knees and feet pointing straight ahead.
2. Place an 8- to 9-inch (20- to 23-cm) diameter ball (soft foam, lightweight) in front of his preferred kicking foot.
3. Say "kick" and praise him and clap for him when he kicks the ball.
4. Stand at his side to assist him as needed so he is successful. He will need to figure out how to balance himself and use his strength to maintain his balance and kick the ball. He will also need to learn to swing his leg rather than just lifting it. Watch him closely to prevent tripping if his foot becomes stuck on the ball.
5. Practice with siblings or friends so he can watch them kick the ball, imitate them, and take turns with them.
6. Practice kicking for several repetitions so he develops the balance and strength to kick the ball easily and consistently without support.
7. When he kicks the ball easily on a level surface, practice on a variety of surfaces, like grass.
8. The final challenge will be to teach your child to kick the ball for 10- to 20-foot distances. To achieve this, he will need to learn to swing his leg and extend his knee as his foot hits the ball. You can model this movement and see if he imitates it. If he needs support to learn this movement, then hold his leg and help him with speed, momentum, and impact when kicking the ball. He may need hand support temporarily while practicing the new leg movement.

**ACTIVITY #3: Running and Kicking the Ball**

1. When your child is able to kick the ball consistently without support and enjoys the kicking game when you place the ball in front of his foot, then you can start practicing walking to the ball, stopping in front of it, and kicking it (fig. 10.4). Begin with hand support so he learns where to stand to kick the ball, figuring out how close to step and which foot to put in front of it (if he has a preferred foot). When he can do this with hand support, then have him do it without hand support.
2. When he can do step #1, then practice walking and kicking the ball without stopping in front of the ball (fig. 10.5). Provide hand support so he learns the leg coordination to kick with either foot, at the

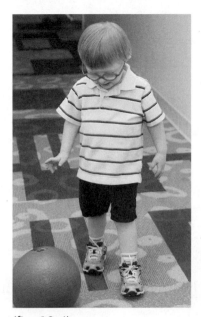

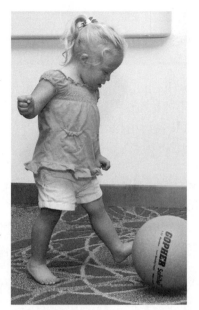

(fig. 10.4)                    (fig. 10.5)

right time (so he does not trip over the ball) as he approaches the
ball. When he is ready, have him do it without hand support.

3. When he can do step #2, practice fast stepping and kicking the
ball. Begin with two-hand and trunk support (as practiced in
Chapter 8; Activity #1) with one person on each side of him, stepping sideways. Move at the fast stepping speed, and he will need to
figure out how to use leg coordination and timing to kick the ball.
Continue fast stepping and kicking for long distances, so he has
many practices of kicking over the distance. This will also improve
his endurance. When he is ready, have him do this with two-hand
support, then one-hand support, and then without hand support.

4. When he can do step #3, practice running and kicking the ball using the same method as in step #3 but at a faster speed. When he
can do this without hand support, he will love practicing on his
own and playing with his siblings.

5. When he can do these skills on level surfaces, then practice on
the grass.

**MOTOR MILESTONE CHECKLIST**

He kicks the ball with two-hand support when the ball is placed in front of his foot:
☐ on level surfaces
☐ on the grass

He kicks the ball with one-hand support when the ball is placed in front of his foot:
☐ on level surfaces
☐ on the grass

He kicks the ball without support when the ball is placed in front of his foot:
☐ on level surfaces
☐ on the grass

He walks to the ball, stops in front of it, and then kicks it
☐ with hand support
☐ without hand support

He walks and kicks the ball, continuously over a 100-foot (30-meter) distance
☐ with hand support
☐ without hand support

He fast-steps and kicks the ball, continuously over 100-foot distance
☐ with two-hand and trunk support
☐ with two-hand support
☐ with one-hand support
☐ without support

He runs and kicks the ball, continuously over 100-foot (30-meter) distance
☐ with two-hand support
☐ with one-hand support
☐ without support

☐ He kicks the ball for 10 to 20 feet (3 to 6 meters), with his knee extending as his foot hits the ball

# 11

# Walking Up and Down Curbs

## Introduction

Now that your child can walk well on level surfaces and has practiced paying attention to the floor to step over obstacles, she is ready to learn the skill of walking up and down "curbs." For the purposes of this chapter, a curb is defined as any single step or raised surface from 1 to 8 inches (2.5 to 20 cm) in height. The goal is to walk up and down a curb (about 8 inches or 20 cm) in the community without hand support. Examples of curbs are: an exercise mat or board on the floor, a step at the front door of your house to the front porch, railroad ties at a playground or park, or any place where there are two adjacent surfaces with one higher than the other. On her own, when your child first encounters a raised surface, her first reaction will be to move to plantigrade and climb up rather than walk up. With your support and structure, she will learn the new strategy of walking up.

Learning to walk up and down curbs will improve her walking pattern, particularly in her hips, knees, and feet. She will learn to balance on one foot and use leg, foot, and abdominal strength to walk up and down. As she balances on one foot, her hip will be in neutral rotation, and she will weight shift to the outside border of her foot. Learning to do this will help her walk with a narrower base, with her knees and feet pointing straight. The strength she will use in her legs and feet to step up and down will help her bend her knees when walking, and use toe push-off for propulsion. This skill will also prepare her for walking up and down stairs as she becomes familiar with the leg motions, and gradually builds up the strength she will need to step up and down the height of the stair.

A prerequisite for this skill is your child's ability to *notice* and *pay attention* to obstacles on the floor or changes in the floor surfaces. If she is not able to do this, she will not notice the raised surface and will trip and fall. You will need to give her cues to point out the changes in the surfaces. With experience, she will learn to pay attention. When she notices that one surface is higher or lower than the other, she will need to stop and plan how to step up or down with control. She will learn depth perception through practicing this skill.

---

### Steps in Learning to Walk Up and Down Curbs

To achieve the goal of this skill area, your child will need to practice the following steps:

1. Walk up and down 1" curb with support; without support;
2. Walk up and down 2" curb with support; without support;
3. Walk up and down 3" curb with support; without support;
4. Walk up and down 4" curb with support; without suport;
5. Walk up and down 5" curb with support; without support;
6. Walk up and down 6" curb with support; without support;
7. Walk up and down 7" curb with support; without support;
8. Walk up and down 8" curb with support; without support.

You will begin with hand support and work toward your child doing it by herself. You will gradually increase the height of the curb when she is ready.

---

## Components

The components to focus on are:

1. one-foot balance strategy (hip in neutral rotation, narrow base, knee and foot pointing straight, weight shifting to the outer border of the foot) in standing to step up and down
2. strength in abdominals, leg, and foot to lift the body up or lower it down
3. weight shifting of the trunk, pelvis, and lower leg *forward* over the foot *with momentum* to step up efficiently (fig. 11.1)
4. eccentric actions (like your child learned when walking down an incline) to move slowly with controlled movements to step down the curb (fig. 11.2)
5. leg strength to step down the curb with the knee and foot (of the balancing leg) pointing straight ahead (fig. 11.3)

## Tendencies

The tendencies are:

1. to automatically climb up and down on hands and knees or hands and feet for safety and speed

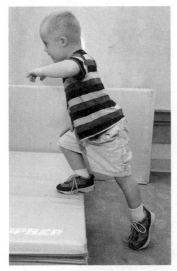 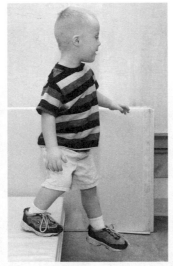 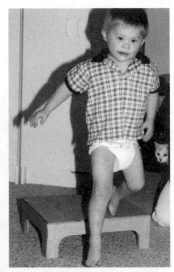

(fig. 11.1)    (fig. 11.2)    (fig. 11.3)

2. to have inadequate strength or balance, or to not know how to use her strength to walk up and down
3. to step up and place her foot on the surface, pause with her ankle/lower leg at 90 degree angle, and then prop on her hands to climb up
4. to step off without attention to the curb, quickly and without control, and then stagger to regain balance
5. to lack control when stepping down the curb (because she likes moving fast and feeling out of control, or does not know how to do it with control)
6. to persist with stepping down sideways with hip external rotation (knee and foot turned outward)

Your child will need to learn how to plan to walk up and down curbs. Since her automatic reaction will be to climb, you will need to set her up to succeed by providing the right support and the right height surface. It is best to start with the easiest setup so she learns how to do it. If you challenge her too soon, it will be counterproductive, and she will choose to climb up and down rather than walk.

## Setup for Learning

**To walk up a curb** (assuming she is leading with her right foot), your child will need to:

1. Stand with her knees and feet pointing straight, and then weight shift onto the outer border on her left foot
2. Maintain her balance with this weight shift, and then lift and place her right foot up on the curb (fig. 11.4)

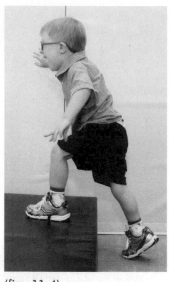 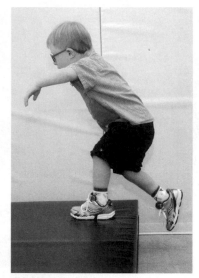

(fig. 11.4)          (fig. 11.5)

3. Maintain her balance with her right foot on the curb and her left foot on the ground
4. Lean her trunk, pelvis, hip, and knee forward over her right foot on the curb, with her knee and shoulders over her toes (fig. 11.5)
5. Straighten her right hip and knee and push off with her right foot to lift her body up on the curb
6. End by placing her left foot on the curb

This is the slow motion, step-by-step sequence of what she needs to do. When she is first learning this skill and does it slowly, it is harder and requires more strength. When she learns to do it quickly with momentum, especially steps 4 and 5, it will be easier and more efficient.

**To walk down a curb** (assuming she is leading with her left foot), she will need to:

1. Stand and balance with her weight shifted over the outer border of her right foot
2. Maintain her balance over her right foot and move her left foot forward (off the curb) to prepare to step down with it (fig. 11.6)
3. Keep her trunk up straight, maintaining her balance, and slowly bend her right knee and hip to lower her left foot to the ground (fig. 11.7)
4. Move her right foot from the curb to the ground

When your child is first learning to step down, she will do best if she partially turns sideways on the curb (fig. 11.8). Or, she may feel more comfortable

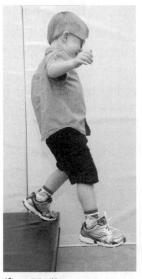
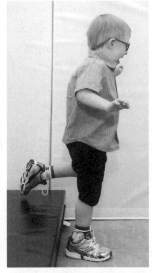
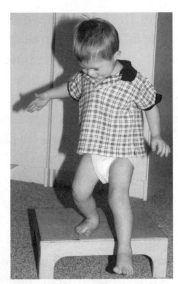

(fig. 11.6)　　　　　(fig. 11.7)　　　　　(fig. 11.8)

doing this skill with her right knee and foot (in the above example) turned outward. When the skill is established, she will learn to execute it in a refined way, with her hip in neutral rotation (hip and knee pointing straight ahead).

She will need hand support to learn how to walk up and down the curb with control. She will first develop the *leg strength* needed to walk up and down curbs while she is holding your index finger. Once she has practiced with hand support and can do the movements effectively, she will need to learn how to *balance* herself, while using her strength, to do the skill on her own.

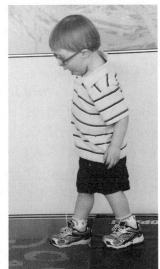

(fig. 11.9)

You will start with a 1-inch (2.5-cm) high "curb" (fig. 11.9). (The best surface is a gymnastics mat. It is a large surface that is safe to fall on and is noticeable because it is a different color than the floor.) In the beginning, your child may not pay attention to the surface, and she may trip when stepping up or down. Or, she may pay attention to the surface but not have the depth perception to judge the height of the surface, causing her to trip. She will learn depth perception through practice with many repetitions using the same surface. She will learn by trial and error, and will develop new strategies based on her mistakes. She will succeed if you systematically practice the height she is ready to learn and gradually increase the height when she is ready.

You can help your child step up by cueing her to march—to do high stepping movements with her legs. She may take bigger steps than needed and will learn to modulate the height of her step to be more efficient through practice. To step down, your child may move her foot forward, with her toes over the edge, and then tilt her foot so her toes feel the ground. Then she will be comfortable with stepping down. If she lunges or trusts that you will catch her, then you need to guide her with a safe method to step down.

Your child's short stature, particularly her short leg length, will influence her ability to achieve the goals in this skill area *without hand support.* She will be able to do 1-3" (2.5-7.5 cm) curbs fairly easily with practice. The higher curbs, 4-8 inches (10-20 cm) , will be more difficult, and she may need to grow taller, as well as gain leg strength and balance, to walk up and down them without hand support. She can still practice this height with hand support to build strength. She will also build strength by practicing walking up and down stairs, toddler size and regular size.

To determine whether a curb is too high for your child to do *without hand support,* look at her leg position from the side, with her foot on the curb. When she places her foot on the curb, if her knee is at the level of her hip, then it is too high for her to do *without hand support* (fig. 11.10). If you challenge your child to do a curb that is too high, she will climb up rather than walk up. Rather than encouraging climbing, it is better to wait for increased leg length before challenging her to do this height curb *without hand support.* To understand the leg strength and balance needed, try stepping up onto a surface where your knee is at or above hip level.

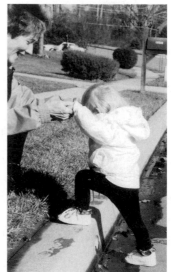

(fig. 11.10)

## *Guidelines*

*Let your child lead with the leg she chooses.* As she practices walking up and down curbs, she may choose to step up with one foot and step down with the other foot. When walking up a curb, the leg that she leads with is usually the stronger leg. When walking down a curb, the leg that stays on the curb is the stronger leg since it needs to lower her body down to the ground. Through practice, she may figure out which leg is stronger and automatically use that leg to step up and lower herself down. For example, if her right leg is stronger, she will step up leading with her right foot and step down leading with her left. When you see her use this method consistently, she is showing you which leg is dominant. Some children lead with the same leg when stepping up and down. If your child does this, she is strengthening each leg, rather than using the strength of her dominant leg.

When she is practicing curbs, observe if she does have a preferred leg to lead with. In the beginning, she will experiment with each leg, and with

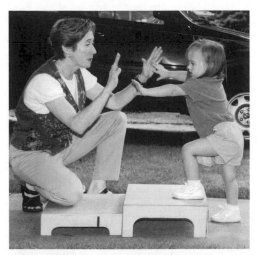

(fig. 11.11)

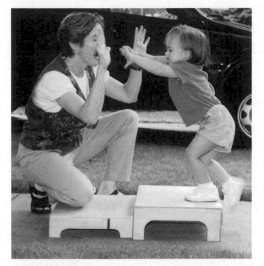

(fig. 11.12)

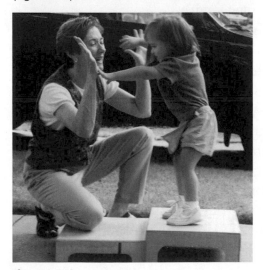

(fig. 11.13)

practice, she will figure out which leg is stronger and use it. If one leg is preferred or easier, guide that strategy so she is successful with learning this skill. Later, when she is familiar with curbs, she may experiment with leading with either leg. When she is ready to practice walking up and down stairs, alternating her feet with one foot on each stair, she will develop strength in both legs. (See page 387 for stairs, alternating feet.) Your child will eventually develop strength in each leg through this stair skill, so let her walk up and down curbs the way that feels best for her.

*Begin with hand support so she develops the strength, and then let go so she develops the balance.* Your child will begin with one-hand support, with you in front of her or at her side. Have her hold your index finger and position her hand in front of her chest, at the level of her shoulder. Your goal is to have her hold your finger and learn to balance herself while holding onto this support.

When she is ready to walk up and down without hand support, the best setup is for you to kneel in front of her at her eye level. She will feel secure with you so close and will be willing to challenge herself. She will be motivated to move to you, and she will feel safe knowing that she can prop against you if she needs support (figs. 11.11–11.13). She also trusts that you will help her, particularly if she falls. By positioning yourself in front of her at eye level, you can encourage her to look forward at you, which will help her step up and down. If she looks down, she will want to climb rather than walk.

*Watch to see whether walking up or down is easier for your child.* This will help you strategize how to help her be successful. You can be sensitive to her reactions to walking up and down and effectively help her learn the parts that she perceives as difficult.

Walking up the curb is generally tolerated with hand support. Your child will feel comfortable learning to use the necessary leg motions and strength with one-hand support. She will be challenged when she needs to walk up without hand support.

Walking down curbs is either viewed as fun (by motor driven children) or is met with resistance (by observers). For some children, walking down is easy at first because they "fall off" the curb. They quickly step off the curb with one leg and then try to recover their balance with staggering steps when their feet land on the ground. For other children, walking down is harder because they do not know how to do it with control. To do it with control, your child will need to slowly bend the hip and knee to lower herself, while balancing on one foot. She may resist this movement because she does not feel stable. She will need hand support to learn the movement and later will be willing to try without hand support if you kneel in front of her. You can also make it easier for her by turning her body partially sideways and having her step down sideways, leading with her preferred foot.

Test your child to see what height curb she is able to step up and down. She may be willing to use a higher surface when moving in her preferred direction. When she is first practicing curbs, if up is easier, she may step up a 3-inch (7.5-cm) curb and step down a 1.5-inch (4-cm) curb. Later, if down is easier, she may step down a 7.5-inch (19-cm) high curb but only be able to walk up a 6-inch (15-cm) curb due to her leg length.

*Provide verbal and visual cues.* You need to be strategic with the setup to help your child be successful.

1. **Make sure the curb is noticeable.** I like to use a mat that is big (4 feet by 6 feet or 1.2 by 1.8 meters) and has a distinct color so it is noticeable. Later, when your child is walking in the community, have her practice walking from the grass to the sidewalk so she notices two distinct surfaces and then can pay attention to the height of the surfaces.

2. **Let her know what you want her to do.** You will need to tell her "up" or "down" and demonstrate it so she can imitate you. If you model the movements needed to step up by making exaggerated marching motions, she will see what you are doing with your legs and imitate you.

3. **Make sure she is motivated to walk up or down and feels secure enough to try it.** Provide a motivator so it is worth challenging herself to walk up or down. For example, she may step up or down to move to a ball or toy, or pop bubbles. Or setup the mat in front of the light switch and then she can turn the lights on and off after she steps up. If there is a toy that she likes to play with, like a kitchen set, you can place the mat in front of it. Then she will practice stepping up and down every time she plays with it. You will need to hold or place the motivator at her eye level so she must be standing to get it. If you are practicing walking up the curb and you place the motivator on the curb, she will climb up to get it rather than try to walk. If you position yourself in front of her with the motivator, she will also feel secure enough to practice walking up or down.

*Choose adjacent surfaces that are firm and level.* When your child is first learning to walk up and down curbs, she needs to feel secure and stable when walking from one surface to another. She will feel most stable on surfaces that are firm and level. The best surface to use is a firm mat. After she learns to step up and down a particular height curb, then you can challenge her by using uneven surfaces, such as a squishy mat, grass, or wood chips. When she is using uneven surfaces, it will be harder to balance on one foot as she is stepping up or down. Her foot will rock and be in a less stable position to balance herself than when she is on a flat, even surface.

*Select adjacent surfaces that are the appropriate size.* When she is first setup to step up onto a surface without hand support, it needs to be large enough that she has adequate space to recover her balance. After she steps up or down with both legs, she will need to take 2 or 3 more steps to stagger and regain her balance. She could stagger in any direction, and the surface must be large enough to allow her to take the additional steps. The ideal surface is a mat 4 feet wide by 6 feet long (1.2 by 1.8 meters), with 2-foot (60-cm) panels. Mats that are 3 feet by 3 feet (90 cm by 90 cm) or 4 feet by 2 feet (1.2 meters by 60 cm) are also acceptable). The mat surface will be about 1.5 inches (4 cm) thick, so it is a good beginning height to use. Later, it can be folded to be 3 inches (7.5 cm) and then 4.5 inches (11 cm) high. If you have 2 mats, you can stack them to increase the height to practice curbs that are 6 inches (15 cm), 7.5 inches (19 cm), and 9 inches (23 cm). When your child develops better balance and control, she will not need to take additional steps.

*Encourage walking up and down curbs rather than climbing.* Now that your child walks and wants to independently explore the environment, when she approaches a curb or raised surface, she will spontaneously move to the plantigrade position to climb up or down the curb (fig. 11.14). She will

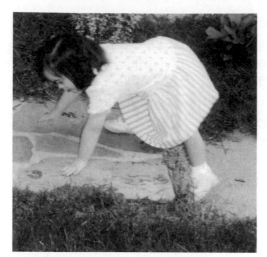

(fig. 11.14)

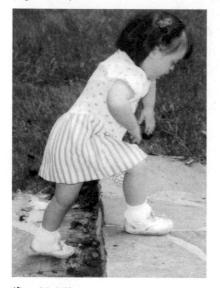

(fig. 11.15)

choose this safe method if she does not feel comfortable walking up and down it. She will need you to teach her to walk up and down, starting with 1- to 2-inch (2.5- to 5-cm) high surfaces. With practice and structure using a mat of this height, she will gain the strength, balance, and confidence to walk rather than climb (fig. 11.15). It is best if you continue to practice the same height until she has mastered it, and she consistently steps up and down with control every time she approaches it.

Increase the height in small increments (1 to 1.5 inches or 2.5 to 4 cm). Realize that she will probably see that the surface is higher and then will use the climbing method rather than walking. If she starts to move to the plantigrade position, let her hold your finger so she walks up and down. When she is ready, see if she will do it without support. If you regularly use a mat for practicing curbs, she may be so familiar with the setup that when you fold the mat, she may not notice the height. She may step up without realizing that it is higher. After she steps up, she will realize the difference, and you will see her reaction in her face! However, she will have demonstrated that physically she can walk up this height curb, and now she just needs to repeat it to feel comfortable and gain confidence with doing it.

***Practice walking up and down a variety of heights of curbs.*** When your child is learning to walk up and down a 3- to 4-inch (7.5- to 10-cm) curb without hand support, you can also practice walking up and down 6- to 8-inch (15- to 20-cm) curbs or stairs with hand support. You will be teaching her to walk rather than climb. When you are at the park and there are railroad ties, if you are walking in and out of your house and there is a step, or if you are walking up and down a standard curb, give her the hand support she needs and encourage her to walk up or down the curb. When she is familiar with walking up and down these curbs in her environment, then you can help her figure out how to walk up or down by herself when possible, by holding onto a nearby support. For example, when walking up or down a step at the front door, help her learn to hold on to the door frame or prop against the wall with both hands to balance herself. If she practices with a variety of heights of curbs, her strength and balance will improve and walking up and down curbs will become easier for her.

## *Temperament*

If your child is an **observer,** walking up a curb will be easier than walking down. She will feel comfortable using her leg strength to walk up the curb, especially with hand support. The leg motions needed to walk down the curb will challenge her, since she needs to lower herself with control and move slowly. At first, she may be fearful or resistant when walking down, and she will want hand support to practice. Since she is detail oriented and attentive to the surfaces, she will notice the change in the surface and will move slowly to lower her foot down to the ground so she is in control. When she is on a 1- to 2-inch (2.5- to 5-cm) curb, she will keep her heel on the curb and slide her toes forward, tipping them downward until they touch the ground. Then she will feel comfortable stepping down with each foot because she will figure out where she needs to go. With practice, she will become familiar with the routine and with what she needs to do and will move faster.

She will prefer to walk up and down with hand support so she feels safe. You will need to wean her from the support when she is ready and show her she can do it by herself. When you are weaning her, you can hold the sleeve of her shirt so she feels a little support. Or kneel in front of her as she is stepping up and down and then she can prop against you if needed, after she steps up or down. She will move slower when she does not have hand support and she will be cautious. You will need to move at her pace so she continues to build confidence rather than lose it. When she is successful with a particular curb height, gradually increase the height of the curb, giving her time to adjust. If you advance her too quickly, she will revert back to climbing up and down rather than walking. With practice and structure, she will walk up and down with control.

If your child is **motor driven,** she will use trial and error to walk up and down the curb. If she trips or falls, she will not be discouraged. Walking down the curb will generally be easier than walking up. She will need to develop the leg strength to walk up the curb but will be willing to just step down off the curb without control and then stagger to regain her balance. She will tend to move fast, so you will need to give her the support she needs to be safe.

When you set her up to walk up the curb surface, she may choose to climb up the curb, if she pays attention to it, or she may keep walking and figure out what to do spontaneously, depending on how it turns out. If she does not step up high enough, she may trip. If she does step up successfully, she may need to take additional steps to recover her balance. You will need to anticipate where to position yourself to guide her to do it safely.

When setup to walk down the curb surface, she probably will just take a step and "fall off" the surface, landing on the ground. On 1- to 3-inch (2.3- to 7.5-cm) curbs, she may be able to take steps to regain her balance after landing on the ground. It is best if you kneel on the ground in front of her. This will help to slow her down and figure out how to lower herself in a limited space with control. If needed, you can give her hand support to help her lower herself to the floor, or she can prop against you for balance after she steps down. With hand support, you can also guide the strategy to step down sideways with control. With practice, she will learn to plan how to step down with balance and control.

## ACTIVITY #1: Walking Up and Down Curbs

1. Pick two firm, adjacent surfaces with one surface raised 1 or 1.5 inches (2.5 to 4 cm). Make sure the surfaces are level and stable, and will not slide or move. Use large surfaces (4 feet by 2 feet or 3 feet by 3 feet) (1.2 meters by .6 meters or .9 meters by .9 meters) so your child can take additional steps to recover her balance. Examples of how you can create 1- to 2-inch curbs are:

   a. Use a firm, foldable gymnastics mat, 4 feet by 6 feet or 1.2 by 1.8 meters (total dimensions when flat on the floor), 1 to 1.5 inches (2.5 to 4 cm) thick, with 2-foot (.6-meter) panels. With this equipment, you can place the mat at the desired height (either flat or folded)

   b. Use a wooden board that is 1 to 1.5 inches (2.5 to 4 cm) thick, 10-12 inches (25-30.5 cm) wide, and at least 3 feet (1 meter) long. Place it on the floor and have your child stand facing the 3-foot length of the board. Have your child step up, walk across the width of the board, and then step down. It is best if the board is on a carpet so it does not slide. The carpet needs to have little or no padding. If it is padded, the board will rock and feel unstable.

   c. Use interlocking squares made of firm, dense foam (2 feet by 2 feet or .6 meters square); they also go by the names "foam floor mats," "kids' mats," "play mats" (Step2 Play Mats). They are durable and lightweight, and the thickness ranges from 3/8 inch to 7/8 inch (1 cm to 2.2 cm). They can be locked together for a 2-foot by 4-foot (.6 meter by 1.2 meter) size, and then stacked to the desired height.

  d. Look everywhere for 1- to 2-inch (2.5- to 5-cm) steps; for example, from the sidewalk to the grass, from the driveway to the grass, or from the garage to the driveway.
2. Once you have setup the curb surface, then model stepping up and down, exaggerating your leg movements by marching. As you walk up and down, say the verbal cues "up," "down," or "march." Then have her take a turn and walk up and down, imitating you.
3. If needed, provide hand support to structure walking up and down. Position yourself in front of her or at her side. Have her hold your index finger, then position her hand in front of her chest, at the level of her shoulder. If she only needs minimal support, you can hold the sleeve of her shirt.
4. If you position yourself in front of her, sit on your heels so you are at eye level to her. If she is ready to step up or down without hand support, place your hands at your chest, to cue her where to prop against you if needed. Encourage her to look at you, rather than looking down. If she looks down, she will probably climb rather than walk.
5. Set up the motivator (either you or a toy) so it is at eye level. For example, you can setup the mat on the floor, against a door, and then hang a motivator on the door handle. Or, setup the mat in front of the wall with the light switch.
6. Once your child is familiar with the setup and game, have her practice on her own for several repetitions. You can model it in the beginning and then see if she will spontaneously play the game on her own. If needed, provide hand support, visual cues, or verbal cues. If she does not pay attention to the surface, pat it to draw her attention to it so she plans stepping up and down.
7. Praise her and clap for her when she walks up or down.
8. Practice this height curb until she consistently and automatically walks up and down with confidence, *without hand support*. When she is ready, try a 2" (5 cm) curb. Follow steps 1-7. Gradually increase the height in 1- to 1.5-inch (2.5- to 4-cm) increments, when she is ready. The folded gymnastics mat is the best surface to use when practicing 3- to 7.5-inch (7.5- to 19-cm) high curbs. The surface that she uses will be 4 feet by 2 feet (1.2 meters by .6 meters) and she will feel confident stepping on and off this large surface.
9. When your child can walk up and down a curb (when placed in front of it or at the edge of it), place her 10 feet (3 meters) from the curb and have her walk to it, and then step up and down. If needed, get her attention by patting the surface to show her where the curb is so she can plan how to do it rather than tripping.

10. Continue to increase the height of the curb, as tolerated, up to about 8 inches (20 cm). Once your child has mastered this height, then she can routinely practice this skill by walking up and down curbs in the community.

11. While she is practicing walking up and down 3- to 4-inch (7.5- to 10-inch) curbs, without hand support, also have her practice walking up and down 6- to 8-inch (15- to 20-cm) curbs with hand support. Work toward having her do it by herself, by holding a door frame, a rail, wall, or something similar.

---

### Strategies for Helping Your Child Master Higher Curbs

When your child is ready to walk up curbs that are 3 inches (7.5 cm) or higher *without hand support*, she will need to learn a new strategy to be successful. She will need to place her foot on the curb and quickly lean her trunk, pelvis, hip, and knee forward over her foot (knee and shoulders over her toes), and then simultaneously straighten her hip and knee and use toe push-off to lift herself up onto the curb. She will need to move fast, holding her knee forward over her toes, to execute this skill. If she moves slowly, or stops after she places her foot on the curb, it will be very difficult for her to step up onto the curb *without hand support*. She will either need hand support, or she will prop her hands on the curb to climb up.

To walk down 3-inch (7.5-cm) and higher curbs with control *without hand support*, she will need to find a method that she feels comfortable using. If she does not figure out a method and continues to try to step off quickly without control, then you need to guide her. The method that many children have used is to turn partially sideways (about 45 degrees), and then step down sideways. For example, if she wants to step down leading with her left foot, she turns 45 degrees to the right with her left foot at the edge of the curb, and then she steps down leading with her left foot. Another method used is to stand with both feet at the edge of the curb, with her right hip, knee, and foot turned outward (for stability) and then step down leading with the left foot. (The left foot will either point straight or turn inward.)

# 🏃 MOTOR MILESTONE CHECKLIST

❑ She walks up 1" (2.5 cm) curb with support
❑ She walks up 1" curb without support
❑ She walks down 1" curb with support
❑ She walks down 1" curb without support

❑ She walks up 2" (5 cm) curb with support
❑ She walks up 2" curb without support
❑ She walks down 2" curb with support
❑ She walks down 2" curb without support

❑ She walks up 3" (7.5 cm) curb with support
❑ She walks up 3" curb without support
❑ She walks down 3" curb with support
❑ She walks down 3" curb without support

❑ She walks up 4" (10 cm) curb with support
❑ She walks up 4" curb without support
❑ She walks down 4" curb with support
❑ She walks down 4" curb without support

❑ She walks up 5" (12.5 cm) curb with support
❑ She walks up 5" curb without support
❑ She walks down 5" curb with support
❑ She walks down 5" curb without support

❑ She walks up 6" (15 cm) curb with support
❑ She walks up 6" curb without support
❑ She walks down 6" curb with support
❑ She walks down 6" curb without support

*(continued on next page)*

❏ She walks up 7" (18 cm) curb with support

❏ She walks up 7" curb without support

❏ She walks down 7" curb with support

❏ She walks down 7" curb without support

❏ She walks up 8" (20 cm) curb with support

❏ She walks up 8" curb without support

❏ She walks down 8" curb with support

❏ She walks down 8" curb without support

# 12

# Walking Up and Down Stairs

## Introduction

Your child can start practicing walking up and down stairs after he walks all of the time on level surfaces. He will be comfortable learning to walk *up* stairs, and this will be the first skill to learn. Walking *down* stairs will be harder, so you will need to test when he is ready to practice this skill. He will do best practicing on stairs that are suitable for his short leg length, using toddler-size stairs, found at toddler playgrounds. Toddler-size stairs are usually 4-5 inches (10-12.5 cm) high, with a low railing, and there are 4 stairs in the set. Regular size stairs are 7.75 to 8.25 inches (19.68 to 21 cm) high, and your child can practice on them after he masters toddler-size stairs. The goals will be to:

1. Walk up and down a flight of stairs, holding the railing, with two feet on each stair (marking time) (figs. 12.1, 12.2);

2. Walk up and down a flight of stairs, holding the railing, with one foot on each stair (alternating).

While your child is practicing walking up and down stairs, he will simultaneously be practicing walking up and down curbs. Some children prefer practicing one skill over the other, so you can practice the preferred skill, knowing that each skill reinforces the other.

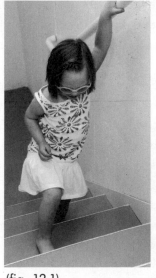 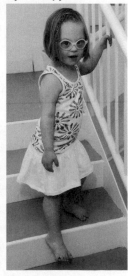

(fig. 12.1)          (fig. 12.2)

The curbs will prepare him to use the leg motions and to develop the strength needed to walk up and down stairs. Walking up and down stairs requires more leg strength and endurance because stairs are higher and several must be climbed in a row.

These goals will take a long time to achieve, especially walking up and down stairs, alternating his feet. He will probably achieve the first goal of walking up and down stairs, marking time, between the ages of 3-4 years. He will achieve the second goal in two stages with walking up stairs, alternating feet, occurring at 4-5 years, and walking down stairs, alternating feet, occurring between 6-8 years. These skills are delayed in children with Down syndrome due to the physical characteristics of shorter legs and arms and smaller hands and fingers. The height of the regular stairs in proportion to the length of the leg puts the child at a mechanical disadvantage since his hip and knee are in more flexion, and therefore more strength is required to step up the stair and lower himself down. With his short arms and legs, it will take time to reach the standard height railing, and his grasp will be compromised with his small fingers and hands, trying to hold onto the large width of the railing.

While your child is working on achieving the goals, there will be times when you will need to be patient and wait for his legs to grow before he can practice the next level skill. For example, if he has mastered walking up and down stairs, marking time, holding the railing but his legs are too short to use the alternating pattern, you will need to wait for his legs to grow before he can progress to the next skill level.

## Steps in Learning to Walk Up and Down Stairs

To achieve the goals of this skill area, your child will practice the following steps:
1. Walk up and down stairs, marking time, holding onto an adult with two-hand support
2. Walk up and down stairs, marking time, holding onto an adult with one hand and to the railing with his other hand
3. Walk up and down stairs, marking time, stepping sideways and holding the railing with both hands (optional)
4. Walk up and down stairs, marking time, with one hand holding the railing
5. Walk up stairs, alternating feet, with one hand on the railing and one hand holding onto an adult
6. Walk up stairs, alternating feet, with one hand holding the railing
7. Walk down stairs, alternating feet, with one hand on the railing and one hand holding onto an adult
8. Walk down stairs, alternating feet, with one hand holding the railing

## Components

The components to focus on are:

1. strength in the arms, abdominals, legs, and feet to lift the body weight up to the next stair, or to lower down, and the endurance to walk up and down the flight of stairs
2. arm and hand strength to assist leg strength and provide balance when stepping up and down the stairs, and the ability to plan advancing the hand on the railing to the most effective place to do these actions
3. weight shifting the head, trunk, pelvis, and knee forward over the foot and toes to step up the stairs

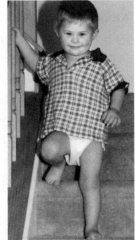

4. eccentric leg and foot actions (also practiced when walking down curbs and inclines) to move slowly, with controlled movements, to step down the stairs
5. leg strength to step down the stairs with the knee and foot (of the balancing leg) pointing straight ahead (fig. 12.3)
6. ability to plan and carry out the sequence of steps necessary to walk up and down the entire flight of stairs

(fig. 12.3)

7. judgment and attention to walk up and down the entire flight of stairs safely on a consistent basis

## Tendencies

The tendencies are:

1. to automatically climb up and down the stairs rather than walk, and to prefer climbing for speed, safety, and independence
2. to have inadequate strength, or to not know how to use his strength to walk up and down
3. to walk up with two-hand support, with an adult holding the child's hands above his shoulders, and to learn to become dependent on the adult's support
4. to walk up the stairs with hand support and to lean his trunk and pelvis back and to straighten his knee (rather than weight shifting his trunk, pelvis, and knee forward over his foot and then straighten his knee), so the adult is lifting and balancing the child
5. to choose to walk down by sliding both feet forward off the stair simultaneously, and totally depend on the adult to manage balance and safety

6. to try to walk down, keeping the knee (of the standing leg) straight, and resist bending the knee to lower himself to the next stair
7. to feel insecure with just holding the railing, and to want to hold onto an adult's hand even though he is ready to do it by himself
8. to persist with stepping down the stairs with the standing leg positioned with the knee and foot turned outward
9. to become distracted when walking down the stairs, causing him to trip and fall

## Setup for Learning

When you start practicing on the stairs at home, your child may initiate standing on the stairs spontaneously on his own. Even though he is competent using his usual safe method of climbing up and down the stairs, he will experiment with this new method since you have introduced it to him. Also, if he has siblings, he has seen them do it and wants to be like them. Until he can safely walk up and down stairs by himself, you need to plan a strategy for stair safety when he is unsupervised.

Practice stairs often and find motivating ways to incorporate them into your child's daily routine. Walk up stairs to take a bath or to find siblings playing in their bedrooms. Walk down stairs to play with the dog or to eat, or to go to a playroom in the basement. Look for ways to modify your stairs, such as by installing a lower railing or CareRails® Bannister Kit, so your child can be successful walking up and down safely by himself. Practice on a variety of stairs in the community so your child learns to adapt to different railings, heights of stairs, and stairs with and without risers (open space in between the stairs). You will have lots of time to practice the goals since stairs are everywhere. When your child learns to walk up and down stairs by himself, he will be independent at home, school, and in the community. It is urgent to achieve the final goal— walking down stairs, alternating his feet while holding the railing—since he will need to be competent if there is a fire drill at school or in the community. He needs a safe and efficient way to move with a group of people in an emergency situation.

Each of the steps in learning to walk up and down stairs will be described in the following sections. The terms for the various parts of stairs can be confusing, so for the purposes of this chapter, we will use the following definitions:

1. **Banister:** the handrail or the diagonal (angled) bar that everyone uses.
2. **Spindles:** the vertical posts that hold up the banister, also referred to as the baluster.
3. **Railing:** the place your child holds on; it could refer to either the banister or the spindles.

It will be important to use a railing that is the right height for your child to reach, and small enough in diameter so he can grip it and hold on effectively. When your child is young, spindles will be easier because they are often narrow enough for his hand to grasp and he can choose the height that works best for him. The banister is usually too high and so wide that it is hard for him to hold onto it. You will

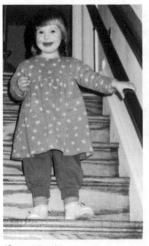

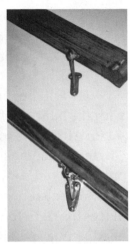

(fig. 12.4)                    (fig. 12.5)

need to find a railing your child can use so he is successful in learning to walk up and down stairs. You could use CareRails® toddler stairway handrail products (banister or rail mount kits). Or, like Sarah's father, you can add a lower and smaller railing to help your child master the stairs (figs. 12.4, 12.5). Here is how he describes installing the rail:

"We bought the narrowest banister rail at Home Depot. I brushed on stain/polyurethane and let it dry. We mounted the brackets directly underneath the higher ones (since we knew there had to be a stud there). Apparently, you don't tighten down the upper part of the bracket (attached to rail) until you've fitted the rail onto the lower part of the bracket. The whole process of mounting the rail took us less than fifteen minutes!"

In the following sections, the descriptions will use the example that your child is stepping up leading with the right leg and stepping down leading with the left, which would be seen if his right leg was dominant. If your child is left leg dominant or if he prefers to step up and down leading with the same leg, you will need to adjust the instructions accordingly.

### Walk Up Stairs, Marking Time, Stepping Forward

To walk up stairs, your child will need:
1. to hold on with one or both hands
2. to lift his right foot up on the stair and balance himself using his arms while holding your finger(s) or the railing
3. to lean his head, shoulders, trunk, pelvis, and knee forward over his right foot and toes
4. to straighten his right hip and knee, and push off with his foot, to lift his body weight up on the stair. He will simultaneously use his arms and hands for balance, and to pull his body weight up on the stair.

5. to place his left foot on the stair so both feet are together
6. to advance his hand forward on the railing
7. to repeat these steps until he walks up the flight of stairs.

He will begin with two-hand support, holding an adult's index fingers with his hands in front of his chest at shoulder level (fig. 12.6). (See Activity #1A.) After he is comfortable walking up holding your index fingers, then you can test when he is ready to progress to holding an adult's index finger with one hand and a railing with the other, as detailed in Activity #1B (fig. 12.7).

You also need to watch your child's posture and movements after he places his right foot on the stair. He will need to learn how to weight shift his head, trunk, pelvis, and knee forward over his foot and toes, and then use hip, knee, and ankle strength to lift his body up onto the stair. He will need to follow the two-step movement sequence of weight shifting forward, and then moving upward. A common mistake is for the child to place his foot on the stair and then straighten his hip and knee without doing the weight shift forward, so the result is that he leans his trunk back, and you need to manage his position and balance on the stair.

Once he learns how to step up one stair using the right sequence, then see if he uses the marking time pattern with two feet per stair. The marking time pattern is the beginner's method so you would anticipate that he would use this pattern first. Some children will use the alternating pattern with one foot per stair, since they have two-hand support for balance, and they have adequate leg strength to use either leg. If your child alternates his feet, check your hand support to see if you are providing too much support; for example, holding his hands above his head. Also, check to see if he is leaning back rath-

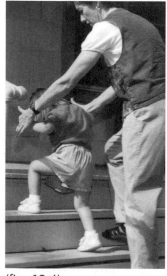

(fig. 12.6)

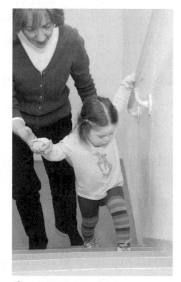

(fig. 12.7)

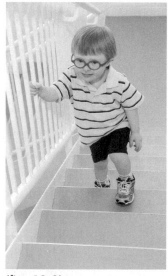

(fig. 12.8)

er than leaning forward. If your child is alternating his legs because of these problematic methods, then guide him to use the proper methods. If the hand support and position of his arms is right and if he is doing the two-step movement sequence to step up the stair with balance and control, then allow him to use the alternating pattern since it will develop leg strength in both legs. However, when he is ready to walk up stairs just holding the railing (with only one-hand support), he will use the marking time pattern. When his legs are long enough, then he will learn to use the alternating pattern.

When your child easily walks up the flight of stairs, marking time, with one hand on the railing and one hand holding an adult's finger, test to see when he is ready to walk up the flight, just holding the railing (fig. 12.8). When he first tries to walk up the stairs using only the railing for support, he may compensate by propping one hand on the next stair. If he does this, provide minimal support to promote walking up the stairs rather than allow this climbing method. You can let him hold your finger so he has two-hand support, but lower your hand to provide the least support. Or, you can let him hold the railing with both of his hands until he is confident with maintaining his balance with one hand. Another option is to hold the sleeve of his shirt, above his shoulder, so he feels your support and has the confidence to walk up rather than prop his hand.

### Walk Down Stairs, Marking Time, Stepping Forward
To walk down stairs, your child will need:
1. to hold on with one or both hands
2. to straighten his trunk and lean slightly to the right, and then move his left foot forward to prepare to step down to the next stair
3. to maintain his balance with his trunk up straight and using his arms, slowly bend his right knee, hip, and ankle to lower his left foot to the next stair
4. to step down with his right foot so both feet are together
5. to advance his hand forward on the railing
6. to repeat these steps until he walks down the flight of stairs

Walking down is usually harder to teach, and your child may be fearful, so you need to proceed slowly until he is familiar with the knee, hip, and ankle actions he needs to use. He will not know how to lower himself and will resist you when you try to bend his knee (Step 3 above). His strategy will be to keep his right knee straight so he feels stable and then take a wide step sideways with his left foot to move down to the next stair, relying on you to control his balance. Or, he will keep his knees straight and slide both feet forward off the stair together. You will need to provide maximal support, as described in Activity #2, so he feels stable learning to slowly bend his right hip, knee, and ankle to lower his left foot to the next stair. Once he is familiar with the necessary movements and feels comfortable using them, walking down stairs will be easy.

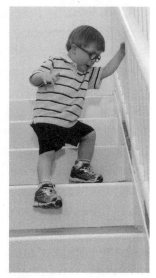

(fig. 12.9)

With the stress of learning this challenging skill, your child may use movements to stabilize until the skill becomes easier (fig. 12.9). For example, if he steps down leading with his left foot, he may position his right knee and foot turned outward and his left foot and knee turned inward. You also might notice that he slides the back of his lower left leg against the stair as he moves it down to the next stair. These compensations will decrease with practice and increased leg length, and he will learn to step down with both knees and feet pointing straight ahead.

### Walk Up and Down Stairs, Marking Time, Stepping Sideways

Walking up and down stairs sideways can be practiced if you have spindles or a lowered railing. It can be practiced at the same time as walking up and down stairs, marking time and facing forward, with one hand on the railing and one hand holding an adult's hand. You can practice this skill if your child shows interest. Some children want to practice this setup, and it prepares them to walk up and down stairs independently. When setup to practice this skill, make sure your child is positioned to use the railing that allows him to lead with his preferred leg.

To walk up the stairs, he will need:
1. to hold onto the spindles or banister with both hands and stand sideways, facing the railing. (For example, if he prefers to lead with his right leg, he will hold the railing on the left side of the staircase so his right leg can lead.)
2. to step sideways and lift his right foot up on the next stair and balance using his arms
3. to lean his trunk sideways and weight shift his body over his right foot
4. to straighten his right hip and knee, and push off with his foot and lift his body weight up on the stair. He will simultaneously use his arms for balance and to pull his body weight up on the stair
5. to place his left foot on the stair so both feet are together

6. to advance his hands forward on the railing
7. to repeat these steps until he walks up the flight of stairs

To walk down the stairs, he will need:
1. to hold onto the spindles or banister with both hands and stand sideways, facing the railing. (For example, if he prefers to lead with his left leg, he will hold the railing on the right side of the staircase so his left leg can lead.)
2. to lean his trunk and weight shift his body over his right foot
3. to step out with his left foot
4. to maintain his balance and slowly bend his right hip, knee, and ankle to lower his left foot to the next stair. He will simultaneously use his arms to lower himself and for balance.
5. to lean over his left leg and step down with his right leg, using his arms for balance
6. to advance his hands forward on the railing
7. to repeat these steps until he walks down the flight of stairs

At first, you will need to hold your child's hands on the railing to assist his grip and advance them as he walks up or down. When he is walking up the stairs, you will position yourself behind him so you can easily reach his hands. When walking down the stairs, you will position yourself in front of him, one to two stairs below him, facing him. When he is ready, you will decrease your support.

You will need to supervise your child until he learns to do this skill safely on a consistent basis. When he is ready, he will spontaneously let go with one hand and begin stepping forward with only one hand on the railing. By practicing walking up and down sideways, he will learn what he needs to do to control his own body rather than learning to do it with another's support.

### Walk Up Stairs, Alternating Feet

To walk up stairs, he will need:
1. to hold on with one or both hands
2. to lift his right foot up on the stair and balance using his arms, by holding on to your hands or the railing
3. to lean his head, shoulders, trunk, pelvis, and knee forward over his right foot and toes
4. to straighten his right hip and knee, and push off with his foot, to lift his body weight up on the stair. He will simultaneously use his arms and hands for balance and to pull himself up on the stair
5. to advance his hand forward on the railing

6. to hold on and balance while lifting his left foot up two stairs from where it was
7. to lean his head, shoulders, trunk, pelvis, and knee forward over his left foot and toes
8. to straighten his left hip and knee and push off with his foot, to lift his body weight up on the stair. He will simultaneously use his arms and hands for balance and to pull himself up on the stair
9. to advance his hand forward on the railing
10. to hold on and balance while lifting his right leg up two stairs from where it was
11. to repeat steps 3 to 10 until he walks up the flight of stairs

Your child will usually show you he is ready to practice this new method of walking up stairs by spontaneously using an alternating pattern when he walks up the top one or two stairs of the flight. He will need two-hand support to learn to use the alternating pattern for the entire flight. Through using his old method of walking up stairs, marking time, holding the railing, he gained the leg strength in his dominant leg for the alternating pattern, and now he needs to improve the strength and endurance in his nondominant leg, to walk up a flight of stairs. Each leg will need to have adequate strength to lift his body weight up onto the next stair. When marking time, only one leg, the leading leg, needed to have that degree of strength.

If your child does not initiate practicing the alternating pattern, and he is proficient with walking up stairs, marking time, holding the railing, then you need to figure out when to teach him the new method of alternating his feet. Since the average age for children with Down syndrome to walk up stairs, alternating feet, holding the railing is 4.5 years (according to my data), you can introduce the skill around 4 years as long as his leg length is adequate. You can test if your child will automatically alternate his feet if given two-hand support. If not, you can have him step up with his dominant leg, and then assist his nondominant leg. In the beginning, you just want to introduce the new method with whatever support he prefers, hand or leg support, or both. Once he is familiar with the new method with support, he will work on improving the strength in his nondominant leg to lift his body weight up each stair and to do this for several repetitions to walk up the flight.

### Walk Down Stairs, Alternating Feet
To walk down stairs, he will need:
1. to hold on with one or both hands
2. to straighten his trunk and lean slightly to the right, and then move his left foot forward to prepare to step down

3. to maintain his balance using his arms, and slowly bend his right hip, knee, and ankle to lower his left foot to the next stair
4. to advance his hand on the railing
5. to straighten his trunk and lean slightly to the left, and then move his right foot forward to prepare to step down
6. to maintain his balance using his arms, and slowly bend his left hip, knee, and ankle to lower his right foot two stairs below where it was
7. to advance his hand on the railing
8. to straighten his trunk and lean slightly to the right, maintain his balance with his arms, and then slowly bend his right hip, knee, and ankle to lower his left foot two stairs below where it was
9. to repeat steps 4-8 until he walks down the flight of stairs

Walking down stairs this way will be harder to learn than walking up stairs and occurs much later. For children with Down syndrome, the average age to achieve this skill is 6 to 8 years (according to my data). Your child will need to have additional leg strength and length in order to do it successfully. Some children will be fearful of the combination of lowering the body so far with each leg, and of looking down the flight of stairs. You will need to be sensitive to your child's reaction, and figure out the best time and method to practice this skill when he is ready.

If your child is still using the marking time pattern to walk down stairs when he is 7.5 to 8 years old, you need to figure out when to introduce this new method. Consider when he mastered walking up stairs, alternating his feet, holding the railing and compare his age to the average age for children with Down syndrome. Also consider his leg length. If his legs are very short, then he may need more length before he will be successful. Any depth perception problems will also make him more sensitive to practicing this skill. These parameters will guide you in figuring out when and how to practice this skill in a way that works best for your child.

When you practice walking downstairs, alternating legs, you need to provide whatever support is needed to help your child become familiar with the new pattern. His habit will be to lead with the same leg, based on leg dominance, so he will resist moving his other leg. Be patient with this process and experiment with setups that make this new method easier to tolerate. For example, start with a set of two stairs, letting him lead with his usual leg, and then assist his other leg down the bottom stair. Whatever you can do to help him participate with the new method will start the process of changing his habitual way of walking down stairs, marking time.

Your child will need to practice this skill for many repetitions to learn to do it quickly and automatically. At first, he will move slowly and focus on one stair at a time. You can give verbal cues ("one, two" or "left, right") and visual cues (such as modeling how to kick each foot forward and then lowering it down to the next stair). If he pays attention, he will use the new method. However, if he is distracted, he will use his old habit of walking down, marking time. Continue to persevere with practicing this skill until it is consolidated into his daily repertoire. It is an important skill to master for safety in school settings and in the community, in the event of a fire drill evacuation.

## Guidelines

*Let your child lead with the leg he chooses.* As discussed in the last chapter, your child will generally prefer to lead with a particular leg when stepping up and use the opposite leg when stepping down. If he does not show a preference, watch him to see if he develops one. Generally, he will learn to step up leading using his stronger, dominant leg and step down leading with his other leg.

Allow him to lead with the leg he chooses so he feels stable walking up and down the stairs. Later, when he is ready to learn to use the alternating pattern, you can encourage him to do the opposite of what he is familiar with in order to strengthen his non-dominant leg.

*Observe your child and identify if walking up or down stairs is easier.* Up is generally easier because he is more familiar with straightening his hip and knee, and he feels secure with the next stair being so close that he could prop on it if he needed to.

Down is generally harder because he needs strength to lower himself to the next stair. A standard size stair will seem like a long way for him to have to lower himself. It will also require more control than stepping off the curb since he cannot "fall off" and then catch his balance. Stepping down is hard for many children, but particularly those who have tended to move with stiff knees.

Be sensitive to your child's reactions to walking up and down the stairs and provide the support he needs to be comfortable learning these skills.

*Give your child hand support and, when he is ready, let go.* He will need your hand support until he can walk up and down by himself, holding the railing. How to provide hand support is outlined in the Activity section below. Children with the observer temperament will want to continue holding your hand to feel secure, and you will need to wean your support.

When your child has mastered walking up and down stairs with his hand on the railing, I recommend continuing to use the railing for safety, especially in crowded settings like school and community environments. When stairs in the community do not have a railing, like in a stadium, then it will be functional for him to learn to walk up and down without a railing.

***Help your child learn to balance himself.*** Try not to offer your child more hand support than he needs. If you hold his hands rather than teaching him to hold your fingers, he will become dependent on you and not learn to hold on and balance himself. Another common mistake is to hold your child's hands above his head when walking up stairs. With this support, you lift him up onto the next stair and control his balance. When this is done, he does not learn the arm and leg movements nor develop the strength and balance needed to walk up the stair. Later on, if he does not use the railing effectively, it could be because you are providing too much support, or he is relying on your hand support. Remember that the purpose of your support is to help him balance himself, and to work toward weaning your support rather than creating dependence on your support. How you provide hand support will be critical in developing the actions, strength, and balance needed to walk up stairs.

***Give verbal, visual, and tactile cues.*** When your child is learning to walk up and down stairs, you will say "up" or "down." When he is practicing walking up or down a flight of stairs, you can focus him on each stair by counting them as he steps on each one. When he is ready to learn to alternate his legs, you can say "big step" or "one and two," or "left and right." He will probably repeat the words you say, and this will help him focus on what he is doing.

Give him visual cues to model, like having his sister walk up the stairs in front of him. Or, his sister can stand at the top of the stairs and hold a toy for motivation. To help him move his hand forward on the railing, you can slap the railing with your hand (or tap your ring on a metal railing for the sound effect). This will focus him on where you want him to put his hand. When he is ready to alternate his legs, you can stand beside him, and he can watch you do it, and then imitate you.

You will initially provide tactile cues by giving him hand support so he feels the motions needed for walking up and down stairs. Later, you can give specific cues to his hands to help him hold onto the railing, and to his legs to help him use an alternating pattern.

***Use spindles if they are available, or add a lowered railing.*** If your stairs have spindles, use them to initially practice walking up and down stairs. It will be easier for your child to hold the spindles because he will be able to reach them at a height that is comfortable for him, and the width is narrow enough to grasp. When he is taller and can comfortably reach the banister, he will use it instead of the spindles.

If your stairs do not have spindles, then add a lowered railing that is a good diameter for his hand size. Your child will make the best progress in learning to do stairs by himself if he can hold on to a railing.

***Use a railing that is small enough for your child to grasp.*** Your child probably has short fingers and small hands, which will make it hard for him to hold onto many railings. If you can find a railing that is small enough for him to hold and grip with his hand, he will be more successful. With a small diameter railing, he will be able to use his arms more effectively to pull up, lower, and balance himself when walking up and down stairs. If he cannot hold onto the railing, he will need to hold onto your hands to effectively use his arms, and he will become dependent on you. Look for small railings at toddler playgrounds, use spindles or CareRails®, or add a lower railing (using a narrow dowel or banister) to your stairs. Later, when your child's legs are stronger and he only needs to use his arms and hands for balance, he can prop his hand against the wall to walk up and down the stairs.

*Begin with walking up and down a few stairs and work toward doing a flight of stairs.* When possible, begin with a set of three to six stairs so he is successful in reaching the top or bottom before he is fatigued. You can also use the top three to six stairs when walking up a flight of stairs or the bottom three to six when walking down. When he is ready, gradually increase the number of stairs until he can walk up and down the entire flight of stairs.

When practicing new challenging skills, such as decreasing hand support from two-hand to one-hand or when beginning to learn the alternating pattern, practice at the top or bottom of the flight.

*Use carpeted stairs, if available.* Your child will generally feel more secure on carpet because it will not be slippery. You will probably feel more comfortable, too, knowing he will not hurt himself if he falls. When he is not using a carpeted surface, supervise him more closely until you feel comfortable with his ability to walk up and down the stairs safely.

*Start with toddler-size stairs with a height of 4-5 inches (10-12.5 cm), if available.* Your child will be ready to walk up and down stairs earlier if he can use shorter stairs with a lower railing (fig. 12.10). The major difficulty in using standard size stairs is your child's height and short leg length relative to the 8-inch (20-cm) high stair and the standard height banister (fig. 12.11). To understand the challenge, consider the following: If you measure your child's leg when sitting in a chair, from the crease in his knee to the bottom of his heel, it will be approximately 8 inches (20 cm). If you are 5 feet 3 inches (157 cm)

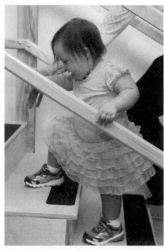
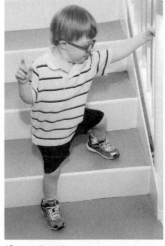

(fig. 12.10)          (fig. 12.11)

tall and do the same measurement on your leg, it will be approximately 16 inches (40.5 cm). If you were to walk up 2 stairs at a time, you would be exerting the same degree of effort that your child needs to do for an 8-inch (20-cm) stair.

If shorter stairs are not available, your child will need to practice on standard size stairs with support until he has adequate strength, balance, and height to use them by himself. Some brick front porch stairs are shorter, and you may also find sets of shorter stairs at toddler playgrounds, at parks, and in your neighborhood.

*Provide supervision appropriate to your child's skill level.* In the beginning, you may be reluctant to practice walking up and down stairs in the home due to your fear of your child falling down the stairs. You will realize that once he has the idea of standing on the stairs, he may try it when you are not there. So, once you start practicing walking up and down stairs at home, you will need to setup the house so your child is safe. You can use gates so he can only be on the stairs when you are with him. You will need to manage his safety on the stairs until you know he has developed the physical skills and judgment to walk up and down the flight of stairs safely on a consistent basis.

*When stepping sideways up or down the stairs, set him up to lead with his preferred leg.* He will need to use the railing on a particular side of the staircase in order to lead with his preferred leg. For example, if he prefers to lead with his right leg, he will need to use the railing on the left. If there is only one railing for the staircase and it is not on the side your child needs it to be, he will not be able to practice walking up and down sideways on that staircase. You will need to practice walking up and down, facing forward, with one hand holding the railing and his other hand holding your finger. When he has adequate leg strength and only needs to prop his hand(s) against the wall for balance, then he can walk up sideways with his hands against the wall.

*Encourage your child to carry a small toy in one hand when he is ready to use one hand on the railing.* Your child will be reluctant to have you let go of his hand. When he is ready to learn to walk up and down the stairs with only one hand on the railing, give him a small, lightweight toy to hold in his other hand. This may help him forget about holding your hand. You can play a game where he needs to take the toy and give it to someone at the top or bottom of the stairs.

*Practice stairs often with siblings so your child has the desire to do them, wants to walk rather than climb, and learns to do them independently.* Encourage your child to walk up and down stairs at home with support so he develops the strength for stairs. If there are railings that work for his size, then he will have the ideal setup to learn to walk up and down stairs. He will want to imitate and model his siblings, and walk up and down like they do, so this environment will motivate him to learn this skill.

If the railing does not work for his size, then his habit will be to climb, since this is the only method he can use independently. You can help him practice walking up and down when you are with him, but he will not be able to choose to do it on his own and will not be motivated to learn it. Later, you will need to teach him to walk up and down, and change his preferred habit of climbing.

*You may need to wait for your child to grow in order to learn the next goal.* Because of his short stature, there will be times when you need to wait for his legs to grow before he can master the next level skill. In the meantime, his strength will improve by repeating the skills that he can do, and then when he is the right size, you can practice the skill when he will be successful using it. For example, if your child can walk up and down the stairs at home independently with your lowered railing, he may not be able to use stairs in some community settings until he is tall enough to hold the standard railing. In any setting, when he can walk up and down the stairs, marking time, holding the railing, his legs may be too short to learn the next goal of walking up the stairs, alternating his feet.

## Temperament

If your child is an **observer,** he will want to feel safe, secure, and in control when walking up and down the stairs. He will prefer his old method of climbing up and down the stairs because he knows how to do that, and it is easier for him. He will need to be motivated to walk up and down the stairs, but with hand support, he will cooperate. He will pay attention to each stair and will be careful with each step he takes and where he places his foot. He will intuitively focus on being safe, and you will need to focus on helping him learn to do the movements easily, efficiently, and quickly.

After he has learned to walk up and down the stairs with hand support, he will be reluctant to change to only holding the railing. He will prefer holding your hand because he will feel more stable and safe.

When it is time to learn to use an alternating pattern, your child will probably need to be taught. Walking up and down the stairs using a marking time pattern will be effective for him, and it is a habit he has used for awhile, so he may not initiate using an alternating pattern.

Taurean could walk up the stairs well using an alternating pattern. He was seven years old, very tall, and ready to learn to walk down using an alternating pattern. When I first began teaching him to walk down the stairs, he told me, "I'm scared." He would step down with his left foot easily and then I would move his right foot down to the next stair. Every time I moved his right foot, he said "hurts." We kept repeating the leg motions together and after several repetitions, he no longer said "hurts" or "I'm scared." Then I started counting "1, 2," and on "1," he would move his left foot, and on "2," I would move his right foot. By practicing this way, the movements were tolerated and became familiar. He learned he was safe and could trust what I was doing to his right foot. With practice, he learned to alternate his legs by himself.

If your child is **motor driven,** you will need to supervise him closely until he learns how to move his legs safely. He will learn to walk up the stairs safely before he learns to walk down. When walking down, he may slide both feet off the stair or be resistant to bending his knee to move slowly with control. He may try to move fast and "fall off" the stair. You will need to slow him down so he learns to lower himself safely, with control. He may not pay attention to where he places his feet and place his foot on the edge of the stair so it easily slides off. He may let go of the railing and rely on you to balance him. He will learn by experience how to walk up and down stairs safely, and you will need to provide strategic support to help him make the necessary corrections.

## ACTIVITY #1: Walking Up Stairs, Marking Time, Facing Forward

If your child is a new walker, use a set of toddler-size stairs, found at a toddler playground. When your child is comfortable with walking up toddler-size stairs with two-hand support, then use a set of regular-size stairs. Begin with a set of 4-6 stairs or use the top half of the flight. When your child is ready, use the entire flight of stairs.

## Activity #1A: Walking Up Stairs, Marking Time, with Two-Hand Support

1. Place a motivator at the top of the stairs on the landing or have your child follow a sibling walking up the stairs.
2. Position yourself behind him, leaning your trunk forward, over him.
3. Place your index fingers horizontally in front of his chest and have him hold onto them. His right hand will hold your right index finger, and his left hand will hold your left index finger. Position his hands at the level of his shoulders. You can hold his wrists if needed for stability. Lessen your wrist support whenever possible.
4. With this support, say "up" and wait for him to lift his foot up on the stair.
5. After he lifts his foot and places it on the stair, then with the hand support, lean his shoulders, trunk, pelvis, and knee forward over his foot. Once he is weight shifted forward, wait for him to hold on and use his leg and foot strength to lift his body up onto the stair, and then place his other foot on the stair.

6. Encourage him to repeat this sequence to walk up the stairs to the landing. Clap for him, praise him, and give him the motivator.

7. Continue to practice the above steps until your child is familiar and comfortable with walking up the entire flight of stairs easily.

## Activity #1B: Walking Upstairs, Marking Time, with Hand & Rail Support

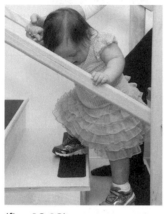
(fig. 12.12)

1. When your child can do step 7 of Activity #1A, guide him to hold the railing with one hand and hold your index finger with his other hand (fig. 12.12).

2. Use a railing that he can reach and grip; for example, spindles or a low banister.

3. Set him up so the hand holding the railing is opposite to the leg he leads with.

4. Stand behind him, and have him hold your index finger with his other hand. Position his hand in front of his chest, at the level of his shoulder.

5. Assist his hand holding the railing, providing hand over hand guidance. At first, help him grasp the railing and advance his hand forward with each stair to model the movements that he needs to learn. Later, see if he can do these actions by himself.

6. Follow steps 1-2 and 4-7 in Activity #1A, except he will hold the railing with one hand and hold your index finger with his other hand. When he is doing step 5, use his hand holding your index finger to guide him to lean his shoulder, trunk, pelvis, and knee forward over his foot.

7. When he is comfortable with this setup and can do it easily, then lower his hand (holding your index finger) toward waist level to decrease the support.

## Activity #1C: Walking Up Stairs, Marking Time, Holding the Rail

1. When your child can do step 7 of Activity #1B, test when he is ready to practice only holding onto the railing.

2. Use a railing that he can reach and grip; for example, spindles or a low banister.

3. Set him up so the hand holding the railing is opposite to the leg he leads with.

4. Stand behind him and assist his hand with **holding the railing,** if needed, by providing hand over hand guidance, or wrist support. If he feels stable with that hand, he may be able to walk up the stairs with this support. Also, see if he will **advance his hand forward** on the railing as he walks up the stairs and assist if needed. With practice, he will do both of these actions by himself.

5. If he does not feel ready to walk up just holding the railing, he may prop his unsupported hand on the stair. If he does this, hold the sleeve of his shirt, or above his shoulder, to give slight support to his unsupported arm. He may feel secure enough with this amount of support. You can also try giving him a small, lightweight toy to hold in his free hand to see if this eliminates the propping.

6. If he chooses to hold the railing with both hands to walk up by himself, turning partially sideways, let him. With practice, he will let go with one hand and then face forward, walking up with only one hand on the railing.

7. Continue to practice until he can walk up the flight of stairs just holding the railing, safely, on a consistent basis.

## ACTIVITY #2: Walking Down Stairs, Marking Time, Facing Forward

If your child is a new walker, use a set of toddler-size stairs, found at a toddler playground. When your child is comfortable with walking down toddler-size stairs with support, then use a set of regular-size stairs. Begin with a set of 4-6 stairs or use the bottom half of the flight. When he is ready, use the entire flight of stairs.

These instructions are written for a child who prefers to step down leading with the left foot. Adjust the instructions if your child prefers to step down leading with his right foot.

## ACTIVITY #2A: Walking Down Stairs, Marking Time, with Trunk Support

1. Place a motivator at the bottom of the stairs, or have your child follow a sibling walking down the stairs.

2. Position yourself standing behind him, and hold his trunk under his armpits, leaning his trunk back against your legs.

3. Turn him sideways about 45 degrees, setting him up to lead with his preferred leg. (In this example, he prefers to lead with his left

leg, so turn him to the right so it is easy to step down with his left leg.) Place his feet at the front edge of the stair.

4. With this support, say "down" and wait for him to step out with his left foot and then bend his right hip and knee to lower his left foot down to the next stair. If he keeps his right knee straight, then lean over him and place your hand behind his knee to bend it, and guide him to lower his left foot with control to the next stair. Then he will move his right foot down beside his left foot. Continue to practice until he can do all of these leg actions by himself, with you supporting his trunk.

5. Encourage him to repeat this sequence to walk down the stairs. Clap for him, praise him, and give him the motivator.

6. Continue to practice the above steps until he is familiar and comfortable with walking down the entire flight of stairs easily with this method.

 ## Activity #2B: Walking Down Stairs, Marking Time, with Two-Hand Support

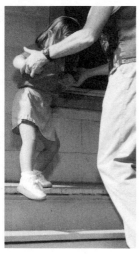

1. When your child can do step 6 of Activity #2A, begin practicing walking down the stairs, with him holding your index fingers with two-hand support (fig. 12.13).

2. Position yourself standing in front of him, facing him, about 1-2 stairs below him, and you will step backwards. By standing in front of him, you will also block the view down the flight of stairs, which will allow him to focus on stepping down one stair at a time.

3. Turn him sideways about 45 degrees, setting him up to lead with his preferred leg. (In this example, he prefers to lead with his left leg, so turn him to the right, with the railing on his right side, so it is easy to step down with his left leg.) Place his feet at the front edge of the stair.

(fig. 12.13)

4. Place your index fingers horizontally in front of his chest, at or below shoulder level. Have him hold onto your fingers and hold his trunk up straight.

5. With this support, say "down" and wait for him to step out with his left foot and then bend his right hip and knee to lower his left foot down to the next stair. If needed, assist him with bending his right knee, and lowering his left foot with control to the next stair. Then he will move his right foot down beside his left foot. Continue

to practice until he can do all of these leg movements by himself, holding your index fingers.

6. Follow steps 5-6 of Activity #2A.

## Activity #2C: Walking Downstairs, Marking Time, with Hand and Rail Support

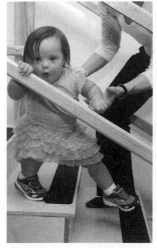

1. When your child can do Activity #2B, then practice walking down the stairs with one hand holding the railing and one hand holding your index finger.
2. Use a railing that he can reach and grip, for example spindles or a low banister.
3. Set him up so the hand holding the railing is opposite to the leg he leads with.
4. Position yourself standing in front of him, facing him, about 1-2 stairs below him.
5. Turn him sideways about 45 degrees, setting him up to lead with his preferred leg. (In this example, he prefers to lead with his left leg, so turn him to the right, with the railing on his right side, so it is

(fig. 12.14)

easy to step down with his left leg. Place his right hand on the railing.) Place his feet at the front edge of the stair.
6. Place your right index finger horizontally in front of the left side of his chest, at or below shoulder level. Have him hold onto your finger with his left hand and hold his trunk up straight.
7. If needed, stabilize his right hand to hold the railing with your left hand, providing hand-over-hand guidance. Lessen your support when he can grip it by himself.
8. With this support, say "down" and wait for him to step out with his left foot and then bend his right hip and knee to lower his left foot down to the next stair. If needed, assist him with bending his right knee, and lowering his left foot with control to the next stair. Then he will move his right foot down beside his left foot. Continue to practice until he can do all of these leg movements by himself, holding your index fingers.
9. Wait for him to advance his right hand on the railing; assist if needed.
10. Follow steps 5-6 of Activity #2A.
11. When he is comfortable with this setup and does it easily, lower his hand (holding your index finger) to waist level to decrease support.
12. You can also try standing on his left side, stepping sideways down the stairs, with his left hand holding your left index finger (fig. 12-14).

## Activity #2D: Walking Down Stairs, Marking Time, Holding the Rail

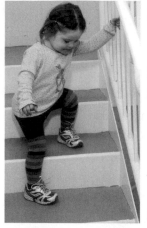

(fig. 12.15)

1. When he can do step 11 of Activity #2C, test when he is ready to walk down the stairs, only holding the railing (fig. 12.15).
2. Follow steps 2-5 in Activity #2C.
3. Your child will hold the railing with his right hand, and you can provide hand over hand support if needed. If he feels stable with that hand, he may be able to walk down the stairs with that support.
4. Encourage him to step down with his left and right legs with control.
5. Watch to see how he advances his right hand on the railing, and assist if needed.
6. If he does not feel ready to walk down with one hand holding the railing, hold the sleeve of his shirt, or above his shoulder, to give slight support to his unsupported arm. You can also try giving him a small, lightweight toy to hold in his free hand.
7. If he chooses to hold the railing with both hands to walk down by himself, turning partially sideways, let him. With practice, he will let go with one hand and then face forward, walking down with only one hand on the railing.
8. Continue to practice until he can walk down the flight of stairs, just holding the railing, safely and consistently.

## ACTIVITY #3: Walking Up Stairs, Stepping Sideways

Start with toddler-size stairs, and then progress to regular size stairs, starting with 4-6 stairs, and then work toward walking up the entire flight.

1. Place a motivator at the top of the stairs on the landing, or have your child follow a sibling walking up the stairs.
2. Position your child on the bottom stair, facing the railing, so he can lead with his preferred leg. (In this example, he prefers to lead with his right leg. He will hold the railing on his left, so he is setup to lead with his right foot.) Use spindles or a low banister so he can hold on and reach the railing.
3. Position yourself behind him.
4. If needed, place his hands on the railing and provide support to help him hold on.

5. Say "up" and wait for him to step sideways and lift his right foot up onto the stair.

6. After his right foot is placed on the stair, he will need to hold on and balance with his arms, weight shift sideways over the right foot, and then straighten his right hip and knee, and push off with his foot, to lift his body up onto the stair. Once his body is lifted onto the stair, he will place his left foot next to the right.

7. See if he advances his hands forward on the railing, and assist him if needed.

8. Encourage him to repeat this sequence and walk up the stairs to the landing.

9. Continue to practice until he can walk up the entire flight easily using the arm and leg motions required.

## ACTIVITY #4: Walking Down Stairs, Stepping Sideways

Start with toddler-size stairs, and then progress to regular size stairs, starting with 4-6 stairs, and then work toward walking down the entire flight.

1. Place a motivator at the bottom of the stairs, or have your child follow a sibling walking down the stairs.

2. Position your child on the top stair, facing the railing, so he can lead with his preferred leg. (In this example, he prefers to lead with his left leg. He will hold the railing on his right, so he is setup to lead with his left foot.) Use spindles or a low banister so he can hold on and reach the railing.

3. Position yourself in front of him, facing him, one to two stairs below him. (You will step backwards down the stairs.)

4. If needed, place his hands on the railing and provide support to help him hold on.

5. Say "down" and wait for him to balance himself on his right leg and step sideways with his left foot. Then he will slowly bend his right hip, knee, and ankle to lower his left foot to the stair below. Once his left foot is placed on the stair, he will move his right foot next to it. He will use his arms to assist with balance and lowering his body.

6. See if he advances his hands forward on the railing, and assist him if needed.

7. Encourage him to repeat this sequence and walk down the set of stairs.

8. Continue to practice until he can walk down the entire flight easily using the arm and leg motions required.

## Activity #5A: Walking up Stairs, Alternating Feet, with Two-Hand Support

1. Place a motivator at the top of the stairs, or have your child follow a sibling up the stairs.
2. Position your child at the base of the stairs. Begin with a set of 4-6 stairs or use the top half of the flight.
3. Say "up," and then use words to cue the alternating pattern—for example, say, "big step" or "one and two" or "left and right."
4. Test the best method to elicit the alternating leg pattern. Since you want to introduce a new method, provide whatever support makes it easiest for your child to alternate his legs. Then use the method for several repetitions so he feels the pattern by stepping up the flight of stairs. Once he is familiar with the movements, then you can decrease your support. To figure out the best setup, begin with these ideas:
    a. Provide two-hand support with one adult on each side of him. Each adult will hold one of the child's hands forward of his shoulders, and above his shoulders if needed. Observe whether holding his hands above his shoulders makes it easier to alternate his legs. Once he knows how to alternate his legs, then you can lower his hands to the level of his shoulders.
    b. Provide two-hand support, with one hand holding the railing and his other hand holding an adult's hand. Test where to hold his hand for the best results.
    c. Provide hand and leg support on the side of the nondominant leg. For example, if he prefers to step up leading with his right foot, place him on the right side of the stairwell, holding the railing on the right. You stand on his left side, and hold his left hand. After he steps up onto the stair with his right foot, then you move his left leg to alternate up to the next stair, moving his left arm forward and upward to assist the alternating pattern. Test the best method of moving his left leg. You could lift his thigh, support behind his knee at the crease, or lift his foot. When tolerated, lessen your support to just tapping the thigh or calf area to cue it to move.
5. When he can alternate his legs with one of the methods listed above, then continue to use that method for many repetitions to build leg strength in both legs.

## 🏃 Activity #5B: Walking Up Stairs, Alternating Feet, with Hand and Rail Support

When alternating his legs is easy and automatic, then provide less support.

1. Have your child hold the railing with one hand, and hold your index finger with his other hand.
2. Stand behind him, and after he holds your index finger (placed horizontally), position his hand in front of his chest, at the level of his shoulder.
3. He will hold onto the railing and your finger, and learn to lean his body forward and balance himself as he uses the alternating pattern up the flight.
4. He will also advance his hand on the railing.
5. Practice this method for several repetitions to improve leg strength with this decreased support.
6. Continue to practice until he can walk up the entire flight of stairs easily and automatically, alternating his legs, with one hand on the railing and his other hand holding your finger. Then, lower his hand (holding your finger) toward waist level to further decrease the support.

## 🏃 Activity #5C: Walking Up Stairs, Alternating Feet, Holding the Rail

When your child can do Activity #5B, test when he is ready to practice only holding onto the railing (fig. 12.16).

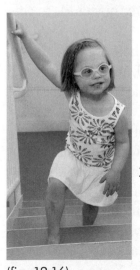

1. Stand behind him, and assist his hand with holding the railing, if needed, by providing hand-over-hand guidance, or wrist support. If he feels stable with that hand, he may be able to walk up the stairs with this support. Also, see if he will advance his hand forward on the railing as he walks up the stairs, and assist if needed. With practice, he will do both of these actions by himself.
2. If he does not feel ready to walk up just holding the railing, hold the sleeve of his shirt, or above his shoulder, to give slight support to his unsupported arm. He may feel secure enough with this amount of support. You can also try giving him a small, lightweight toy to hold in his free hand (to distract him from wanting to hold your finger).

(fig. 12.16)

3. If he chooses to hold the railing with both hands to walk up by himself, turning partially sideways, let him. With practice, he will let go with one hand and then face forward, walking up with only one hand on the railing.

4. Continue to practice until he can walk up the flight of stairs, alternating his feet, with one hand holding the railing, safely and consistently.

## Activity #6A: Walking Down Stairs, Alternating Feet, with Two-Hand Support

1. Place a motivator at the bottom of the stairs, or have your child follow a sibling down the stairs.

2. Position your child at the top of the stairs. Begin with a set of 4-6 stairs or use the bottom half of the flight.

3. Say "down," and then use words to cue the alternating pattern. For example, say "big step" or "one and two" or "left and right."

4. Test the best method to elicit the alternating leg pattern. Since you want to introduce a new method, provide whatever support makes it easiest for your child to alternate his legs. Then use the method for several repetitions so he feels the pattern by stepping down the flight of stairs. Once he is familiar with the movements, then you can decrease your support. To figure out the best setup, begin with these ideas:

   a. Provide two-hand support with one adult on each side of him, holding your child's hands forward of his shoulders. Observe whether holding his hands above his shoulders and forward makes it easier to alternate his legs. Once he knows how to alternate his legs, then you can lower his hands to the level of his shoulders.

   b. Provide two-hand support, with one hand holding the railing and his other hand holding an adult's hand. You hold his hand to give added support and test where to hold his hand for the best results.

   c. Provide hand and leg support on the side of the nondominant leg. For example, if he prefers to step down leading with his left foot, place him on the left side of the stairwell, holding the railing on the left. You stand on his right side, and hold his right hand. After he steps down the stair with his left foot, then you move his right leg to alternate down the next stair, moving his right arm forward to assist the alternating pattern. Test the best method of moving his right leg. You could move his calf area, or move his foot. When tolerated, lessen your support to just tapping the calf area to cue him to move it.

    d. Provide two-hand support, with one hand holding the railing and his other hand holding your hand and give verbal and visual cueing. Have him look at your feet and then say "kick" and kick your foot forward. Have him imitate you and do the same motion. Then say "down" and move your foot down to the next stair, and have him do the same. Continue these actions, alternating your feet, down the flight of stairs. As he learns the movements, then you can move faster.

5. When your child can alternate his legs with one of the methods listed above, then continue to use that method for many repetitions to build leg strength in both legs.

## 🏃 Activity #6B: Walking Down Stairs, Alternating Feet, with Hand and Rail Support

When alternating his legs is easy and automatic, then provide less support.

1. Have your child hold the railing with one hand, and your hand with his other hand.
2. Stand beside him, and after he holds your hand, position his hand in front of his chest, at the level of his shoulder.
3. He will hold onto the railing and your hand, and he will learn to balance himself as he uses the alternating pattern down the flight.
4. He will also advance his hand on the railing.
5. Practice this method for several repetitions to improve leg strength.
6. Continue to practice until he can walk down the entire flight of stairs easily and automatically, alternating his legs, with one hand on the railing and his other hand holding your hand. Then, lower his hand (holding your hand) toward waist level to further decrease the support.

## 🏃 Activity #6C: Walking Down Stairs, Alternating Feet, Holding the Rail

When your child can do Activity #6B, test when he is ready to practice only holding onto the railing (fig. 12.17).

1. Stand in front of him, facing him, and walk backwards down the stairs. Help him hold the railing, if needed, by providing hand-over-

hand guidance, or wrist support. If he feels stable with that hand, he may be able to walk down the stairs with this support. Also, see if he will advance his hand forward on the railing as he walks down the stairs, and assist if needed. With practice, he will do both of these actions by himself.

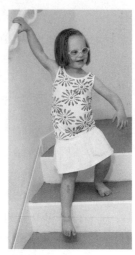

(fig. 12.17)

2. If he does not feel ready to walk down just holding the railing, hold the sleeve of his shirt or above his shoulder, to give slight support to his unsupported arm. He may feel secure enough with this amount of support. You can also try giving him a small, lightweight toy to hold in his free hand.

3. If your child chooses to hold the railing with both hands to walk down by himself, turning partially sideways, let him. With practice, he will let go with one hand and then face forward, walking down with only one hand on the railing.

4. Continue to practice until he can walk down the flight of stairs, alternating his feet, with one hand holding the railing, safely and consistently.

# 🏃 MOTOR MILESTONE CHECKLIST

❏ He walks up a set of toddler-size stairs, marking time, with one hand holding the railing and his other hand holding an adult's index finger

❏ He walks down a set of toddler-size stairs, marking time, with one hand holding the railing and his other hand holding an adult's index finger

❏ He walks up a set of toddler-size stairs, marking time, stepping sideways, with both hands holding the railing

❏ He walks down a set of toddler-size stairs, marking time, stepping sideways, with both hands holding the railing

❏ He walks up a set of toddler-size stairs, marking time, facing forward, with one hand holding the railing

❏ He walks down a set of toddler-size stairs, marking time, facing forward, with one hand holding the railing

❏ He walks up a flight of stairs, marking time, stepping forward, holding onto an adult with both hands

❏ He walks down a flight of stairs, marking time, stepping forward, holding onto an adult with both hands

❏ He walks up a flight of stairs, marking time, stepping forward, with one hand on the railing and one hand holding an adult's finger

❏ He walks down a flight of stairs, marking time, stepping forward, with one hand on the railing and one hand holding an adult's finger

❏ He walks up a flight of stairs, marking time, stepping sideways, with both hands holding the railing

❏ He walks down a flight of stairs, marking time, stepping sideways, with both hands holding the railing

❏ He walks up a flight of stairs, marking time, stepping forward, with one hand holding the railing

❏ He walks down a flight of stairs, marking time, stepping forward, with one hand holding the railing

❏ He walks up a flight of stairs, alternating his feet, with one hand on the railing and one hand holding an adult's finger

*(continued on next page)*

- [ ] He walks up a flight of stairs, alternating his feet, with one hand on the railing

- [ ] He walks down a flight of stairs, alternating his feet, with one hand on the railing and one hand holding an adult's hand

- [ ] He walks down a flight of stairs, alternating his feet, with one hand on the railing

# 13

# Jumping

## Introduction

After your child walks, she is ready to practice bouncing to prepare for jumping. Once she is familiar with the new movement and the equipment used, she will enjoy the feeling of the upward and downward motions. You will need to teach her how to stand and bounce with hips and knees bending or else she may try other methods that will not lead to jumping. It will be fun to do with her siblings, and their enthusiasm for jumping will motivate her to do it often. You can do it to music if her dance movements are similar to the bouncing movements.

The first goal will be to jump on the floor with toe push-off (fig. 13.1). After your child can do this, then she will be ready to learn to jump forward (fig. 13.2), and then jump off a step with both feet together (fig. 13.3). Jumping takes time to develop, and the average age of jumping on the floor for a child with Down syndrome (according to my data) is four years old, although some children can

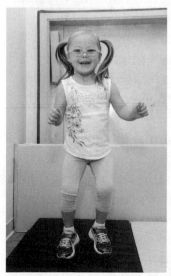
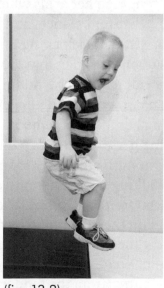
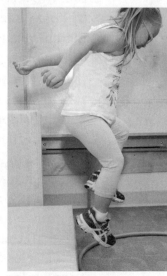

(fig. 13.1)     (fig. 13.2)     (fig. 13.3)

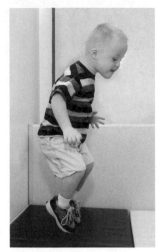
(fig. 13.4)

do it when they are three. Each child will need to be playful and motivated to persevere with figuring out how to generate lift-off.

There are three parts to jumping on the floor. To prepare, your child will need to bend her hips, knees, and ankles to move into a mild squat. Then she will need to quickly straighten her hips and knees, and push off on tiptoes. She will need to do this upward movement with speed and momentum to generate the power needed to jump, lifting both feet off the surface simultaneously (fig. 13.4). The third part is the landing, and she will need to learn to land with hips, knees, and ankles bending to decelerate and land with control on the floor. She will need to land on her feet and regain her balance.

Each of these steps requires finesse and coordination. If they are not done correctly, they will limit your child's successful performance of the skill. If she bends too far into a squat, she will not have the strength to do the second step. If she rises up on tiptoes, but without momentum and speed, she will not achieve lift-off. If she tries to land with her knees locked, she will land with a jolt and too much impact on her knee joints. She will learn to do the refined movements of each step with practice and your guidance.

There are many physical benefits from learning to jump:

1. Your child will strengthen her whole body, particularly her abdominals, calf muscles, and muscles on the inside borders of her feet, which tend to be weak in children with Down syndrome.
2. She will also strengthen her arms when she is learning to jump, by holding onto a bar for balance, and later, holding on and pulling upward to assist with achieving lift-off.
3. The jumping motion will elicit upward movement with toe push-off in her walking pattern, adding a lightness to her stepping. This is in contrast to her tendency to use a heavy-footed pattern, slapping her feet on the floor.
4. By strengthening her calf muscles to generate toe push-off, she will use ankle strength efficiently for propulsion when walking, running, walking up inclines and on uneven surfaces (like sand), walking up stairs and curbs, and even pedaling a tricycle (to keep her feet on the pedals and push to pedal).
5. By strengthening the muscles on the inside borders of her feet, the muscles of her arches will be strengthened, which will balance her foot posture (from the tendency of stronger muscles on

the outer borders of the feet, which turn the feet outward and flatten the arches) and improve alignment for walking and post walking skills (Calais-Germain, 2007, page 289).

6. As she jumps for many repetitions, she will use her abdominal muscles to stabilize her core and for balance.

---

## Steps in Learning to Jump

To achieve the goals of this skill area, your child will need to practice the following steps:

1. Bouncing on a springy surface with her hips and knees bending and feet flat, holding onto a bar for balance
2. Bouncing, as above, on tiptoes
3. Jumping on a springy surface (for example, a mini-trampoline with a bar), with lift-off using toe push-off, holding onto a bar for balance
4. Jumping on the floor with lift-off using toe push-off, with hand support; without hand support
5. Jumping forward 6-8 (15-20 cm) inches with both feet together with hand support; without hand support
6. Jumping off a 4-8 inch (10-20 cm) high step with both feet together with hand support; without hand support

---

## *Components*

The components to focus on are:

1. standing leg posture with knees and feet pointing straight ahead (neutral hip rotation), weight bearing toward the balls of the feet, and a narrow base
2. abdominal strength to hold the trunk and pelvis erect and tucked, and to maintain balance (fig. 13.5)
3. leg and ankle strength for generating bouncing movements and coordination to maintain the rhythm, moving feet simultaneously
4. leg, ankle, and abdominal strength to execute the 3 steps of jumping: bending, lift-off, and landing
5. arm strength to hold onto a bar for balance, and later, to pull upward to assist with generating lift-off
6. perseverance and motivation to figure out how to generate lift-off

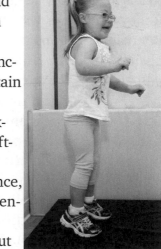

(fig. 13.5)

## *Tendencies*

The tendencies are:

1. to stand with knees and feet pointing out (hip external rotation), weight bearing toward the heels, wide base, knees stiff and straight, trunk and pelvis arched, and flat arches
2. to activate the back muscles and not use the abdominals
3. to bounce using one of these variations:

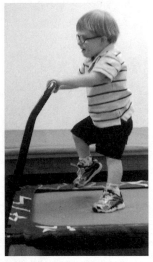

(fig. 13.6)

   a. rocking the head and trunk forward and then upward, keeping the knees straight while bending and straightening the hips
   b. rocking head and trunk from side to side with knees stiff
   c. making marching or galloping movements, alternating the feet (fig. 13.6)
4. to have weakness in legs, ankles, and abdominals, or to not understand how to use strength to execute the three parts of jumping
5. to learn to jump with full-sole weight bearing, rather than using toe push-off
6. to land with her knees stiff and straight, with excessive impact
7. to learn bouncing and be unable to work on learning to generate lift-off due to timid temperament or difficulty with figuring out how to do it

## *Safety Precautions*

Jumping is a difficult gross motor skill for children with Down syndrome to learn, and they need the right setup to learn how to do it. In my experience, if they practice on a *springy surface,* they begin to understand the concept of bouncing and jumping, and eventually learn how to generate lift-off using toe push-off to jump. While practicing the trunk and leg movements for bouncing and jumping, they need to hold onto a *bar/handle* to maintain their balance.

I use a mini-trampoline with a handle to teach this skill using a structured training program. However, if this type of equipment is used*, it is vital to understand these precautions:*

1. The American Academy of Pediatrics (AAP) has thoroughly examined and reviewed children's usage of trampolines, and they have published a policy statement on trampolines. In 2012, the AAP reaffirmed its recommendation against any home or other recreational usage of trampolines and recommended use only

as part of a structured training program with appropriate safety measures employed (Sept. 2012).

2. Since children with Down syndrome have ligamentous laxity and are at risk for AAI, they need additional supervision and safety measures to make sure they practice bouncing and jumping on this equipment using safe methods, specifically watching the neck position and avoiding forward/backward motions.

I use the mini-trampoline as a training device while a child is learning to jump in my clinical setting. After the child can jump well on the floor, I stop using the mini-trampoline. If you use a mini-trampoline at home to teach your child to jump, it is critical to understand the risks of using a trampoline. For the safety of all your children, you need to regard the mini-trampoline as training equipment and not as a toy. It is imperative to put it away in a secure place so that it is not accessible when you are not there to assist and supervise using it.

The following *safety measures* are recommended when you are practicing bouncing and jumping:

1. Use a mini-trampoline that is well designed, in good condition, and has a safety pad around the edge (to cover the springs and frame).
2. Ensure adult assistance is provided when carrying out the structured training program (Activities #1-3) and provide constant, direct supervision for safety.
3. Only one child should be on the mini-trampoline at a time.
4. Use this setup for practicing:
   a. Have your child stand in the center on the mini-trampoline surface (away from the springs and frame).
   b. Ensure that your child stands and bounces/jumps with her neck erect while holding onto the handle with both hands for balance.
   c. Only allow standing, bouncing, and jumping; do not permit roughhousing, falling to sitting, or stunts.
5. If a sibling participates in the practice sessions, have her model what you are teaching your child with Down syndrome (including holding the handle).

## Setup for Learning

You will need to use the right setup to teach your child to bounce and later, jump. She will need a springy surface, like a mini-trampoline, so she feels the upward and downward movements. She will learn to generate force into the surface to increase the magnitude of the movement and to produce upward momentum for lift-off. She will need to hold on for balance, so the

## Choosing a Mini-Trampoline or Other Springy Surface

The best surface to use is a mini-trampoline with a bar. Since jumping takes a long time to develop, having the ideal equipment to practice on is important and a worthwhile investment. Mini-trampolines can be easily put away and stored in between practices for safety, if need be.

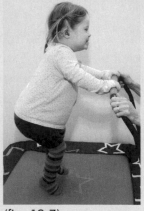

(fig. 13.7)

Before you buy a trampoline, test your child on different trampolines to see how she responds to the tautness and springiness of the various types of surfaces (fig. 13.7). Some children prefer a taut surface since it feels more stable when first standing on it. However, with a taut surface, a child needs to move her legs more vigorously to move the surface. Check the springiness of the surface, since this is critical to assist jumping with lift-off. Some mini-trampolines have minimal springiness and the surface sags; these trampolines are ineffective and should be avoided. With the right surface, your child will feel the bouncing rhythm and learn to generate it.

***The height of the bar is also important.*** If your child is using the bar for balance, it needs to be at the level of her chest. If she is pulling herself up with the bar to assist with jumping with lift-off, it needs to be at the level of her shoulders or chin. Make sure that the diameter of the bar is small enough that she can grip it easily.

If you do not have access to a mini-trampoline, other surfaces to use to practice jumping or bouncing are:

1. Bed or crib
2. Sofa
3. Sofa cushion or mattress placed on the floor
4. "Swinging bridge" playground equipment
5. BOSU balance trainer (dome side)
6. Sometimes a child needs supportive equipment that she can bounce in, such as an activity jumperoo, or bouncer. In my clinical setting, I use the Infant Swing with the Vertical Stimulation Device (available from Southpaw Enterprises at www.southpawenterprises.com) as a bouncer (fig. 13.8). It is a safe way to practice bouncing and jumping, pushing off with both feet simultaneously.

With each of these surfaces, you will need to provide hand support.

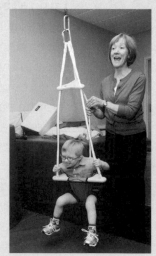

(fig. 13.8)

most stable setup is to use a mini-trampoline with a bar. If she holds the bar, she will learn to balance herself and later use it to pull upward to assist with generating lift-off. If she holds your hands, she will tend to rely on you rather than produce the movements herself. She will learn to jump on the springy surface for many repetitions, then jump on a mat surface, and then jump on the floor. After she jumps in place on the floor, then she will learn jumping forward and then jumping off. She will learn to jump in three directions: upward, forward, and downward.

When practicing bouncing and jumping, the position of your child's trunk and pelvis, arms, legs, and feet is critical. The desired posture is described in the Components section above. If this posture is used, then she will strengthen the right muscles for jumping. If your child uses orthoses (SureStep) and shoes with flexible soles, she will need to wear them so her knees and ankles are aligned properly for efficient muscle actions. Once she learns to jump, she can practice barefoot, if desired.

### Bouncing with Feet Flat on the Surface

You will prepare your child for jumping by teaching her to bounce. Your first job will be to introduce her to bouncing and make it fun so that she is interested and willing to participate. It is best to use a mini-trampoline with a bar. If she learns to hold the bar, then she will be responsible for balancing herself and feel in control. If she learns to hold you, she will become dependent on you to bounce her and balance her.

Once you introduce the equipment, have your child climb onto it and stand on it. Then watch her and see how she reacts to the springy surface. If she is comfortable, proceed with teaching her to bounce. If you stand in front of her and model bouncing with your hips and knees bending, see if she will imitate you. If you add music, she may dance using bouncing motions. Let her experiment with bouncing and using the springy surface. Watch how she imitates you and see if she is happy to bounce or afraid. If she is engaged in bouncing, you can provide strategic support to improve her bouncing pattern. If she is scared, provide support so she feels safe. Make sure the mini-trampoline is stable, and if the handle or base moves, hold it firmly. Keep the experience fun and take turns with siblings to motivate her to practice.

At first, you will help her explore the movements of the springy surface and how she can move her body to bounce on it. With your guidance, she will become familiar with this new game and then will initiate her own playful movements. You will watch her reactions and guide her to learn what's next. Let her choose when she wants to stop and climb off rather than impose long practices. After she takes a break or her sibling takes a turn, then she will want to take her turn again. The first goal is for her to want to be on the mini-trampoline and bounce. At this point, if you impose or interfere too much with her bouncing, she will resist playing the game. For now, let her learn to climb on and off, hold onto the bar when standing on the mini-trampoline, and do whatever bouncing motions she chooses.

When your child enjoys being on the mini-trampoline, holding onto the bar for balance, then you will provide strategic support to teach the trunk and leg movements for bouncing (fig. 13.9). Her standing posture is critical to learning to activate the right muscles.

1. She needs to stand with her trunk and pelvis up straight with her abdominals activated, not with her low back arched and the top of her pelvis tilted forward.
2. Her hips need to be in neutral rotation with her knees and feet pointing straight ahead, with her feet 2-3 inches (5-7.5 cm) apart (narrow base). Her feet need to be placed in the middle of the mini-trampoline, so her weight is shifted forward toward the balls of her feet.
3. With this trunk and leg posture, she will learn to bend her hips and knees to bounce on both legs simultaneously.

On her own, she may choose to stand as discussed under Tendency #1. With this standing posture, then her knees will be straight and locked, and she will not be able to learn to bounce by bending her hips and knees (fig. 13.10). She will want to play the bouncing game, so if her posture blocks the right bouncing pattern, then she will figure out a new method. She will pick one of the variations listed under Tendencies. If these variations are allowed to persist, she will not learn how to jump. You will need to guide her to learn the posture needed for bouncing and jumping.

After she is familiar with the setup for bouncing and is comfortable and playful standing on the equipment, then you need to find a way to help her learn the bouncing movements. Watch her posture and the movements she initiates and then figure out what is needed to teach her to bounce. Focus on supporting her posture first and see what movements she uses after you make these adjustments.

If she is very fearful, she might like you to stand behind her on the mini-trampoline and gently bounce with her, supporting her trunk so she feels stable. If she likes moving on the mini-trampoline but is using the wrong method (variations under Tendencies #3), then support her to train her to use the right method. If she marches (#3c), then support both legs and bounce her with both feet moving together (or use a bouncer or jumper). If she bends her hips with her trunk arched and her knees stiff and straight (#3a), then bend her knees and support her trunk if needed to guide bouncing. If she rocks from side to side (#3b), support her trunk to have her feel bouncing vertically.

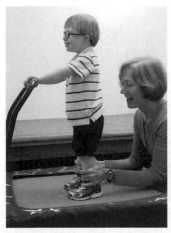
(fig. 13.9)

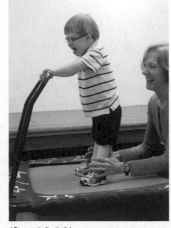
(fig. 13.10)

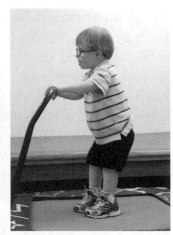
(fig. 13.11)

With practice and your strategic guidance, she will learn the **bouncing game**. Watch her to see if she has learned the right method that will lead to jumping. If not, give support to shape her method toward jumping.

To set her up, see Activity #1, Step 5. After you set her up with the standing posture described, the primary areas to focus on are her trunk and knees. Start with supporting her knees and bending them; this may improve her trunk posture if it is arched. If her trunk continues to be stiff and arched, you will also need to support her abdomen so she can feel the new posture that she needs to learn. See Activity #1, Step 7, for instructions on providing the needed support. You will need to be creative to figure out what your child needs to learn to bounce, and then strategically add that component.

If you need another method to practice jumping, here is a playful way to teach your child the three steps of bending, lift-off, and landing. You can stand your child on a squishy raised surface, like the bed, with you holding her trunk. (She can face you or her back can be against you.) Say "bend" or "down" to cue your child to bend her knees toward a squat. Then say "up" or "stand." After she stands, pick her up to feel lift-off. Then have her catch with her feet and land in standing, with hips and knees slightly bent. After she learns this method on the bed, she can also practice it on the mini-trampoline, holding onto the bar. When practicing this method, watch her knees to make sure she is bending them to squat and when landing.

When your child is able to bounce with the right method, encourage bouncing for many repetitions (fig. 13.11). When she has mastered bouncing with full-sole weight bearing for several repetitions, she will be ready to go to the next skill, bouncing on tiptoes. Since children with Down syndrome have the tendency to learn to jump on the floor with full-sole weight bearing, it is important to work on the next skill to build the foundation of jumping on tiptoes.

### Bouncing on Tiptoes

By now, your child knows the bouncing movements and rhythm and can bounce for several repetitions on the mini-trampoline, holding the bar. The next component to teach is bouncing on tiptoes. First, you need to place her feet back in the middle on the trampoline surface so her pelvis is over her tiptoes (side view), and her weight is shifted onto the balls of her feet. With her feet in this position, she may automatically bounce on tiptoes, while holding onto the bar for balance. If she needs support to stay on her tiptoes and bounce, you can place your hands under her heels or hold her lower legs (calf areas) and lean them for-

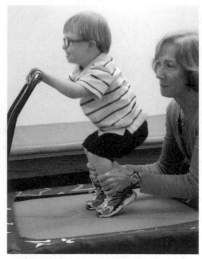

(fig. 13.12)

ward (fig. 13.12). Then bounce her with this support so she feels the movement and becomes comfortable with it. You can also give the verbal cue "tippy toes" and the visual cue of her sibling bouncing on tiptoes.

Your child may know how to rise up on tiptoes when standing on the floor in order to reach up for something, like the door handle lever. She will

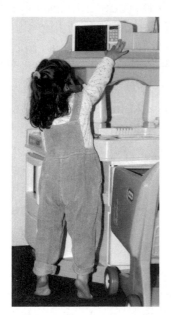

(fig. 13.13)

prop against the wall for balance and use her calf muscle strength to rise up on tiptoes and hold the position while trying to grab the handle and turn it. Practicing this will help her learn the skill of being on tiptoes and improve her strength to rise up high on tiptoes and maintain the position (fig. 13.13). It will prepare her for the stationary skill to stand on her tiptoes on the mini-trampoline, but it will not teach her the dynamic skill of bouncing on tiptoes. To bounce on tiptoes, she will need to do quick bounces, for several repetitions, and generate a coordinated rhythm.

When she can bounce on tiptoes repeatedly, begin to encourage more energetic and vigorous bouncing so she depresses the springy surface with her bounces. Until now, she has primarily used the *lift* provided by the springy surface to bounce up and down. Now we want her to push into the surface to generate more lift and bounce. To do this, she will need to increase the strength in her legs and feet and begin using speed and momentum as she is bouncing up and down.

## Jump on a Mini-Trampoline, Holding onto the Bar

When your child can bounce vigorously on tiptoes on the mini-trampoline, she will be ready to learn to jump on it, lifting both feet off the surface. You will need to show her the new game and siblings can model it in an exaggerated way so she knows what to imitate. She will need to feel "lift-off" so she is comfortable with it and tries to repeat it. You will also need to label the new game and can call it "big jump." Once she understands what jumping with lift-off is, then she will need to experiment to figure out how to do it.

To jump with lift-off, your child will need to be very comfortable with bouncing, love the feeling of moving up and down with a coordinated rhythm, and be willing to challenge herself to go to the next level (figs. 13.14– 3.16). She will need to figure out how to bounce with momentum and speed to generate lift-off. She will need leg strength used in a quick, dynamic way. She will hold onto the bar for balance as she is attempting many strategies to generate lift-off. She will also benefit from holding the bar and pulling her body upward to assist with lift-off. The height of the bar will be critical to her success (see box above on choosing a mini-tramp).

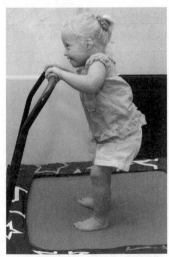 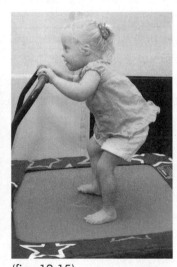 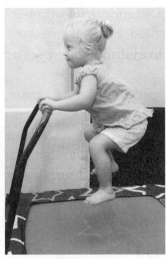

(fig. 13.14)     (fig. 13.15)     (fig. 13.16)

To progress from bouncing on tiptoes to jumping with lift-off will be a huge challenge. During that period, keep stimulating her with the experience of lift-off. When she is bouncing, you can add lift-off by:

1. Holding her lower legs and lifting her feet off the surface, while moving within her bouncing rhythm. She will be holding the bar for balance, and you can kneel on the floor behind her.
2. Holding her under her armpits and lifting her feet off the surface, while moving within her bouncing rhythm (fig. 13.17). She

will be holding the bar for balance, and you can stand in front of her, facing her.

3. Standing behind her on the mini-trampoline and gently bouncing her (while supporting the front of her trunk) so she feels lift-off, while holding onto the bar for balance.

4. Taking turns with her sister and seeing how high her sister's feet move when she jumps.

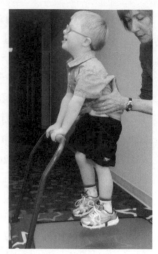

(fig. 13.17)

You will continue to add the experience of lift-off with excitement until she initiates using it in her bouncing routine.

At first, she will accidentally lift her feet one time while doing a series of bounces. It will usually happen on the first bounce. Or, she might lift one foot but not the other. When she feels the lift and sees your excitement and praise, she will keep trying to do it again. With continued practice, she will figure out how to generate lift-off (figs. 13.18–13.20). Then she will gain the strength and endurance to do many repetitions, producing lift-off consistently. She will need to hold onto the bar for balance and safety while jumping on the mini-trampoline.

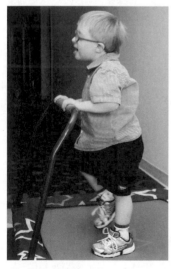

(fig. 13.18)

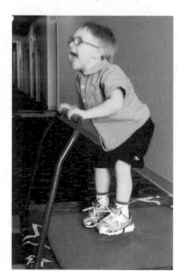

(fig. 13.19)

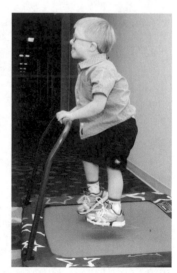

(fig. 13.20)

### Jumping on the Floor

When your child can jump on the mini-trampoline for many repetitions, holding the bar, she will be ready to learn to jump on a padded surface like a mat with two-hand support, and then on the floor. The springy surface of the mini-trampoline assisted the upward lift to jump. Now she will need to learn to generate lift-off using the strength of toe push-off. To jump on the mat or floor, she will need to push off with her toes against the surface with enough strength and speed to lift her body upward.

While she is gaining the leg and foot strength, she will also use arm strength for balance and to assist with lifting her body upward. She can hold onto a 1-inch (2.5-cm) diameter pole, like a broom handle, to simulate the bar she used on the mini-trampoline. Hold it at the level of her shoulders or chin, and hold it firmly so it is stable. With practice and this hand support, she will figure out how to jump with toe push-off on the new surfaces. The next challenge will be to develop the balance and leg strength to do it without hand support. She will need to use her legs and feet to land effectively and maintain her balance in standing. She will enjoy practicing jumping and she will be proud to be able to jump by herself.

### Jumping Forward and Jumping Off, with Both Feet Together

When your child can jump on the floor, she will use toe push-off in a vertical direction. The next game to teach her is to jump forward. When she can jump forward for 6-8 inches (15-20 cm), then she will be ready to learn to jump off a 1-2 inch (2.5-5 cm) high mat, which will combine moving forward and downward. Her tendency will be to lead with one foot rather than moving both feet together. Continue to provide hand support until she can do each skill with both feet together.

You will first practice *jumping forward with two-hand support.* To help her jump forward, follow the steps in Activity #4. Anticipate that moving forward will be a surprise for her since her habit is moving vertically. In the beginning, it is best to give a visual cue, like jumping from the yellow mat to the blue mat, or from the carpet to the hardwood floor. The surfaces need to be level and close together, without any space in between them.

With practice, she will be familiar with this new game and want to participate with jumping forward without hand support. When she can consistently jump forward with both feet together, then you can practice jumping longer distances. You can also use advanced setups like jumping over a rope, jumping in and out of a hoop, or jumping from one shape (spot marker) to another.

When your child can jump forward 6-8 inches (15-20 cm), you can start teaching her to *jump off a 1-2 inch (2.5-5 cm) high mat.* You will provide the same support as jumping forward, and she will experience the new direction of moving downward. Watch her reaction and use a 1-inch (2.5-cm) surface if 2 inches (5 cm) scares her. When tolerated, gradually increase the height of the step to an 8-inch (20-cm) stair. With each height surface, start with hand support and then have her learn to do it without hand support. She will need hand support to adjust to the motion of jumping off the height of the step and to regain her balance when she lands. Continue to provide hand support until she jumps off easily with both feet together. The surface that she jumps off will need to be stable to elicit her best performance. She will feel insecure if it rocks, wobbles, or slides.

### Other Jumping Activities

When your child achieves the goals in this skill area, she will have learned the basics of jumping. Now, she can jump for fun and exercise! It is recommended that jumping activities be continued for the benefits described in the introduction. She can practice jumping at home with her siblings, at school with her classmates, in her physical education program at school, and in community rec center gym programs. Here is a list of possible jumping activities:

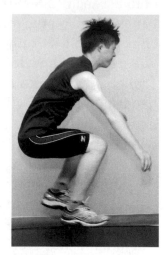

(fig. 13.21)

1. jump in place for multiple (20-50) repetitions (fig. 13.21);
2. broad jump;
3. successive jumps across a room (10-30 feet) using big jumps; repeat using small jumps;
4. jump forward and then backward over a line; begin with one repetition of this sequence and practice until she can do 10 repetitions without pausing in between jumps
5. jump side to side over a line; begin with one repetition of this sequence and practice until she can do 10 repetitions without pausing in between jumps
6. jump in a square: Have your child stand at number 1, facing number 4. Have her jump sideways to number 2, then forward to number 3, sideways to number 4, and then backwards to number 1. Do in one direction and then repeat in the opposite direction.
7. jumping jacks: begin with leg motions alone; then do jumping jacks with only the arm motions; when she can do the arm and leg motions in isolation, then practice arm and leg motions together;
8. hopscotch;
9. jumping rope;

These activities will continue to improve your child's strength, balance, coordination, and endurance.

# Guidelines

*Use the best motivators, which are music and other children.* When your child is first learning to bounce, she will automatically bend her hips and knees to dance if she hears music. The livelier the music, the more energetic she will be. When she is able to bounce and is working on jumping, you can use songs that include the word "jump," such as "Five Little Monkeys Jumping on the Bed." You can also use action songs such as "Pop Goes the Weasel." If you have videos of children jumping, your child will love watching them as she practices bouncing and jumping.

Your child will also love bouncing and jumping with her siblings and friends. She will see it as fun since everyone is excited and laughing when they are on the mini-trampoline. She will practice longer, for more repetitions, and more vigorously and will try to imitate what they are doing. The best setup is to take turns, first the sibling or friend, and then your child. You can say "your turn" to prompt each child when it is her turn to jump. Supervise the sibling or friend and have them do what you want your child to practice, such as bouncing on the trampoline while holding the bar. Or, have the sibling or friend do it in an exaggerated way so your child sees what you want her to imitate; for example, jumping with lift-off. By taking turns, your child will get a break but will stay engaged watching the other child. She will be ready for her next turn and will continue practicing for several repetitions, as long as her sibling or friend wants to play this game.

With all jumping activities, praise your child and clap after each series of bounces or jumps. If she is doing it with siblings and friends, both you and your child will clap for them too. The praise and clapping will let everyone know they are doing a great job and will motivate them to do it more!

*Provide verbal, visual, and tactile cues.* You will need to provide these cues for your child to fully understand and practice each jumping activity.

*Verbal Cues:* Whether your child is bouncing or jumping, say and sign "jump" to help her learn the word and to label the game. At first, it will mean the motion of bouncing up/down, and later it will mean jumping with lift-off. As she practices each jumping skill, she will learn new words to distinguish the new movements—e.g., "down" or "bend" to bend the knees to bounce, bouncing on "tiptoes," "big jump" (jumping with lift-off and later jumping forward), and "jump down."

See what verbal cues work best for your child as she does each of the jumping activities. Your child may like you to count while she is bouncing or jumping. She also may like you to be a cheerleader. For example, Lily loved her mother to say or sing "jump, Lily, jump" as she was practicing jumping. You also can use other words to engage your child in the jumping activities. For example, Elizabeth would jump her best if her mother said "Jump like

Charlie" (her brother) or "show me how Charlie jumps." When your child is practicing jumping forward or jumping off, you can say "Ready, go" or "1, 2, 3, bend, and jump."

*Visual Cues:* Your child will need to *see* each jumping activity in order to practice it. She will imitate what she sees, and you will need to help her *see* and *pay attention* to what you want her to imitate. For example, it will be easy for her to see bouncing up and down with hips and knees bending with feet flat. It will be harder for her to focus on her brother's feet when she needs to pay attention to bouncing on tiptoes. You will need to point to her brother's feet and say "toes" and then when your child takes her turn, you will need to support her on her toes and give the same verbal cue. When her brother jumps with lift-off, he can exaggerate how high he jumps to draw attention to the lift-off, and you can give the verbal cue "big jump."

Since your child will imitate what she sees, whoever is jumping needs to model it the way you want your child to do it. If you want your child to jump on the trampoline, holding the bar, her sibling needs to do it that way when she is jumping. Your child will also enjoy watching herself jump by watching herself in a mirror. She will see what she is doing and then may try new or more vigorous movements.

*Tactile Cues:* Your child will need to *feel* the movement you want her to imitate. Each jumping activity will have new movements to experience. She will need to feel bouncing with knees bending with feet flat, bouncing on tiptoes, jumping with lift-off, jumping with toe push-off, landing on her feet after she jumps, jumping forward, and jumping off. After she feels the movement, she can then try to imitate it. Examples of how to provide the tactile cues are included in the Steps and Activities sections of this chapter.

**Use a springy surface to practice bouncing and jumping (while holding onto a bar for balance).** When learning to bounce and jump, a springy surface is needed for these reasons:

1. To give your child the *feeling of moving up and down* while standing on the surface. The more vigorous she is, the more the surface moves. When she practices on the floor, she feels nothing but a firm surface. When she practices on a springy surface, there is a cause and effect reaction. She pushes down and the surface moves down and up so it is a fun game to explore, to feel the distance the surface moves.
2. To *assist with propelling her upward,* to promote jumping with lift-off.

A springy surface will help her feel the up/down motions more dramatically, and she will be motivated to practice. As she practices, she will increase the distance she moves up and down, increase the number of repetitions she can do within a set of bounces, and later she will use the spring to assist jumping with lift-off. She will feel successful because she is feeling and generating the movements.

See the box on page 414 for information on choosing a mini-tramp or springy surface for your child.

***Make sure that your child's neck is maintained in the normal, upright position when she is practicing bouncing and jumping.*** Since children with Down syndrome are at risk for atlantoaxial instability, for safety's sake they need to be ***constantly supervised*** when using a mini-trampoline or other springy surfaces. You need to prevent wild, sudden movements of the head, either forward or backward. You must make sure she learns to use the springy surface safely. Since she will imitate what others do, you will need to make sure her siblings and friends use it safely also. You will need to setup the rules early so only standing, bouncing, and jumping are allowed, with no roughhousing or falling. It is also best if only one child is on the mini-trampoline at a time. When your child has learned to jump on the floor, then she no longer needs to practice on the mini-trampoline. For more information on atlantoaxial instability, refer to pages 83-84 in *Babies with Down Syndrome: A New Parents' Guide* (third edition/2008).

***Large trampolines are not recommended and are considered dangerous.*** Children tend to move wildly with the increased space and spring provided by the surface. A child will jump and land on her head, buttocks, and back and can easily bump into other children. Children may even fall off the trampoline and injure themselves. It is hard to manage children on a large trampoline and accidents happen easily and quickly. These possibilities are even more dangerous for a child with Down syndrome, so large trampolines are strongly discouraged.

***Provide two-hand support while your child is learning each jumping activity.*** With hand support, she will be able to use her hand and arm strength to *hold on* for balance, *pull herself upward* to jump with lift-off, and *pull herself forward* to jump forward or off the step. She will challenge herself by increasing the power and range of her leg movements if she has hand support for balance. This will be especially critical when she is ready to learn to jump with lift-off.

When she is practicing bouncing and jumping using a springy surface, the best, most stable setup is the mini-trampoline with a bar. She learns to hold the bar for balance and then tries to figure out how to self-initiate bouncing movements. If she is setup to hold your hands, then she will rely on you to bounce her and balance her. She will look to you to entertain her, and she will participate passively rather than actively.

If you do not use a mini-trampoline with a bar, some possible setups are:

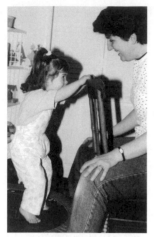

1. Place the back of a chair directly next to the mini-trampoline or springy surface, and your child holds the top of the back of the chair (fig. 13.22).
2. Place a chin-up bar in a doorway with the mini-trampoline or springy surface underneath it.
3. Hold a dowel, plastic pole, or broom handle horizontally at the level of your child's chest as she is standing on the mini-trampoline, springy surface, or bed.
4. Hold the horizontal crib railing while bouncing in the crib.
5. Place the mini-trampoline under the horizontal bar at the end of the metal swing set.

(fig. 13.22)

6. Place the mini-trampoline, springy surface, or sofa cushion under the armrest of the sofa.
7. Have your child hold the headboard while bouncing on the bed.
8. Have her hold the top of the back of the sofa while bouncing/jumping on the seat.
9. Use a "swinging bridge" at the playground and bounce while holding onto the railing.

If you choose setup #1 above, a "sled base" chair is ideal because the base slides under the mini-trampoline and then your child can stand in the middle rather than near the edge of the trampoline (fig. 13.23). Check the height of the chair so it is best for the skill being practiced. The top edge of the back of the chair needs to be thin enough for your child to grip easily. You will need to stabilize the chair to prevent it from sliding, and the best solution is to have someone sit on it. Try a variety of chairs to see what works best— kitchen chairs, dining room chairs, metal folding chairs, and patio/deck chairs.

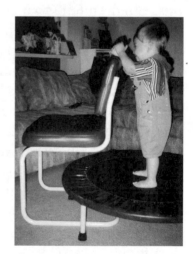

(fig. 13.23)

Whatever she uses for hand support will need to be stable and she will need to be able to hold it effectively with her small hand size. Check the diameter to make sure it is small enough to grip. You will need to vary the height of the support depending on what she is practicing. When she is bouncing with her feet flat, the support can be at the level of her chest. When she is learning to jump with lift-off, experiment to find the height that works best, and frequently shoulder to chin height is best.

When she is learning to jump forward and jump off, then she can hold your thumbs for support. Place your thumbs horizontally and hold her wrists for extra support if needed. Since she has learned to jump, she will use your support for balance and to learn the skill. When she can do the skill on her own, she will not want your support since she will be proud to do it independently.

***Practice jumping with the footwear she uses to walk and run.*** Her leg and foot posture is critical to learning to jump. If she wears orthoses (in particular, the dynamic type—SureStep orthoses), inserts (for example, Cascade Dafo HotDogs), or athletic shoes, then it is best for her to practice jumping in them. The shoes will need to be flexible in the toe box area so she can move onto tiptoes and use toe push-off for lift-off to jump. When she can jump and is practicing jumping forward and off the stair, the shoes will also reduce the force of impact when she lands on her feet in standing.

***Practice jumping for short periods of time or within your child's tolerance.*** Jumping requires a lot of strength, stamina, and endurance. You will notice how strenuous it is for you as you practice doing several repetitions with your child. Look for signs of fatigue in your child and give her a break. Taking turns with a sister works well because she can bounce ten times and then take a break and recover while her sister takes a turn. Your child will be able to practice longer if she does a series of bounces or jumps and takes a break in between each series.

When she first learns to jump with lift-off, she may not be able to repeat it because she will fatigue quickly. You can try again later and look for it in the beginning practices when she is strongest and most active.

Your child will build strength and endurance through practice. As her strength improves, she will be able to do more repetitions of bouncing and jumping. When she is able to do more repetitions, her endurance will also improve and she will be able to jump for longer periods of time before she fatigues.

***If your child resists your support when learning to bounce or jump,*** focus on making jumping fun and intermittently and briefly add strategic support to have her feel the component she needs to learn. Be creative and playful when providing the support. Watch and see if she starts to use the new movement or if she begins to tolerate your support.

***Children are interested in learning to jump at different times.*** Start practicing after your child learns to walk and keep it fun and familiar. She will show you when she is interested and then you can practice more. If her sibling does it, she will want to do what he or she does.

***If your child wants to learn to hop (on one foot), watch her leg and foot posture.*** If your child is interested in hopping, you can teach her using the methods in this chapter for jumping with lift-off. I do not recommend it if your child is not interested, and you can substitute jumping (on both feet) when others are hopping. Jumping will strengthen both legs and ankles, while in good alignment, and this is beneficial. Hopping primarily strengthens the dominant leg, and since she has to balance on one leg, she will tend to stand with her weight shifted over the inside border of her foot (flatten her arch), and then her knee will also tilt inward. She will then hop with this posture, which will produce impact on her knee and ankle. Her knee and ankle posture is due to her lax ligaments, and the alignment is worsened when she is trying to balance on one foot. For these reasons, I do not focus on teaching hopping.

## Temperament

If your child is an **observer,** move slowly when introducing bouncing and jumping. She will first need to adjust to standing on the springy surface and will feel unstable and off balance because the surface will move. She will also need to assimilate the new movement of bouncing on the springy surface. In the beginning, she may need to be convinced that this is fun!

You will need to setup the experience of bouncing and jumping so she feels safe and in control as much as possible. With each change in the routine, she will need time to adjust and practice until she feels comfortable. She will prefer small bounces for a couple of repetitions. She will need to build up her tolerance to bouncing by increasing the *distance* of the up/down motion, the *speed* of the bounces, and the number of *repetitions*. If you watch how she responds and let her adjust gradually, she will be willing to practice. If you overwhelm her, she may avoid it.

Practice bouncing and jumping when she shows you she is interested. Never force or impose jumping. Keep it fun and find ways to motivate her to try it. Have her brother jump and then see if she will take a turn. Look for other ways to motivate her if this does not work. For example, Lily became motivated when she practiced jumping with her baby doll. We would take turns with Lily in charge. She would say "baby jump" and then "Lily jump." She would also tell me when she was "done."

Your child will learn to jump with lift-off on the mini-trampoline, holding the bar, when she is willing to be vigorous with her leg movements. With practice, she will gain confidence and then she will be comfortable using the mini-trampoline and challenge herself to generate lift-off. When she does jump, she will be very proud.

If your child is **motor driven,** she will love the feeling of bouncing and jumping. She will be ready to practice when she is placed on the springy surface. She will easily adjust to the surface, and she will like the up/down motions.

You will need to supervise her so she is safe. She may let go or try some "wild" movements. For example, she may be standing and bouncing and then lift her legs up, landing in sitting and bouncing on her buttocks. You will need to manage her safety with each bouncing or jumping activity that she is practicing.

She will be motivated to practice bouncing and jumping, and will increase the repetitions if encouraged. If she is using one of the variations described in the Tendencies section, she may be impatient with you supporting her if she feels like you are interfering with her movements. If you provide support with movement, she will probably like it. You can motivate her by counting, clapping, or simultaneously jumping on the floor when she is jumping on the mini-trampoline. She will repeat the up/down rhythm as long as she is motivated. After she does a series of bounces or jumps, let her take a break and then repeat it again. She will enjoy taking turns with her sibling or friend.

When she knows how to bounce and feels comfortable with the setup, she will experiment with moving her legs more vigorously and increasing the speed of the bounces to work on jumping with lift-off. She will see you jump, feel how you assist her with jumping, and she will try to do it by herself. Once she does it, she will work on repeating it again and again, until she can do it all the time. After she does it on the springy surface, she will want to try to do it on the floor. Both of you will be surprised when she does her first jump on the floor. She may do it when she is practicing, or, like Michael, she may do it when she is having a tantrum!

When she is ready to learn to jump off, she will not be scared. You will need to set her up with the right height surface and increase the height until she can jump off the bottom stair. She will need to hold your thumbs for balance and then will do it on her own. You will need to clear the area and supervise her so she is safe and does not bump into furniture. You will also need to watch her and make sure that she does not try to jump off surfaces that are too high.

## 🏃 ACTIVITY #1: Bouncing on a Springy Surface with Feet Flat

The best method is using a mini-trampoline with a handle such as the One Step Ahead—Kids Safety Trampoline with a handle (www.onestepahead.com). This activity will be described using this equipment. Refer to the Guidelines for other possible setups.

1. Setup the mini-trampoline and have a sibling demonstrate climbing on and bouncing, holding onto the bar. If a sibling or another child is not available, then you do it.
2. Sign "jump" and encourage your child to climb onto the trampoline, move to stand, and hold onto the bar for balance. Watch her reaction to the springy surface and help her feel comfortable on it if she is afraid.

3. Stand in front of her on the floor and bounce with hips and knees bending, exaggerating the movements so she knows what to imitate. Have her sibling join you. See if she tries to imitate you. Let her bounce using any method she initiates.

4. Make it fun by practicing with other children, by singing "Monkeys jumping on the bed," with rhythmical music, or watching a jumping video.

5. When she is comfortable standing and moving on the trampoline, then adjust her posture:
   a. place her feet 2-3 inches (5-7.5 cm) apart, pointing straight, in the middle of the trampoline, with her weight shifted toward the balls of her feet
   b. have her hold onto the bar, and make sure the height is at chest or shoulder level and the diameter of the bar is narrow enough for her to grip
   c. have her trunk vertical, not arched or leaning forward so her face is close to the bar
   d. watch her knees and assist bending if needed

6. With these adjustments to her posture, repeat steps 3 and 4 and encourage her to bounce. If she resists the adjustments to her posture or quits practicing when you support her, then let her use her method to keep the game fun. Keep testing when she will allow the postural support, and also be creative and playful with how you provide the support so she will accept it.

7. When she is comfortable with bouncing, give support where needed:
   a. If her knees are stiff and straight:
      - You can kneel behind her with your thumbs horizontally behind her knees (the crease behind the knees). Then, press forward to unlock her knees and help her bounce in this position (fig. 13.24).
      - You can also sit in front of her on a bench with your hands behind her knees and do the same movements.
      - Or, you can kneel on the floor behind her and hold her lower legs in the calf area. Then press forward to unlock her knees and bounce her with her weight shifted forward toward her tiptoes (fig. 13.25).
   b. If her trunk is arched and her knees are stiff and straight, kneel at her side and place one hand on her lower abdomen and your other hand behind her knees to guide activating her abdominals to tuck her belly and unlock her knees. With this support, you can then assist bouncing with this posture.

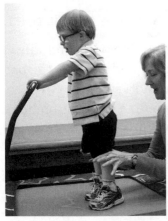 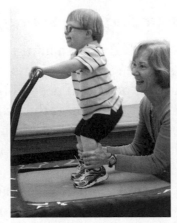 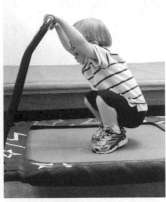

(fig. 13.24)          (fig. 13.25)          (fig. 13.26)

    c. If her chest leans forward so her chin is too close to the bar when she bounces, then support her chest with your hand to keep it vertical.

    d. If she needs support to grip the bar, provide hand over hand assistance.

8. Encourage bouncing for 5-10 repetitions, and then take turns with siblings.

9. Provide verbal and visual cues, and use the motivators that work best for your child.

10. Continue to practice with strategic support until she uses the right bouncing method. Then gradually decrease your support until she can do it by herself. Then practice for several repetitions, 20-30 times.

11. If needed, use this alternative method to teach the three steps of bending, lift-off, and landing:

    a. Place your child standing on a squishy raised surface, like a bed.

    b. You stand on the floor and hold her trunk, either so she is facing you or has her back to you.

    c. Say "bend" or "down" to cue your child to bend her knees toward a squat. Assist her if needed.

    d. Say "up" or "stand," and after she stands up, playfully pick her up to feel lift-off.

    e. Then have her catch with her feet and land in standing, with hips and knees slightly bent.

    f. After she learns this method on the bed, she can also practice it on the mini-trampoline, holding onto the bar. When practicing this method, watch her knees to make sure she is bending them to squat and when landing (fig. 13.26).

    g. You can also try a jumper, jumperoo, or bouncer (p. 414).

## ACTIVITY #2: Bouncing on a Springy Surface on Tiptoes

This activity will be described using a mini-trampoline with a handle.

1. Have your child stand on the mini-trampoline, holding onto the bar for balance. Adjust her posture if needed (Activity #1, step 5).
2. Place her feet back in the middle of the trampoline so she is on her toes, with her pelvis over her tiptoes and her knees bent. If needed, support her feet to maintain them in this position.
3. Encourage her to bounce on tiptoes.
4. If she needs support to learn to bounce on tiptoes, try the following methods to shift her weight onto the balls of her feet:
    a. lift her heels with your hands by putting your fingers under her heels or cupping your hands under her heels
    b. hold her lower legs (calf areas) with the palms of your hands and tilt them forward
    c. once you provide the support, assist the bouncing movement while your child is on tiptoes
5. Provide support until she can bounce on tiptoes by herself.
6. Have her sibling do it in an exaggerated way and help your child watch the feet. Give the verbal cue saying "tippy toes," "tiptoes," or "toes."
7. Encourage bouncing for 10-20 repetitions; take turns with siblings.
8. When she bounces well on tiptoes for several repetitions, encourage her to be more vigorous and bounce harder, increasing the movement of the springy surface. You can teach her how it feels by:
    a. holding her lower legs and pushing them downward to exaggerate pressing her toes into the surface
    b. standing on the surface with her and gently bouncing to move the surface (while supporting the front of her trunk)
9. Also practice standing on tiptoes on the floor during playtime. Encourage your child to reach up to food on the counter, or for toys on a raised table, while propping against the surface. She will need to learn to rise up high on her tiptoes and hold the position for a few seconds. Also give the verbal cue to label the game.
10. You can also try a jumper, jumperoo, or bouncer (p. 414).

## Jumping with Lift-off

### Activity #3A: Standing on a Mini-Trampoline, Holding the Bar for Balance

1. Encourage your child to bounce on tiptoes (holding the bar for balance) and add the experience of lift-off to her bouncing rhythm by:

a. kneeling behind her on the floor, holding her lower legs

b. standing in front of her, facing her, and holding her trunk under hers armpits

c. standing behind her on the trampoline and gently bouncing her (while supporting the front of her trunk)

2. Say "big jump" and sign "jump."

3. Take turns with a sibling; have the brother or sister hold the bar and do an exaggerated jump, lifting her feet high off the surface.

4. Practice in front of a large mirror so she sees lift-off when you help.

5. Look at the height of the bar on the trampoline. If it is at chest level or lower, experiment with having her hold a 1-inch (2.5-cm) diameter pole (or broom handle) at the level of her shoulders or chin. See if she will hold on and pull her body upward to assist with lift-off when using a higher bar.

6. Clap for her and praise her, especially when any lift-off is achieved.

7. If she is on the verge of lift-off or does one bounce with lift-off, continue to practice to see if she can figure out what she needs to do to consistently generate lift-off. Take turns with her sibling so she has time to regain her strength to practice again.

8. Continue to practice on the mini-trampoline, holding the bar for balance, until she can do 50 jumps with lift-off.

9. When she is practicing jumping on the mat and floor (B & C), she will still practice jumping on the mini-trampoline, holding the bar. Encourage this, since it will improve her strength and endurance for jumping on the floor.

## Activity #3B: On a Mat, Bed, or Sofa Cushion

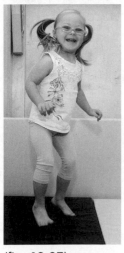

1. When jumping with lift-off is established on the mini-trampoline, holding the bar, then encourage jumping on a mat (or bed or sofa cushion), holding onto a 1-inch (2.5-cm) diameter pole. You will need to hold the pole very still (to simulate the stability of the bar on the mini-trampoline). She will do best if the pole is held at the level of her shoulders or chin. An alternative is for her to hold your index fingers.

2. When she can do several jumps on the mat, holding the pole or your fingers, see if she can do it without support.

3. Continue to practice until she can jump with toe push-off for several repetitions (fig. 13.27).

(fig. 13.27)

## Activity #3C: Jumping on the Floor

1. When jumping with lift-off is established on the mat, then encourage jumping on the floor, holding the pole or your fingers. You will need to hold the pole very still (to simulate the stability of the bar on the mini-trampoline). She will do best if the pole is held at the level of her shoulders or chin.
2. When she can do several jumps on the floor, holding the pole or your fingers, see if she can jump with lift-off without holding on.
3. Continue to practice until she can jump on the floor with toe push-off, without hand support, for several repetitions.

 ## ACTIVITY #4: Jumping Forward, Both Feet Together

1. Stand her on a surface with two distinct adjacent colors (like a mat with colored panels, interlocking foam squares, or at the border of the carpet and hardwood floor). Place her toes at the edge of one color.
2. Kneel in front of her, leaving enough space between you so she has room to jump to the next color.
3. Have her hold your thumbs (placed horizontally), while you hold her wrists. Support her hands at her shoulder level. Or, hold a 1-inch diameter pole at the level of her shoulders, with your hands over hers to assist her grip.
4. Say "1, 2, 3, bend, and jump." When you say "jump," wait for her to initiate the jump and then quickly and gently pull her forward so she feels the forward motion. It is important to coordinate the timing of the jump so you move together. You want to build on her jumping action rather than passively move her forward.
5. Practice for several repetitions so she becomes familiar with the forward motion and participates with moving in that direction.
6. Watch her feet and provide support so she moves both feet together.
7. Test when she can jump forward with both feet together, without hand support.
8. Measure the distance that she can jump and practice until she can jump forward 6-8 inches (15-20 cm).
9. When she can consistently jump forward with both feet together, without hand support, you can use advanced setups like jumping over a rope, jumping in and out of a hoop, or jumping from one shape (spot marker) to another.

**Activity #5: Jumping Off, Both Feet Together**

Your child will be ready to learn to jump off when she can jump forward 6-8 inches (15-20 cm).

1. Pick two firm, adjacent surfaces, with distinctly different colors, with one surface 1-2 inches (2.5-5 cm) higher than the other. Examples are: a firm mat on the floor, a mat with three panels with one panel folded over the other two, interlocking foam square on the floor, or a wooden board on the carpet. Stabilize the surfaces so they do not slide or wobble.
2. Stand her on the raised surface, with her toes at the edge.
3. Kneel in front of her, leaving room for her to jump to the other surface.
4. Have her hold your thumbs (placed horizontally), and you hold her wrists. Support her hands at shoulder level. Or, have her hold a 1-inch (2.5-cm) diameter pole shoulder level, with your hands over hers to assist her grip.
5. Say "1, 2, 3, bend, and jump." When you say "jump," wait for her to initiate the jump and then quickly and gently pull her forward and downward so she feels the motions. It is important to coordinate the timing of the jump so you move together. You want to build on her jumping action rather than passively move her forward.
6. Practice for several repetitions so she becomes familiar with jumping off and participates with moving in that direction.
7. Watch her feet and provide support so she moves both feet together.
8. Test when she can jump off with both feet together, without hand support. Practice until she can do it for several repetitions.

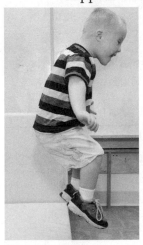

9. When she can consistently jump off the 1-2 inch (2.5-5 cm) high surface with both feet together, without hand support, start increasing the height of the surface in 1-inch (2.5-cm) increments. With each higher surface, start with hand support and then have her learn to do it without hand support (fig. 13.28). Provide hand support until she can jump off with both feet together.
10. Practice with a sibling, having them stand together on the surface and taking turns jumping off.
11. If your child is timid about jumping off, kneel on the floor in front of her and catch her after she jumps and lands on the floor.

(fig. 13.28)

12. Continue to practice until she can jump off the bottom stair (7-8 inches or 18-20 cm high) with both feet together.

## 🏃 MOTOR MILESTONE CHECKLIST

She bounces on a springy surface, holding onto a bar for balance, with hips and knees bending, and feet flat:
- ❑ 1-5 repetitions
- ❑ 10 repetitions or more

She bounces on her tiptoes on a springy surface, holding onto a bar for balance:
- ❑ 1-5 repetitions
- ❑ 10 repetitions or more

- ❑ She jumps with lift-off occasionally while bouncing on a springy surface, holding onto a bar for balance
- ❑ She jumps with lift-off consistently on a springy surface, holding onto a bar for balance
- ❑ She jumps on a mat with lift-off, holding onto a bar for balance
- ❑ She jumps on a mat, with lift-off using toe push-off, without hand support
- ❑ She jumps on the floor with lift-off, holding onto a bar for balance
- ❑ She jumps on the floor, with lift-off using toe push-off, without hand support
- ❑ She jumps on the floor, with lift-off using toe push-off, for several repetitions
- ❑ She jumps forward 6-8 inches (15-20 cm) with both feet together, without hand support
- ❑ She jumps off a 2-inch (5-cm) step with both feet together, without hand support
- ❑ She jumps off a 4-inch (10-cm) step with both feet together, without hand support
- ❑ She jumps off an 8-inch (20-cm) stair with both feet together, without hand support

# 14

# Riding a Tricycle or Bicycle

## Introduction

After your child walks, he will enjoy learning to scoot around on a ride-on toy. He will practice climbing on and off, and then figure out how to move forward. When his leg scooting movements are strong, he can progress to using the motorcycle, cozy coupe, and car, van, and truck models. It will be fun to do this activity with other children and ride around the neighborhood. Your child can also pretend that he is driving to the store or the park.

When your child sees other children riding tricycles and bicycles, he will become interested in riding a tricycle since he will want to do what the other children do. He will sit on the tricycle and probably try to put his feet on the pedals. If they do not reach, then he will use his leg scooting movements to move forward. If his feet do reach, he will place them on the pedals but not be able to make the trike go. He will need support to learn the leg pedaling movements, and he will be ready to start practicing when his legs are long enough to fit a tricycle.

The goal will be to pedal and steer the tricycle on level surfaces for at least 15 feet (4.5 meters). This goal will take time for your child to achieve. The average age for a child with Down syndrome to achieve this skill (according to my data) is 4-5 years old. Once your child can ride that far, he will know the basics for riding a tricycle, and, with practice, will increase the distance if motivated. After he learns to ride the tricycle, he will continue progressing to riding a bicycle.

You want your child to have the fun experience of being independent on a ride-on toy first. When his legs are long enough to reach the pedals of a tricycle and he is interested, then you can begin practicing riding a tricycle with support, usually around the age of 2½ to 3 years. You will need to find a tricycle suitable for his short arms and legs. Then the training will begin to teach him the alternating leg movements for pedaling. You will need to push him with his feet supported on the pedals and do the steering. Through feeling the leg movements, he will learn how to pedal. After he learns to pedal, you can teach him to steer. When he can do each skill, then you can teach him to do them simultaneously in a coordinated way.

Since it will probably take your child one to two years to learn to ride a trike well, practice as tolerated and always have it be a playful time. If your child has a negative experience or is frustrated with it, he may avoid learning it later.

Riding a tricycle will benefit your child in many ways, socially and physically. He will enjoy playing outside with other children. He will be proud and feel "big" to be riding his tricycle with his siblings and the neighborhood kids. His physical skills will also improve as he develops the strength and coordination needed for pedaling and steering. To pedal, he will strengthen both legs and ankles and integrate the movements into a smooth, rhythmical alternating pattern. He will strengthen his core to hold his trunk stable to efficiently move his legs to pedal and his arms to steer. Besides developing the arm and hand strength needed for steering, he will also need to constantly pay attention and look forward without being distracted, to have the sense of timing to know when to turn, to be quick in his reaction time to execute turning, and to use spatial awareness to understand when turning is needed. Once he can do the individual skills of steering and pedaling, he needs to coordinate these skills and use them simultaneously to ride his tricycle in the neighborhood with the other children.

When you think of all the components needed for riding a tricycle, you appreciate how complex it is and why it is a process that takes time to fully develop.

### Steps in Learning to Ride a Tricycle

To achieve the goal of this skill area, your child will need to practice the following steps:

1. Climb on and off the ride-on toy or tricycle;
2. Scoot forward on a ride-on toy;
3. Ride a tricycle with full support to pedal and steer;
4. Pedal a tricycle for 15 feet (4.5 meters);
5. Steer and pedal a tricycle on level surfaces.

## Components

The components to focus on are:
1. leg posture with neutral hip rotation (knees and feet pointing straight ahead), knees in line with feet, and feet maintained straight on the pedals

2. leg pedaling movements, with each leg having the strength to bend and straighten the knee, and the ankle strength to keep the foot on the pedal and push the pedal with the ankle moving up and down

3. leg coordination and strength to maintain the pedaling rhythm continuously over the distance

4. trunk strength to sit erect with the pelvis up straight, so he has a stable base for pedaling and steering

5. arm and hand strength to hold handlebars and steer

6. arms, legs, and trunk moving together in an integrated way to simultaneously pedal and steer

7. perseverance to increase distance, speed, and endurance

## Tendencies

The tendencies are:

1. to position his legs with his hips in external rotation so his knees turn out and are wider than his feet, and his feet turn outward on the pedals

2. to stiffen one or both knees when trying to pedal and become stuck

3. to have weak or inactive ankles so he does not push his feet to pedal

4. to hold one or both feet on the pedals with his toes turned outward, and then when he pedals, his heel hits the pedal hardware and falls off the pedal

5. to have a strong leg and a weak leg so that when he pedals, he has difficulty using coordinated leg movements to achieve a continuous pedaling rhythm

6. to sit with his trunk rounded and his pelvis tilted back, which makes pedaling and steering more difficult

7. to resist holding the handlebars firmly to turn them to steer, or to resist using the combination of trunk rotation and arm movements to turn effectively

8. to be able to pedal or steer but have difficulty coordinating both skills

9. to lose interest in riding the tricycle and only ride for short distances and then be done

## Setup for Learning

### Climbing On and Off

You will need to teach your child how to climb on and off the ride-on toy or tricycle. If you teach him how to do it from the beginning, he will do it by himself rather than rely on you to put him on or take him off. He will learn quickly and be motivated to do it because he will want to be independent and in control.

When he is climbing on or off, you will need to hold the ride-on toy or tricycle to prevent it from sliding or moving. To climb on, his initial position will be critical to his success. He should stand next to the seat, with his body facing the handlebars. He will hold onto the handlebars with both hands and then lift the leg closest to the seat over the seat. He will probably bend his hip and knee to lift his leg in front of his body. You can help him lift his leg if needed. Once his legs are positioned on each side of the seat, he can sit down. His first strategy to climb off will probably be to slide his buttocks off the seat sideways to the floor. You can guide him to climb off from standing. To climb off, he will stand up, hold onto the handlebars, and lift the leg he chooses over the seat.

With practice, your child will climb on and off by himself and will only need you to stabilize the ride-on toy or tricycle. Later, depending on how easily the tricycle moves on the surface it is on, he will learn to climb on and off without your support.

### Scooting Forward on a Ride-on Toy

The ride-on toy has to fit your child properly so he can be successful using it (fig. 14.1). Try a variety of styles and test which one works best for your child. You need to check the following features:

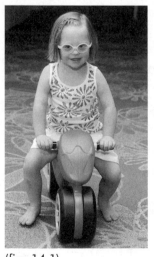

(fig. 14.1)

1. *Seat height:* your child's feet should be flat on the floor with his hips and knees bent approximately 90 degrees.
2. *Rear wheels:* look at how close the rear wheels are to the seat and how wide they are positioned. It is best if they are under the base or far enough behind the seat that your child's feet do not touch them when he is scooting forward, pushing off with his feet. If his feet bump into the wheels when he is pushing off, he will be frustrated and will not be successful using the ride-on toy.
3. *Seat width:* it is better if it is narrow so your child learns to scoot his legs with his thighs closer together rather than very wide apart.
4. *Back support:* your child will feel more stable on the seat if it has a back support. It will help him hold his trunk up straight and tilt the top of his pelvis forward, which is the ideal position for scooting himself forward with his legs.
5. *Handlebars:* buy a toy with handlebars so your child has a firm surface to hold onto while scooting.

In the beginning, your child will probably learn to push himself backwards. He will place his feet on the floor, and push off with his feet while straightening his knees. He will be happy he is moving, and continue this easy method.

You will need to help him learn to move himself forward because it is more difficult. If you show him the method, he will learn quickly. You will need to show him how to move his legs. You will hold his lower legs and bend his knees, pushing his feet into the floor so he weight shifts from his heels to his toes and moves the ride-on toy forward. To demonstrate the scooting motion, you can move his legs together or one at a time. With practice, he will learn to bend his knees and push off with his toes to scoot forward. You may need to motivate him and encourage him to try to move forward rather than backward.

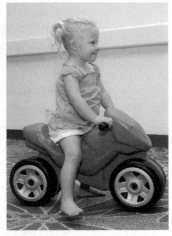

When he learns to scoot, he will either move both legs together or move one foot at a time. Either method is acceptable. Begin with short distances and increase the distance when he is ready, until he spontaneously rides the toy to play. When his legs are longer, he can use a ride-on toy with a higher seat, such as the Step2® Free Wheeling Motorcycle (fig. 14.2). The seat is narrower, so it will be easier to scoot with his legs. He will enjoy scooting fast, for long distances. Since the seat and width of the base are narrow, he will also need to balance himself while scooting.

(fig. 14.2)

In addition to learning how to move his legs, your child will also need to learn how to position his trunk and pelvis to use his legs effectively. He will need to hold his trunk up straight with the top of his pelvis tilted forward. You can support his low back if needed to help him maintain the position while he works on the leg movements. If he sits on the ride-on toy with his trunk rounded and the top of his pelvis tilted back, it will be much harder to do the leg motions required to move himself forward and much easier to move backwards.

When your child has mastered scooting forward on a ride-on toy, you can try using the car, van, truck, and cozy coupe models. It will take him time to learn how to use them because they are heavier and require more leg strength to push. You also need to check the shape of the seat and his trunk posture when sitting on the seat. If he leans his trunk and pelvis back in the seat, he will not be able to use his legs effectively to scoot forward. He needs to lean his trunk forward toward the steering wheel to effectively use his legs to move forward. In the beginning, he may prefer to play with the steering wheel, beep the horn, open and close the door, and climb in and out of the car. You can help him learn to scoot and go for a ride in the car when he is motivated.

## Riding a Tricycle with Full Support to Pedal and Steer

When your child shows an interest in a tricycle and his legs are long enough for his feet to easily reach the pedals, you can begin practicing pedaling a tricycle with full support. The initial setup and fit of the tricycle is critical for his success. You need to use the tricycle that fits him the best and has the accessories that teach him the leg pedaling movements. These features are important to consider in the tricycle you use:

1. ***Pedals:*** Since your child's leg length is short, you need to find a tricycle with the shortest distance from the seat to the foot pedal. To check the fit, have him sit on the seat and then place one foot on the pedal, with the pedal in the farthest position from the seat. Make sure his leg is long enough to fit, with his foot flat and resting on the pedal, for a complete revolution.

2. ***Footpedal attachments:*** To feel the leg movements for pedaling, your child will probably need to use footpedal attachments to stabilize his feet on the pedals (fig. 14.3). Then you will push him with his feet secured on the pedals, so he will feel the continuous movements of his hips, knees,

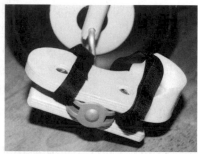

(fig. 14.3)

   and ankles and will feel the pedaling rhythm. From this experience, he will eventually learn to keep his feet on the pedals, and use alternating leg motions to pedal.

3. ***Seat:*** The seat will support his pelvis best for pedaling if it has a contoured edge at the back of the seat, or if it has a back, like a bucket seat. If the seat is flat, his pelvis will slide back as he tries to pedal with his legs, and then his pedaling will be ineffective. With his pelvis stabilized, he will be successful with moving forward every time he pushes with his legs and feet.

   a. The *height* of the seat is also important. Your child will feel more stable if the seat is low and his feet can touch the ground. It will also be easier for him to climb on and off.

   b. It is helpful to have an *adjustable seat* so the same equipment can be used from the beginning stage of being pushed, to the later stage when he can pedal and steer it by himself.

4. ***Base:*** The base of the tricycle needs to be wide so it is stable and does not tip over easily or feel wobbly. Measure the width be-

tween the outside edges of the rear wheels. The wider it is, the more stable it is.

5. *Handlebars:* Since your child's arm length is short, the handle bars need be positioned close to his trunk or angled toward his trunk as he sits on the seat of the tricycle. If the handlebars are too far to reach, it will be harder for him to steer.

6. *Weight:* Plastic is preferable to metal. When your child is first learning to pedal, a plastic tricycle will be easier since it is lighter and requires less strength to move forward. After he has mastered pedaling a plastic tricycle, he can use a metal tricycle and he will challenge himself to access the strength needed to pedal.

7. *Diameter of front wheel:* Pick a tricycle with a larger diameter (8.5-10-inch; 20-25-cm) front wheel (for example, the Fisher Price Rock Roll n' Ride has a 10-inch front wheel). In my experience, this is the size that children with Down syndrome can use most effectively.

My favorite tricycle is the Fisher Price Rock Roll n' Ride (fig. 14.4). It works well for three-year-olds with Down syndrome and has the special features described above, as well as a push handle for easy maneuvering by the parent.

Once your child is setup with the right-size tricycle, with his feet secured to the pedals with footpedal attachments, then you will further check the position of his legs, especially his knees,

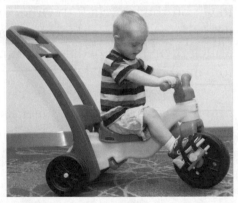

(fig. 14.4)

while pushing him. If his knees are fully straight when the pedal is in its farthest position, then the seat-to-footpedal length is too long, and his pelvis needs to be moved forward on the seat or the seat needs to be adjusted to a shorter setting (if possible).

If the seat is already in its shortest setting, then you can stabilize his pelvis on the seat using grip liner. Place the grip liner on the seat and then move his pelvis forward to the desired position on the seat. After you make this adjustment, then push him again and see if his knees are maintained in the slightly bent position. If so, then he is ready to go for a ride and feel the leg pedaling movements.

The pedaling rhythm flows best if the knees are slightly bent. If one or both knees straighten, then your child will tend to lock his knee in the straight position and hold it stiffly, which will block the pedaling motion. Also check the handlebars, because if they are turned, one knee will be straight. If your child persists with locking one or both knees even after you have moved his pelvis forward on the seat, stabilized it with grip liner, and turned the handlebars so he moves straight, then you may need to wait for his legs to grow a little before practicing this skill. (See Activity #2A, Step 6.)

If you introduce your child to the tricycle at around 2 ½ to 3 years old, footpedal attachments will help him succeed. Otherwise, it will be too difficult for him to keep his feet on the pedals while you push him. He may be able to place his feet on the pedals while sitting on the tricycle, but they will slip off easily when the pedals are moved. He does not know how to push his foot against the pedal yet, and he will learn this detailed movement later, after he masters the complex alternating leg pedaling movements.

You can purchase footpedal attachments from Equipment Shop (www.equipmentshop.com). These footpedal attachments are sturdy and conveniently attach to the pedals, and then your child's foot is easily strapped in place and held with Velcro straps. With the Velcro straps, his feet can be quickly released, which is very important when your child is done and wants to get off the tricycle fast. Other alternatives are to use masking tape, make a homemade version of footpedal attachments, or use old Velcro sandals and attach them to the pedals. You can see which type of support will work best for you and your child.

When you use the footpedal attachments, you will need to stand beside him for his safety. With his feet secured to the pedals, if he tips over, he will not be able to put his foot out to catch himself. You will need to supervise him closely to keep him from tipping over or to catch him if he begins to tip over.

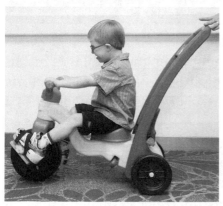
(fig. 14.5)

Once you have provided the best set-up, your child is ready to ride the tricycle with your support (fig. 14.5). As described in Activity #2A, you will push him and steer the tricycle, and he will hold onto the handlebars and experience the leg pedaling movements. You will have fun together going for walks, going fast and slow, riding with siblings and neighbors, and chasing them. If you make it exciting, he will enjoy it and want to do it often. Follow his lead and practice when he wants to, and for as long as he wants to. If he wants to stop, try again another time. It may help to motivate him if his brother rides his bicycle or tricycle at the same time. Practice with the goal of having fun and gradually increase the time he will ride the tricycle with support.

He will need a lot of practice to learn to use the leg and foot motions needed to pedal the tricycle. Be patient with the process and expect to push him for a few months. He will need time to become familiar with the leg motions since he has never used them before in other skills. In the meantime, he can enjoy the other aspects of riding a tricycle. For example, Yehuda explored the handlebars, looked down at his feet, watched the sidewalk go by, watched his siblings, and looked sideways at the grass and flowers while he was being pushed. Your child can take in the full experience now, and then later when he is ready to practice pedaling and steering, he will pay attention and focus on these skills and moving himself forward.

When your child is familiar with the leg motions and likes riding the tricycle, try letting him ride down a 1-2 degree inclined driveway or sidewalk as described in Activity #2B. Gravity will make it easier for him to pedal, and he will be motivated to do it because he will be successful. He will love playing this game with his siblings, as they take turns riding down the "hill."

While you are pushing him on the tricycle, he can explore steering if he shows an interest, but it is not a priority. He may have experimented with steering when using his ride-on toy or coupe. At this time, have him focus on pedaling, and when pedaling is mastered, then he can learn to steer.

If your child shows an interest in riding a trike but his legs are too short to fit one, try to find a way to practice pedaling to encourage his interest. *His* solution may be to scoot with his legs to move forward on the tricycle, and this may satisfy his interest. If he wants to try pedaling, test other products available such as the VTech Ride and Learn Giraffe Bike. This will give him a fun alternative to enjoy while waiting for his legs to grow. Also check all available tricycle models, as you may be able to find a tricycle that fits his leg length.

### Pedaling a Tricycle for 15 Feet (4.5 Meters)

When your child is familiar with pedaling and tries to pedal while you are pushing him, then you can begin to let go to see if he will continue pedaling on his own for short distances. Since this will be difficult for him, make sure the setup is ideal with the right-size tricycle, grip liner on the seat, foot-pedal attachments, his trunk and pelvis up straight, and a smooth surface to ride on. Begin with 1-2 foot (30 to 60 cm) distances, progressing to 3-5 feet (.9 to 1.5 meters) when he is ready. You will need to start the forward movement and then see if he can continue it. You can push him from behind or you can be in front of him and push one foot to start him moving forward.

Practice in an open space so steering is not necessary. Provide intermittent support so he is successful (fig. 14.6). Clap when he reaches the endpoint so he understands the new game and is proud that he did it. Keep him moving because if he struggles too much, he may become frustrated and avoid the activity. As you practice, try to keep a balance between challenging him to do it by himself and enjoying the skill while being pushed.

To pedal, your child will need to:

1. Bend and straighten his hips and knees, pushing one leg forward at a time in an alternating pattern
2. Move his ankles up and down and press his feet against the pedals to maintain his feet on the pedals and push them in a circular motion.

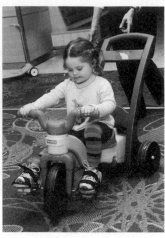

(fig. 14.6)

He will need to combine the hip, knee, and ankle movements to move the wheels in a full revolution (fig. 14.7). The hip and knee movements move the pedals forward and back, and the ankle movements provide the circular motion to do a full revolution. Once he learns the hip and knee movements, then he will need to focus

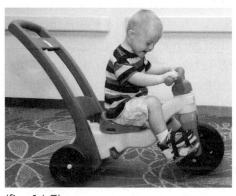

(fig. 14.7)

on pushing with his feet to pedal on his own. Each leg and ankle will need to be strong to create a balanced alternating rhythm. Figuring out how to move his legs and feet to move the tricycle forward is something he will need to grapple with. While he is working on this challenge, he will need his feet secured to the pedals so he can focus on pushing with his feet rather than wrestling with trying to keep his feet on the pedals.

When practicing pedaling on his own, a common problem is to have one knee straight and the other bent and be stuck in that position. He will remain stuck because he will continue to straighten the knee that is straight, rather than pushing with his other foot to straighten his other knee. Or, he will contract the muscles of both legs simultaneously (called co-contraction) causing him to be stuck in that position.

You will notice that this "stuck" position repeats itself often, frequently with the same leg. When you see this occurring, position yourself on the side of the knee that he straightens and place your fingers under his knee to unlock it. With this strategic support, he can move his other leg and keep the pedaling rhythm flowing. He will need to strengthen both legs equally and coordinate his leg movements to use the pedaling rhythm effectively. Also check the handlebars to see if they are turned because this will cause one knee to straighten. If the tricycle is a little small for him, his knees will stay slightly bent, and then you will avoid this common problem.

To use his strength to push with his legs and feet, his trunk and pelvis will need to be stable and strong. He will need to sit up straight with his pelvis held firmly on the seat, using grip liner. If additional support is needed, you can **put a belt around the back of his pelvis** and the vertical post below the handlebars. I use a 2-inch (5-cm) wide belt made with cotton webbing, and it has a buckle closure. (It is called a gait belt and is available through the Posey Company (www.posey.com).) It is comfortable and easily tolerated, and it stabilizes the low back so he can push better with his legs and feet.

When he participates with pedaling 3-foot (1-meter) distances and knows this game, you will gradually increase the distance until he can pedal 15-foot (4.5-meter) distances consistently. As he practices working up to 15 feet, you need to start the forward motion of pedaling, provide intermittent support to move to the endpoint, and steer when urgently needed. Learning to pedal is challenging enough so you do not want to make it too hard or he will quit or just avoid practicing the skill.

When a child is practicing this skill with me in my setting, we are in a big open space (20 by 30 feet or 6 by 12 meters) with a linoleum floor, and a sofa against one wall. I set him up on the linoleum floor and I sit on the sofa about 3-5 feet (90 cm-1.5 meters) in front of him. We play the game that he pedals to me and then crashes into the sofa. Then I clap for him and take him for a fast ride for the length of the room and then back to the starting position for him to pedal to me again. This makes the game exciting and breaks up the work of pedaling with a fun ride, which reinforces the pedaling motions.

When a child is ready to start pedaling to me, I lean forward off the sofa to start the forward movement with his leading leg by pushing his foot. Then, as he is moving to me, I say "push," move my hands signing tricycle (which simulates the leg pedaling movements), and keep repeating the word "push" until he pedals the distance to me. This game encourages him to practice the distance for short periods, and we do it as long as he participates. When I see his performance improve, then I increase the distance. With this experience, he gains confidence with pedaling specific distances.

You will need to figure out what verbal cues work best for your child. I usually use the word "push" and combine it with the tactile cue of pushing his foot or pushing his thigh, depending on which movement he needs to learn. Try to understand how he interprets your verbal cue. He may imitate you and use his hand to push his thigh or foot. If so, you need to help him understand that he needs to push with his leg or foot rather than with his hand. You can also try saying "push your foot" or "push" with a grunt to exaggerate pushing hard. You can also try "1, 2, 3, go" or simply "go, feet, go." Experiment with what to say and do to help your child understand how to pedal.

When your child can pedal 15 feet, see if he can initiate pedaling forward from the stopped position. Since he knows pedaling and has gained confidence, he will be willing to challenge himself because he will want to move.

### Steering and Pedaling a Tricycle on Level Surfaces

To ride a tricycle, your child will need to learn:

1. to hold the handlebars and steer;
2. to pedal by moving his hips, knees, and feet in a smooth, continuous rhythm;
3. to keep his feet on the pedals.

So far, he has learned to pedal for 15 feet (4.5 meters), to sit up tall, to hold the handlebars, and to initiate the forward motion. The remaining skills are to pedal longer distances, steer, and keep his feet on the pedals (without the footpedal attachments). Pedaling should be established and automatic before teaching steering. When he can pedal and steer easily, then you will be able to remove the footpedal attachments.

To pedal longer distances, he will need increased leg and ankle strength. His ankles will also need to move with finesse, with his toes moving up and down while pressing against the pedals, to produce the circular motion. Practicing distances is the best way to improve his strength and efficiency. Since the focus is distance, practice in an open space so steering is not required. Have him pedal as far as he can rather than go to a specific place that requires steering to move there. I do not recommend pedaling on the sidewalk because steering is needed to ride straight and stay on the sidewalk. Practice in a gym, the garage, the basement, or any large space without furniture. Walk behind your child as he pedals, and provide intermittent support so he has fun and is successful. He will be motivated if he keeps moving and will be frustrated if he moves slowly with frequent stopping and starting. When he feels comfortable pedaling, he will spontaneously improve his distance, speed, and endurance.

When he can pedal long distances, you can test when he is ready to learn steering. For example, when Peter was pedaling 25-foot distances, he wanted to look at his legs and feet. If he concentrated on them, then he could pedal and continue moving forward. However, if he looked up to steer, his leg motion stopped, and it was hard for him to get started again. At that time, he was not ready to learn steering because pedaling was not automatic yet. Later, when he could pedal well, he was able to look ahead while pedaling and so was ready to learn steering.

To begin practicing steering, your child needs to learn how to turn the handlebars. It is best to teach him when it is functional, like when he bumps into an obstacle and is stuck. At that moment, you can say "turn" to label the action. While he grips the handlebars, hold his forearms and move the handlebars to turn. When you move his forearms, exaggerate the motion so he rotates his trunk too. With this dramatic movement, he will easily feel what he needs to do to turn. As he continues to pedal, follow him and repeat this support every time he needs to turn. With practice, you can lessen your support and only provide what he needs to turn. He will learn to initiate the movement and eventually turn the handlebars as he approaches an obstacle. He will learn how to steer and how to plan ahead to turn before he gets stuck.

When your child can effectively steer and pedal using the footpedal attachments, you can experiment with removing them. This will be the last component for him to learn. He will need to learn to press against the pedal while moving his ankles to pedal. It will be easier to keep his feet on the pedals when he is riding straight ahead, and it will be harder when he is turning. With practice, he will easily learn to keep his feet on the pedals whether he is moving straight or turning.

## Guidelines

*Choose the plastic style tricycle for beginners.* The style of the Fisher Price Rock Roll n' Ride tricycle is ideal, and, since it is plastic, it requires less strength to learn to pedal. The seat is low to the ground so your child's feet are on the floor and he feels stable when sitting on the seat. He also can climb on and off easily with the low seat. With this style, when he pedals, his legs will push in the forward and downward diagonal, which is easy to learn.

More strength is needed to pedal the traditional red metal tricycle and many other metal models, due to the weight of the metal. The seat is also usually higher so his feet will not touch the ground when he sits on the seat, and he may feel unstable with this setup. With the high seat, it will be very difficult to climb on and off until he is taller. When he pedals, he will push more downward than forward. He will be ready to learn to pedal this type of tricycle after he can pedal the plastic type, like the Fisher Price Rock Roll n' Ride.

The "Big Wheels" style tricycle is the most challenging type to learn for the beginner and can be used after he knows how to pedal the plastic tricycle (described above). With this style, he will lean his trunk back in sitting and push his legs more horizontally to pedal. This position requires more abdominal strength to pedal than the other tricycles.

*Use a tricycle that is small (for his leg length) rather than large.* With a small tricycle, his knees will remain bent when he is being pushed and when he is pedaling so you will avoid the common problem of one or both knees locking in the straight position, blocking the pedaling motion. Later, when he is able to pedal independently, it will be easier for him to keep his feet on the pedals when he steers, especially when turning. If you use a tricycle that is large so he can grow into it, it will be difficult for his feet to rest on the pedals comfortably, particularly when the pedal is in the farthest position from the seat. If he needs to use his toes to touch the pedals, it will be very difficult to keep his feet on the pedals and make it harder to pedal.

*When he is learning to ride a tricycle, limit the accessories.* If the tricycle has streamers, a horn, or fancy decorations around the handlebars, your child will want to play with them rather than focus on learning to ride the tricycle. The accessories will distract him, and he will want to explore them rather than practice pedaling. It may be hard to divert his attention to pedaling and steering. It is best if the tricycle is plain at first, and, later, you can add the accessories.

*Teach him pedaling and steering separately, and focus on pedaling first.* If you try to do both when he is beginning to learn to ride the tricycle, you will overwhelm him, and he will lose interest or quit. You will be giving him too many instructions, and he will not be successful. You will be saying "push, feet, push," "turn," "push," "look up," etc., and then riding a tricycle will be frustrating for him. Focus on pedaling first while you manage the steering. While he is practicing pedaling, if he wants to be playful and turn the handlebars occasionally while you push him, let him, but you continue to manage the steering. After he masters pedaling, you can teach him to steer.

*Practice when he wants to, and for as long as he chooses to ride the tricycle.* Provide the right tricycle setup and the best motivators to make riding the tricycle a fun experience. The best motivators are siblings or neighborhood friends riding their tricycles with him. Your child will especially want to ride when other kids are doing it. For example, Allison was very motivated to learn to ride a tricycle when she started attending a daycare where the children routinely rode tricycles and ride-on toys in the gym. She observed the "big kids" flying by on their tricycles and kept plugging away until she too could pedal her tricycle forward.

When you use the footpedal attachments, it is critical that you stop when your child communicates that he is done. When his feet are secured to the pedals with the footpedal attachments, you need to keep him moving so he benefits from using them. After he has practiced pedaling with this support, whenever he indicates that he is done, whether through behavioral cues, signing "all done," or using words, release the Velcro straps immediately. If he is stationary or struggling to move and his feet are secured with the footpedal attachments, he will feel confined and restrained, and will become upset. As a result, he may resist this skill the next time you try to practice.

*Provide verbal, visual, and tactile cues.* Your child will learn to ride the tricycle through feeling it, seeing others doing it, or watching himself do it, and if you give him simple and direct verbal cues. He will learn to pedal by feeling the leg motions when someone pushes him, watching others or his own feet, and with the verbal cues "push, feet, push." He will learn to steer through feeling the trunk, arm, and hand motions when you help him turn and give him the verbal cue "turn." As you teach each component, experiment and find the verbal, visual, and tactile cues that work best for your child. These cues will help him understand each activity so that he can try to do each part by himself. Examples of using these cues are included in the Steps and Activity sections of this chapter.

*Use a smooth, level surface and large, open space in the beginning.* Your child will be able to pedal more easily on a smooth surface like linoleum, hardwood floors, or concrete. You want him to slide easily on the surface with minimal strength and effort. If the surface is rough or uneven or has a slight incline, it will require more strength due to the resistance of the surface.

In a large, open space, steering will not be required, so he can pedal further. He will feel successful pedaling longer distances and the endpoint can be wherever he stops. When steering is provided, his pedaling momentum will stop with the turning of the handlebars. This is why it is better to practice in the driveway, garage, or on a gym floor rather than on a sidewalk.

*Practice riding a tricycle with shoes.* Since he will initially have his feet secured to the pedals with footpedal attachments, it will be easier to secure the shoes to the pedals, and it will be more comfortable if he wears shoes. Later, when he rides without his feet secured to the pedals, the rubber soles of his shoes will help him keep his feet on the pedals.

*While he is learning to pedal a tricycle, continue to have fun scooting on the motorcycle ride-on toy, moving fast and scooting for long distances.* Since the width is narrow, he will be using it like a balance bike (see below), so it is good preparation for using a balance bike. I recommend alternating pedaling the trike and scooting on the motorcycle so he can have a variety of experiences with speed, leg movements, and balance while having fun riding outside with his siblings and friends (fig. 14.8).

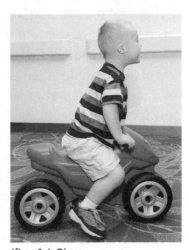

(fig. 14.8)

# After He Masters Pedaling and Steering the Tricycle, What's Next?

Let your child have fun and enjoy riding his tricycle with his siblings and peers. He can also experiment with riding a variety of tricycles, from the red metal tricycles to Big Wheels. With each new type of tricycle, he will need to adjust his pedaling method, either using more strength due to the weight of the tricycle or pedaling with his legs in a new position. Look at the pedals in relation to the seat, and you will see the direction that he needs to pedal, either more downward or more horizontally.

## *No-Brake Bicycles with Training Wheels*

When your child is ready for the next challenge, he can learn to pedal the **no-brake bicycle with training wheels.** In my experience, most children with Down syndrome need this skill to transition to pedaling a regular bicycle with training wheels. This type of bicycle is found in the 10-inch (25-cm) style, and they are frequently referred to as character themed bikes. For example, currently available themes are the Disney Princess bicycle, or Dora, Diego, or CARS bikes.

I recommend the no-brake bicycle because it is easier to learn to pedal than the standard bicycle. It is a fixed-gear or fixed-wheel type, so when the rear wheel turns, the pedals move and turn in the same direction, either forward or backwards. Fixed-wheel bikes do not have coaster brakes. To determine whether a bicycle is a no-brake bike, see whether the pedals move as the rear wheel moves, and look for the "no-brake" label on the frame, just below the seat, toward the rear wheel.

When your child changes from a tricycle to a bicycle with training wheels, he will need to adjust to sitting up higher off the ground and to sitting on a narrower, smaller, and less supportive seat. He will also need to learn a new method of pedaling since the pedals are directly under the seat. He may be fearful about these changes, and, in my experience, this anxiety can make it very difficult to learn to ride with a regular bicycle. If he uses a regular bicycle, he may just rest his feet on the pedals and not move them, or he may move them backwards and put on the coaster brakes.

In contrast, if he uses a no-brake bicycle with training wheels, as the rear wheel moves, the pedals will move, so just keeping his feet on the pedals will teach him the new pedaling movements. (If he learned to keep his feet on the tricycle pedals, with practice, he will generalize this skill to the bicycle. Do not use footpedal attachments because they would be unsafe.) You can stand at his side and push this bicycle and he will feel the leg movements, adjust to pedaling, and may even assist with the pedaling. On some no-brake models, the pedals are on the front wheel, and on other models, the pedals are under the seat. If the pedals are on the front wheel, the pedaling movement will be similar to the tricycle, and he will adapt to pedaling with the new seat position. If the pedals are under the seat, he will learn how to pedal in the vertical direction, which is more similar to a regular bicycle.

When setting your child up on the no-brake bicycle, adjust the seat so his feet are flat on the floor when he sits on the seat. Place both training wheels on the floor and tighten the bolts to maintain them in this position so there is no wobble. He will feel unstable if he feels a wobble and then he will not feel comfortable practicing this skill. (Later, if and when tolerated, you can readjust the training wheels so there is a slight tilt to familiarize him with feeling off balance.) After the seat and training wheels are adjusted, have him sit on the seat and watch his reaction. Some children are uncomfortable on a standard seat and need a larger, more padded seat to tolerate riding.

Before your child actually starts riding his no-brake bike, you will want to make sure he has a comfortable, properly fitted bicycle helmet. Since most children with Down syndrome have smaller head sizes, you may need to try out helmets designed for toddlers or preschoolers, even if your child is over the age of 5. Be sure the helmet fits snugly enough that you cannot wrench it to one side when it is fastened under his chin.

When your child is familiar with sitting on his no-brake bike with training wheels and is ready to learn to pedal, place your hand on the back of his pelvis and the back edge of the seat. Then encourage him to push with his legs to pedal. Since the seat is small, when he pushes downward with his leg, his pelvis will move back on the seat. If you stabilize his pelvis when he is learning to pedal, his pedaling will be more effective, and he will feel more stable. For an alternative way to support his pelvis, you can use the 2-inch (5-cm) wide cotton belt, like you used with the tricycle.

The most difficult part of pedaling will be when his feet are almost vertical. At that point, he will need to learn how to move each ankle up and down to do a full circular revolution. While he is learning to pedal, you will need to steer for him. As his pedaling improves, you can provide intermittent support to keep him moving forward so he enjoys the activity. Once he has mastered pedaling, he can combine pedaling and steering. For safety's sake, you will need to walk next to him while he rides, since this type of bicycle does not have brakes.

## Balance Bicycles

Another option is to use a **balance bicycle**, which is a bike that has two wheels but no pedals (fig. 14.9). The purpose of a balance bike is to teach children how to balance and steer on a two-wheeler without the distraction of hav-

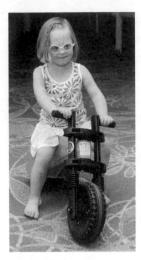

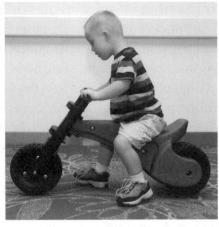

left (fig. 14.9); above (fig. 14.10)

ing to pedal. Your child may love using the leg scooting pattern, so he can use it to scoot on a balance bicycle.

To function properly, the balance bike seat (saddle) needs to be low enough that the child can walk the bicycle while sitting on the seat with both feet flat on the ground (fig. 14.10). The rider starts off walking the bike, then learns scooting, propelling himself forward by pushing off the ground with his feet. With practice, he learns to balance and he increases his speed, progressing to running, gliding, and coasting. Riders use their feet to stop and to control the speed.

Most balance bicycles are made of metal and wood. They are available in a wide range of sizes, starting with toddler size. They are lightweight, small, and easy to maneuver. Examples of brands of balance bikes are: Strider™ (fig. 14.11), YBIKE (three sizes—Pewi Ride On Toy, Original for 2- to 4-year-olds (figs. 14.9-14.10), and Extreme Balance Bike), Kiddimoto, KaZAM™ (fig. 14.12), Wishbone, LIKEaBIKE®, Smart Balance Bikes by Smart Gear, ZUM balance bike, Glide Bike (Ezee Glider, etc.), and Skuut. Go to www.pedalfreebikes.com for more information.

An alternative is to use a regular bike and remove the training wheels, pedals, and chain. You could also just unscrew the pedals (left pedal unscrews clockwise) and remove them.

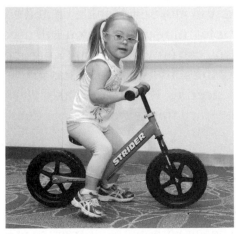

(fig. 14.11)

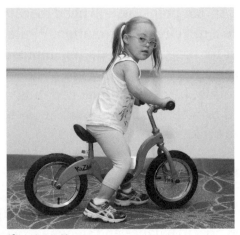

(fig. 14.12)

Using a bicycle without pedals or a balance bicycle will familiarize your child with the higher seat position (compared to a tricycle), and he can practice steering and balancing. You will need to adjust the seat so his feet are flat on the ground when he sits on it. If your child enjoys scooting and is not interested in pedaling a bicycle with training wheels, this is a good intermediate activity. If your child is uncomfortable with the bike tilting, you can add training wheels until he is ready to practice balancing.

## Regular Bicycles with Training Wheels

After your child is comfortable with the seat size, height, and steering of a no-brake bicycle, you can test whether he is ready to learn to pedal a bicycle with training wheels. The big challenge will be learning to pedal. That's because the wheels on a standard bicycle are different than the fixed wheels on a tricycle or no-brake bike. Standard bikes have freewheels, meaning you can coast on the bike, holding the pedals stationary while the wheels are moving. So, if he is pushed, he will not learn to pedal. If he is fearful, he will move his legs backwards and brake.

Before you start your child on a standard bike, adjust the bicycle seat and training wheels just like you did with the no-brake bicycle. To teach him to pedal in the very beginning, you may need to have three people to help him be successful. One person will stand on his right side, another person on his left side, and each person will move the foot on that side to show him how to pedal. The third person will stand in front of him and manage the steering. With this support, he will feel how to pedal, and you can prevent his braking motion. He will also feel more secure with the support, so will not freeze and automatically put on the brakes.

When he is comfortable with pedaling forward with support, you can teach him to keep his feet on the pedals and move his legs and ankles to generate the circular motion. If helpful, you can support the back of his pelvis or use a belt, as discussed with the no-brake bicycle. Until he masters steering, give him intermittent support to keep him moving forward and manage the steering for him.

When he can pedal and steer, the final challenge will be learning to stop. He will need to learn to use the coaster brakes or hand brakes. To use the coaster brakes, he will need to practice the pedal position, timing, and force needed to effectively stop. If he has hand brakes, for safety purposes, it is frequently advised that beginners have the front wheel hand brake disconnected, and only use the rear wheel hand brake. A front wheel hand brake can be dangerous and may cause the rider to take a fall over the handlebars. The hand brake to the rear wheel can be adjusted for gradual slowing to prevent a sudden stop. As the rider gets the feel of the brake, it can be gradually tightened. The front wheel hand brake can be added later when the rider is comfortable with the rear wheel brake function.

Once your child can ride a bicycle with training wheels, he will have fun riding with other children and going on family rides. He will naturally improve his skills by riding longer distances, in a variety of settings, and on various surfaces. He will experiment with going faster, and then will learn to stop more efficiently. His strength and endurance will increase. The more he practices and gains experience now, the more competent he will be later when he learns to ride a bicycle without training wheels.

For family rides or long distance bike rides, you can use bicycle trailers (Weehoo iGo) or tandem bicycles.

# Riding without Training Wheels

When your child is ready to ride a bicycle without training wheels, the challenge will be learning to balance. There are many methods to teach riding a bicycle without training wheels, so you will need to find the best method for your child and customize it to him. In my experience, parents have been successful using a wide variety of methods. If you want ideas, check the Internet—e.g., look at www.ibike.org (under Education). I also recommend the iCan Bike program (formerly called Lose the Training Wheels program), which is available for children eight years and older. For information on the iCan Bike program, contact info@icanshine.org (The 501(c)(3) organization is iCan Shine, and the bike program is called iCan Bike.)

After your child has learned to ride the bicycle and pedal, steer, and brake effectively, the next challenge is to learn to ride safely in a variety of settings, with others. This will be a process and will take time, experience, and lots of practice. There are many details to think about, pay attention to, coordinate, and manage. Some of the details to consider are:

1. Stopping quickly, and then resuming pedaling
2. Moving around other people on the bike path, when they have stopped riding, or if they are riding slower, or if other bikers are passing you
3. Moving within the bike path space, when it is straight or curved, or when another biker is riding in the opposite direction
4. Keeping focused on looking forward **at all times**
5. Having judgment to act and react safely, and do it quickly without delay
6. Consistency in safe behavior, and willingness to follow directions and be obedient

## An iCan Bike Success Story

Despite his parents' occasional attempts to get Connor excited about biking, for many years efforts were unsuccessful to help Connor learn to ride. He liked the idea of riding, but he did not enjoy the uncontrollable side-to-side jerking motion of the training wheels. Trying to learn to ride a bike was scary for Connor and frustrating for his parents. Connor's father, Brian, said, "… We simply couldn't gain his willingness and cooperation often enough or long enough to achieve the necessary minor incremental improvements. As a result, he never enjoyed it enough to see the benefit and rewards that would prompt him to want to practice more. It was unsettling for him, not fun for any of us, and so we made no progress through his elementary and middle school years."

As Connor entered high school, his parents had almost accepted that biking was something he might never do. Connor's fabulous physical therapy consultant, Patricia Winders, urged his parents to keep trying, though. She knew of the iCan Bike camp in Highlands Ranch, Colorado, and reminded the family when the camp came around again in June 2010. Connor's family decided to give it a shot … a few weeks shy of Connor's 16th birthday.

Sherrill, Connor's mom, shared: "We were astonished that in five days with your incredible program, Connor learned—with relative ease—how to balance and pedal a two-wheel bike! It still was a difficult, rather than enjoyable, process for him to coordinate all aspects of bike riding, but the most difficult part of the learning curve was achieved through [the iCan Bike] program…."

After the camp, however, Connor announced to the family that he was "all done with bike riding." Brian and Sherrill knew that, as with many things, if they could just push Connor to where riding became less difficult, he would really enjoy

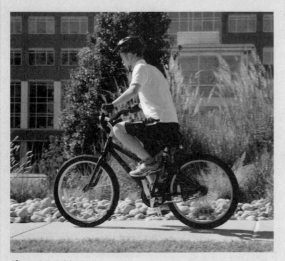

it and it would be a great, fun family activity. After bike camp, they practiced in their cul-de-sac, then moved on to their local high school track, where Connor could just concentrate on building up confidence, speed, and endurance. Initially he would stop every 100 feet, and only ride a lap or two before he tired. Then he built up to 1-2 laps without stopping.

The practice finally paid off. Within a few months the

(fig. 14.13)

family was out riding on flat, wide trails. They knew it was all worth it when they heard Connor exclaim "wheeeeeee!!!" as he furiously pedaled with the wind at his back to race his sister a mile around Harper Lake in Louisville! Today Connor is routinely riding up to 7-8 miles, loves to ride, and asks for more distance and variety of terrain (fig. 14.13). Brian says that Connor really shows a quiet but deep satisfaction and pride when they finish a ride.

According to Connor, "I like being free to go fast and feel the air blasting me. It is fun to be in control and go where I want to go. I sometimes feel like a superhero zooming around. It's a good mix of scary and fun, exciting. The wind keeps me feeling cool (I don't like hot weather too much), just like pool water does when I swim."

For Connor's sister, Karli, biking with him has been fun, as it is a "great equalizer." Brian says of his children: "Biking is a great way to emphasize their alikeness and shared interests and activities, rather than differences. It's wonderful the way they support and encourage each other." Prior to Connor's biking achievement, the Long family loved to swim and hike together. Biking gave them a new family activity and gave Connor another recreational choice to maintain a healthy, active lifestyle throughout his lifetime.

Brian reports, "When Connor took off around the lake and I could hear him yell out 'wheeeeeeee!' it was a very moving moment because of the utter joy he very obviously was feeling. I will never forget that moment or that sweet, wonderful sound. I hope and trust many other parents will experience such a moment for themselves! So we Longs wholeheartedly encourage people to try it! And don't forget to Shine On!!!"

(Excerpted from *iCan Bike Rider of the Month—January 2013,* written by Lisa Ruby, Executive Director of iCan Shine.)

7. Motor planning and control to manage speed, reaction time (to turn or stop), balance, and braking
8. Ability to ride with control even when there are distractions
9. Motivation, strength, and endurance to keep pedaling on level surfaces, uneven surfaces, up hill and down hill

You can assess what he knows and is ready to learn, and based on this, you will select the best settings to use for practice (fig. 14.14). The key will be to keep it fun and do it often, especially with his siblings and friends.

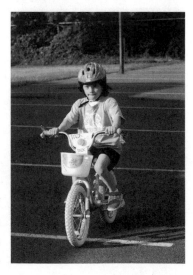

(fig. 14.14)

## Resources for Larger Training Wheels or Adaptive Tricycles

If your child is not ready to ride a bike without training wheels, but traditional training wheels are too small or weak for his size, consider using Fat Wheels training wheels with your bicycle (www.fatwheels.com).

Some children need more specialized equipment to be successful with riding a bicycle, and do best with an adaptive tricycle. This equipment has three wheels, a seating system with a larger seat and a back support, seat belt, larger pedals with foot straps, and a front pulley system that attaches to the pedals and maintains a level pedal position for the child throughout the pedaling cycle. He can use the conventional handlebars and a front hand brake. If needed, additional accessories such as a chest strap, special handlebars, or a steering bar can be added. With the support that this equipment provides, the child feels very stable so he is comfortable with moving his legs to pedal. After he learns to pedal, he learns to steer. For information on adaptive tricycles, see the following resources:

- Rifton Adaptive Tricycle (www.rifton.com)
- Freedom Concepts Mobility Device (www.freedomconcepts.com)
- AmTryke therapeutic tricycles (www.amtrykestore.org) or (www.ambucs.org)

## Temperament

Your child will show you when he is interested in learning to ride a tricycle. Learning to ride a tricycle will depend on his *motivation* more than his temperament. When he is motivated, he will be persistent in practicing it, whether he is an observer or motor driven. He may become motivated because he is around other children who ride a lot, or because his family likes to bike ride. Once he has watched others ride, when he sees a tricycle, he will climb on and try to do it. When he can pedal, he will want to do it by himself and will push your hand away when you try to help him steer, or if you intervene. He will want to be independent, riding his tricycle with others.

When your child needs full support at the beginning, watch his reaction to the footpedal attachments. He will tolerate them best if you secure them quickly and immediately push him so his focus is on the experience of riding the tricycle. When he is done, immediately unfasten the Velcro straps so he can climb off. He will learn the leg pedaling movements best if he uses the footpedal attachments, so be proactive to help him learn to tolerate them until he does not need them any more.

If your child is an **observer,** he will generally be patient and tolerant when sitting on a ride-on toy, riding a tricycle with support, and riding down an inclined surface. Once he learns to scoot with his legs, he will want to use scooting whether he is on the ride-on toy or tricycle. When he learns to ride the tricycle, he will ride at an average, safe speed so he can feel in control.

If your child is **motor driven,** he will want to move fast so may be impatient and impulsive when first learning to scoot on the ride-on toy or to pedal the tricycle. If he cannot make the ride-on toy or tricycle move, he will quit and climb off, but he will be happy when he figures out how to scoot. When he is ready to practice pedaling with full support, you will need to be strategic to help him tolerate using the footpedal attachments. He may react strongly to having his feet secured to the pedals. If he does, then prepare in advance for an ideal setup plan and ride, and make the experience exciting and fun. If you set him up and then push him fast, he will enjoy the ride. This experience will distract him from thinking about his feet. When he shows that he is done riding, quickly unfasten the Velcro straps so he does not feel stuck or confined. If you are proactive and responsive to his reaction, he will learn to tolerate them and use them to learn to pedal.

As your child progresses with pedaling, he will like riding down the inclined surface, if he keeps moving. When he learns to ride the tricycle, he will ride at a fast speed, so you will need to make sure he can steer safely and effectively.

## ACTIVITY #1: Scooting on a Ride-on Toy

As described on page 440, select the ride-on toy that fits him and has the features needed for success.

1. Hold the ride-on toy to stabilize it and encourage your child to climb on. Have him stand beside the seat, facing the handlebars, with both hands on the handlebars. If needed, help him lift his foot over the seat.
2. See if he initiates moving himself backwards. Let him have fun playing on this toy so he is familiar with it and likes it.
3. When he is ready to try a new game, encourage him to move forward for 3 to 5 feet to a motivator. Say "1, 2, 3, go" or practice with a sibling or friend. See if he initiates any movement forward. If he is unable to move forward, help him using these methods:
   a. Hold his lower legs and bend his knees, pushing his feet into the floor so he weight shifts from his heels to his toes, and moves the ride-on toy forward. You can move his legs together or one at a time, to demonstrate the scooting motion.
   b. Place your hand horizontally across his lower back and gently press forward to support his trunk up straight and the top of his pelvis tilted forward.

4. When he moves forward any distance, with or without your help, praise him and clap for him so he learns the game.

5. Continue to practice until he can move forward 3 to 5 feet without support. When he scoots, he will either move both legs together or move one at a time. Either method is acceptable.

6. When he can move forward for 5 feet, increase the distance when he is ready.

7. Continue to practice until he rides the toy spontaneously to play.

8. When he is done and wants to climb off the ride-on toy, hold it still and encourage him to climb off. Have him stand up, hold the handlebars, and then lift his leg over the seat. Assist him with lifting his leg if needed.

9. When he has mastered scooting forward on a ride-on toy, you can try using the motorcycle, car, van, truck, and cozy coupe models. Let him play with the car so he is familiar with it and likes it, and then help him use the scooting method when he is motivated to go for a ride.

##  ACTIVITY #2: Riding a Tricycle

Select the tricycle that fits him and has the features needed for success (type of seat and height, base, handlebars, weight, diameter of front wheel) as discussed in the tricycle sections of this chapter.

##  Activity #2A: Steering and Pedaling a Tricycle while Being Pushed

1. Hold the tricycle to stabilize it and encourage him to climb on. Have him stand beside the seat, facing the handlebars, with both hands on the handlebars. If needed, help him lift his foot over the seat.

2. Set him up with his feet secured to the pedals using footpedal attachments. Use grip liner on the seat and a belt if needed (see page 447). Observe his trunk and pelvis and reposition him if needed so his trunk and pelvis are up straight.

3. Have him hold the handlebars.

4. Push him (with the push handle of the tricycle) and check his knees to make sure they both remain bent as the pedals go around. If not, use grip liner on the seat and move his pelvis forward on the seat so his knees bend when pushed.

5. Take your child for a walk while he consistently holds the handlebars. Make it fun by having him ride with his siblings, playing chase games, and varying the speed. If he is playful with the

steering, let him do what he wants as long as his knees continue to bend while being pushed. You manage the steering so his only focus is the pedaling.

6. If he stiffens one or both knees while you are pushing him, try to figure out why.
    a. Is it because the handlebars are turned, causing that knee to go straight or did the knee straightening cause the handlebars to turn? (For example, if the handlebars are turned to the right, his left knee will straighten.)
    b. Is he stiffening his knee to resist the activity?
    c. If you know the reason for the stiffening, then you can provide the right support.
    d. If he is resisting the activity, then either stop or find a way to motivate him to continue riding.
    e. If the stiffening is due to difficulty coordinating the legs or beginning steering, then you can assist his knee or reposition the handlebars.
    f. If he stiffens one knee, it is usually the same one. The best strategy is to walk beside him (while pushing the handle behind him) and place your fingers under his knee to unlock it. If the knee locking persists, limit the distance practiced because you want to have him feel the smooth leg pedaling rhythm, not the jerky rhythm experienced when one leg keeps stiffening.

7. As you are pushing him, watch the posture of his trunk and pelvis. If his pelvis slides forward on the seat, use grip liner to stabilize it in the right place on the seat. When his pelvis slides forward, the top of his pelvis usually tilts back and then his trunk will be rounded. He will not be able to pedal effectively with this unstable trunk posture. You want him to learn to pedal with his trunk and pelvis up straight, so reposition him as needed when you see this slumped posture.

8. Practice as long as he is interested and stop when he resists or communicates that he is done. With practice, he will increase the distance and length of time he participates in this activity.

## Activity #2B: Riding a Tricycle Down an Incline

1. When your child is familiar with being pushed on a trike and likes it, look for a small incline (1-2 degrees) such as a very gently sloping driveway or sidewalk. Try to set him up in a big space so steering is not needed. If steering is needed for his safety, then you steer for him.

2. Set him up at the top of the incline and let him ride down it. Stand behind him, holding the push handle for safety, since his feet will be attached to the pedals. Use a verbal cue like "1, 2, 3, go" or say "push." Then push him to initiate the forward movement and give intermittent support to keep the momentum going.

3. When he reaches the bottom of the incline, clap for him and praise him.

4. If he likes it, then playfully push him back to the top and let him ride down again. Repeat as tolerated. If he enjoys this game, continue to practice riding down the incline until he uses his legs and feet to pedal the distance.

## Activity#2C: Increasing Distance Pedaled Independently

When your child is interested in pushing his feet to pedal, begin practicing for short distances on a smooth surface. As you are pushing him from behind, feel for when he initiates pedaling and stop pushing when he does it. Keep your hands on the handle and when he stops pedaling, resume pushing so he continues to move rather than stopping and starting. When he initiates pedaling often and can pedal for 3-4 foot (90 cm to 1.2-meter) distances, then practice the following pedaling games.

The purpose of these games is to practice pedaling for a specific distance, beginning with 3-5 feet and increasing as tolerated. Your child is set-up to see the endpoint and continue pedaling the distance once you start the forward movement. The games need to be done in a large space so steering is not needed (since steering will stop his pedaling momentum). It is better for you (or the endpoint) to move to where he is heading than to steer and have him stop pedaling.

### Pedaling Game #1

1. To start, setup a motivating endpoint such as a sibling sitting on a chair. Place your child about 3 feet (1 meter) away, and stand behind him.

2. Give a verbal cue such as "1, 2, 3, go!" or "push" and then push him to begin the forward movement.

3. Have him continue to pedal to his sibling. Provide intermittent support if needed for him to pedal the whole distance. As he is pedaling, say "push" and sign "tricycle" so he stays focused on what to do.

4. When he reaches his sibling, clap for him and praise him so he is excited and knows you are proud of him. Through this experience,

he learns the game and then knows what to do when you set him up to play it again.

### Pedaling Game #2

Try this game when your child can do the first game.

1. Sit on a chair and place him in front of you on the tricycle.
2. Then say "bye, bye" and wave, and push him backwards about 3-5 feet (1-1.5 meters). He may continue pedaling backwards to go further (and laugh).
3. Then give the verbal cues ("1, 2, 3, go" or "come") and lean forward to push his leading foot (and say "push" or "go feet go"). After you start the movement forward, sit on the chair and continue to give the verbal cue "push" while moving your hands to sign tricycle (which gives the visual cue of the leg pedaling movements).
4. Continue to give the cueing until he moves the distance to you. If he stops or becomes stuck (one knee locked straight), give the support needed so he keeps moving to the endpoint. Let him crash into the endpoint if he likes this action. Clap, cheer for him, do high fives, and keep the activity fun.
5. If he likes the game and is participating, do it again. When tolerated, increase the distance. You can sign "more" and see if he responds by signing or saying "more" or "all done."
6. After each repetition, see if he needs a break. If he does, you can take him for a fast ride, which will help him laugh, recover, and feel the ease of the leg pedaling movements. This should refresh him, and then he may want to play the game again.

Through these pedaling games, you can work toward increasing the distance to 15-20 feet (4.5-6 meters). Your child will gain confidence in his ability to pedal and will persevere with moving longer distances to move to the endpoint. He will see the distance to pedal and know that he can do it. Continue to practice until pedaling is easy. Provide intermittent support so he enjoys the ride.

With practice, he will start initiating the forward movement on his own. Practice until he can pedal automatically and easily (using the footpedal attachments) and he can keep the rhythm going without looking down at his feet.

## 🏃 Activity #2D: Combining Pedaling with Steering

When your child has mastered pedaling, then he can practice steering while continuing to use the footpedal attachments. It is best to practice steering when it is functional for him.

1. When he pedals into an obstacle or furniture and is stuck, show him how to steer so he can move again. Have him hold the handlebars firmly, while you hold his forearms (near his wrists).
2. Say "turn" and turn his arms and trunk in a big movement so he feels the fullness of the turning movement. If you exaggerate the movement and make it dramatic, then he will better understand how to steer.
3. If his hands fall off the handlebars, see if he holds more firmly on the next practice. If he continues to let go, then put your hands over his to show him how to grip firmly.
4. Follow him as he pedals and every time he is stuck, practice turning. Over time, he will learn to initiate steering when stuck, and eventually anticipate when he needs to steer as he is approaching an obstacle.
5. When he can pedal and steer for long distances and has mastered both skills, test whether he can do both skills when you remove the footpedal attachments. He will need to learn to push his feet against the pedals and maintain them while pedaling and steering.
6. First, test moving straight, since it is easier to keep the feet on the pedals while moving straight. Second, see if he can keep his feet on the pedals when turning. Put the footpedal attachments back on if he can't do it or becomes frustrated. The goal is for him to be successful, so determine when he is ready to ride without the footpedal attachments.
7. He is now fully independent with riding the tricycle, so give him lots of opportunities to do this activity with siblings and friends.

## 🏃 MOTOR MILESTONE CHECKLIST

He climbs on a ride-on toy/tricycle:
- ❏ while you hold it
- ❏ without support

He climbs off a ride-on toy/tricycle:
- ❏ while you hold it
- ❏ without support

- ❏ He scoots backwards on a ride-on toy for 10 feet (3 meters)

- ❏ He scoots forward on a ride-on toy for 15 feet (4.5 meters)

- ❏ He steers while scooting forward on a ride-on toy for 15 feet (4.5 meters) (optional)

- ❏ He scoots forward using a motorcycle, car, van, truck, or coupe model

- ❏ He enjoys being pushed on a tricycle with footpedal attachments for 100 feet (30 meters)

- ❏ He rides the tricycle down a small incline (1-2 degrees) with intermittent support to assist with pedaling (and steering is managed if needed), using footpedal attachments

- ❏ He pedals the tricycle on a smooth surface, pedaling by himself for 3-5 feet (.9-1.5 meters) (and steering is not needed), using footpedal attachments

- ❏ He pedals the tricycle on a smooth surface for 15 feet (4.5 meters) (and steering is not needed), using footpedal attachments

- ❏ Pedaling the tricycle is established on level surfaces, and he initiates steering intermittently, using footpedal attachments

- ❏ He pedals and steers the tricycle for at least 15 feet (4.5 meters) on level surfaces, using footpedal attachments

(continued on next page)

❑ He pedals and steers the tricycle for 100 feet (30 meters) without footpedal attachments

❑ He pedals and steers a variety of tricycles (metal, big wheels)

❑ He scoots on a balance bicycle and steers (with you controlling his balance or using training wheels) or he scoots on a regular bike without the pedals with training wheels

❑ He scoots, steers, and balances himself using a balance bicycle (if interested in this activity) or on a regular bike without pedals and training wheels

❑ He pedals and steers a no-brake bicycle with training wheels

❑ He pedals and steers a bicycle with training wheels, and uses the brakes effectively

❑ He rides a bicycle without training wheels and is competent with pedaling, steering, and braking

# 15

# Balance Beam Skills

## Introduction

When your child first learns to walk, she will want to walk all over and explore. She will like walking long distances, move fast and slow, and walk on a variety of surfaces. Later, after she has had her fill of walking everywhere in big open spaces, she may show an interest in walking along the curb or walking on a railroad tie at the park. If she sees a line on the floor, she may try to walk on it. This is the perfect time to practice balance beam skills since she is showing you her interest in walking within a narrow boundary.

For the purposes of this chapter, a balance beam will be defined as a board that is ½ to 1½ inches high (about 1.25 to 3.8 cm), approximately 6 feet (2 meters) long, and a variety of widths. I like to use boards that are the following widths: approximately 10 inches, 7.5 inches, 5.5 inches, and 4.5 inches (25, 19, 14, and 11 cm). (For examples of what lumber to use for balance beams, see the box on making a balance beam, page 477.) The goal will be for your child to walk across a 4.5-inch (11 cm) wide balance beam placed on the floor without hand support, with one foot forward of the other.

Walking on a balance beam will help to refine your child's early walking pattern. As a new walker, she will use a wide base, with her hips externally rotated. This causes her knees and feet to turn out, and she will take weight on the inside borders of her feet. By practicing walking on a balance beam, she will learn to walk with her legs and feet in a new position. She will learn to step with a narrower base with her knees and feet pointing straight ahead to walk within the boundary. She will also learn to balance herself to stand and step on the board. With the narrower balance beams, she will weight shift through the centers of her feet.

At first, your child will need to understand the balance beam game, which is to step within the boundary (width) of the board. She will need to look down and constantly pay attention in order to keep her feet on the board as she steps from one end to the other. With each step, she will need to figure out how to balance herself with her feet placed so close together. To achieve the goal of this skill area, she will practice walking across progressively smaller width balance beams (approximately 10, 7.5, 5.5, and 4.5 inches). She will hold your index finger and balance herself with this support until she learns how to move her legs and feet to walk on the balance beams. When she can walk within the width of the balance beam, she can practice without support and develop the balance needed to walk with the narrower base.

Your child will figure out two methods to walk across the balance beams, depending on the width of the board. For the 5.5- to 10-inch (14- to 25-cm) wide balance beams, her first method will be to step by placing one foot beside the other (fig. 15.1). She will take small steps, with her feet side by side, to manage her balance. The narrower the width of the balance beam, the closer together her feet will be. When she is comfortable with walking across the width of a balance beam, she will initiate the second method, which is placing one foot forward of the other (fig. 15.2). She will be ready to advance to the next narrower width board when she easily walks across a board with one foot forward of the other using a longer step length.

For the 4.5-inch (11-cm) wide balance beam, she will not be able to place her feet side by side, since they will not fit, so she will be required to place one foot in front of the other (fig. 15.3). As she is challenged with each narrower width balance beam, she may try her own unique methods to walk across it. She may turn her body sideways and step sideways across

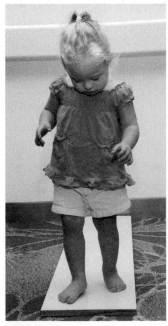

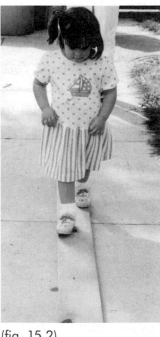

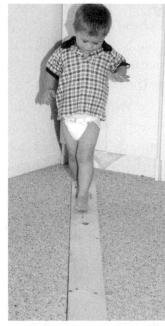

(fig. 15.1)     (fig. 15.2)     (fig. 15.3)

the balance beam. Or, she may step with one foot on the balance beam and one foot on the floor. You will need to help her learn to step forward with both feet on the board.

Using boards that are ½ to 1½ inches (1.25 to 4 cm) high as balance beams will help your child learn to pay attention to walking within a boundary. She will feel the edge of the board and will feel a consequence when she steps off the board with one foot. This will get her attention but not scare her. When balance beams are raised 6 inches (15 cm) or more off the floor, children become frightened of falling off and want more support than they would normally need for that width. It is better to place the balance beam on the floor so she notices the boundary but is not frightened by the height of the board.

---

### Steps in Learning to Walk Across a Balance Beam

To achieve the goal of this skill area, your child will need to practice the following steps:

1. Walk across a 10-inch (25-cm) wide balance beam with support; without support
2. Walk across a 7.5-inch (19-cm) wide balance beam with support; without support
3. Walk across a 5.5-inch (14-cm) wide balance beam with support; without support
4. Walk across a 4.5-inch (11-cm) wide balance beam with support; without support

---

## Components

The components to focus on are:

1. positioning the legs with the knees and feet pointing straight ahead (neutral hip rotation)
2. standing with a narrow base to fit within the width of the balance beam
3. attentiveness to the width of the balance beam, and perseverance and motivation to figure out how to step across the length of it with balance and control
4. ability to use the beginner's method (feet side by side, short steps) and then progress to using the advanced method (one foot forward of the other)
5. leg and ankle strength in combination with balance reactions in the arms, trunk, and legs to walk across the balance beam slowly with control

## *Tendencies*

The tendencies are:

1. to position the hips in external rotation (knees and feet turned outward), with flat arches and weight bearing on the inside borders of the feet
2. to stand with one foot on the balance beam and one foot on the floor because she is uncomfortable using a narrower base
3. to refuse to practice, to lack attention, to move too fast, or to quit because she is not interested or motivated to figure out how to do the skill
4. to persist with using the beginner's method, or require hand support due to inadequate balance and strength

## *Setup for Learning*

### Walking across the 10-inch Wide Balance Beam

Your child will easily adjust to walking across a 10-inch (25-cm) wide balance beam. You want this first size to be easy so you can use this time to teach her the new game of walking across balance beams. You will teach her to pay attention to the board and step within the boundary. She can hold your index fingers for support when practicing the skill. You will also show her how to step on and off the board. When she is ready, you will encourage her to do it by herself.

When she walks across the balance beam without support, she will be more attentive to where her feet are placed on the board. At first, she will position her feet side by side, take small steps, and step with full-sole weight bearing. She will learn to turn her hips so her feet and knees point straight ahead because she will not like the feeling of her toes hanging over the edge of the board. With practice, she will take longer steps, use a narrower base, and consistently step within the boundary. When she is confident with her performance, set her up with the 7.5-inch (19-cm) wide balance beam.

### Walking across 7.5- and 5.5-inch Wide Balance Beams

Once your child knows how to walk across a balance beam, challenge her by using narrower widths, beginning with 7.5" (19 cm) and then 5.5" (14 cm). She will need hand support to adjust to the narrower boundary (fig. 15.4). She will need to learn how to move her legs and feet to consistently walk within the smaller space. When she can do this, then she can practice without hand support.

When she is walking across the balance beams by herself, she will develop the balance to walk with a very narrow base, with the inside borders of her feet very close together. With the 7.5-inch (19-cm) wide balance beam, the inside borders of her feet will be approximately 2 to 3 inches (5 to 7.5 cm) apart. With the 5.5-inch (14-cm) balance beam, the inside borders of her feet will be about 1 inch (2.5 cm) apart. The inside borders of her feet may even touch as she walks from one end to the other, with her feet side by side.

As her balance improves, she will initiate the advanced method of stepping with one foot forward of the other. When she consistently uses this method to step quickly and easily across the length of the balance beam, she is ready to use the next narrower size. When she can walk across the 5.5-inch wide balance beam by herself, she will be ready to use the 4.5-inch (11-cm) wide balance beam.

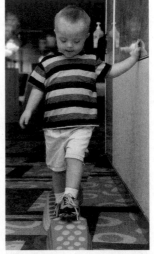

### Walking across the 4.5-inch Wide Balance Beam

(fig. 15.4)

By now, your child has learned how to balance herself to step across a balance beam. She has also demonstrated the motivation and perseverance to accept the challenge and figure out how to do it. With this level of confidence, competence, and drive, she will be ready for the next challenge of walking across the 4.5-inch (11-cm) wide balance beam. With this width, she will need to use the advanced method from the beginning, since the width of the board is too narrow to place her feet side by side. She will need hand support and a lot of practice to learn how to do it by herself. If she shows the attention and motivation to practice this skill, continue to encourage it. However, if she reaches the point where she is no longer interested and prefers to step off the board, then discontinue working on this width board.

To walk across the 4.5-inch wide balance beam by herself, she will need to:

1. Step up on the board, and balance herself in standing with one foot forward of the other (in this example, her right foot is forward of the left)
2. With her legs in this position, she needs to lean her body over her right foot and hold the position
3. While maintaining her balance in #2, she needs to lift and place her left foot in front of her right foot
4. Then she needs to regain her balance in standing with her left foot in front of her right foot
5. With her legs in this position, she needs to lean her body over her left foot and hold the position
6. While maintaining her balance in #5, she needs to lift and place her right foot in front of her left foot
7. Then she needs to regain her balance in standing with her right foot in front of her left foot

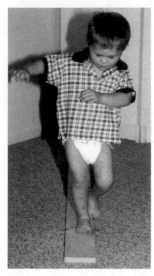

(fig. 15.5)

8. She will continue steps 2-7 until she walks the length of the balance beam.

This skill will challenge your child's balance and her ability to keep her attention focused on the activity until it is completed (fig. 15.5). She will need to move slowly and with control. She will need to concentrate and pay attention as she takes each step, figuring out how to maintain her balance with each movement. If she becomes distracted, she will lose her balance. If she is no longer motivated to do it, she will quit and step off. You will need to see when and if she is ready to practice this activity. She will need a lot of practice and motivation to accomplish it.

## Guidelines

*Setup the balance beam so your child feels stable on it and is comfortable using it.* Your child will be focusing on balancing herself, so she will need to feel safe enough to practice. She will feel more comfortable using a balance beam placed on the floor rather than raised off the floor. Place it on a firm surface such as a linoleum, hardwood floor, or an unpadded carpet. On a padded carpet, it will rock from side to side with each step, and she will feel unstable on it. The balance beam will need to be stabilized to prevent sliding in any direction or any wobbling movement. The easiest way to stabilize it is to have an adult stand on it. Always test the balance beam setup before you have your child practice on it. Make sure it does not tilt because the board is warped or because the underlying surface is uneven. If it is warped or tilts as she steps, she will not demonstrate her best performance because she will feel unstable.

*Provide hand support, and when she is ready, let go and encourage her to do it by herself.* Hand support can be provided in two ways:

1. She can hold your index finger and balance herself.
2. She can prop her hand against the wall (fig. 15.6).

Holding your finger will provide more support because she can use her arm strength to assist with balancing herself in any direction. When she props her hand against the wall, she can only lean in that direction to steady herself.

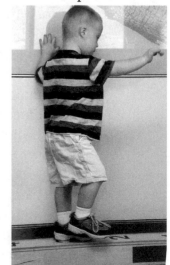

(fig. 15.6)

When she holds your finger, position her arm in front of her chest with her hand at or below shoulder level. She needs to be centered on the board, so make sure you do not lean her to one side with your hand support. It is best if you walk at her side, facing her, so you can be attentive to this.

To prepare your child to walk across the balance beam by herself, begin by having her hold your finger and, later, prop her hand against the wall for support. When she can walk across the balance beam with her hand against the wall, you can reposition the balance beam so half is next to a wall (or furniture) and the other half is in open space with nothing for her to prop against. When she begins to walk across the balance beam without support, position yourself in front of her and encourage her to take steps to you. You can start with taking 2 or 3 steps, then walking across half of the balance beam, and then progressing to walking across the full length of the balance beam.

It will be a challenge for your child to walk across the balance beams without hand support. She will feel stable with support and will prefer to hold on. As soon as possible, you will need to experiment with letting go. Once she does not have support, she will really work on figuring out how to balance herself with her feet closer together. When she learns how to balance herself using a narrower base, her walking pattern will improve.

*Provide verbal and visual cues and motivate her to walk across the balance beam.* Set her up so she knows what to do and is motivated to do it. Give her simple verbal instructions like "march" or "walk." If she walks with one foot on the board and one on the ground, tell her "two feet on the board." Give her the visual cues by having her watch or follow her sibling doing it. She will enjoy playing this game and will like taking turns with others. Help her focus her attention on your feet by exaggerating your leg movements, by marching or stomping your feet as you walk across. She may also like counting each step she takes. If needed, place a motivator at the end of the balance board at eye level. If she is practicing walking across the balance beam without hand support, you can sit at the end of the balance beam and have her walk to you.

*Test whether she walks across the balance beam better when barefoot or with foot support and shoes.* If your child uses foot support with shoes, test her ability to walk across the balance beam with this support or when barefoot. If she does not use foot support, then practice barefoot so she can freely move her feet to effectively balance herself when walking across the balance beam. If she is barefoot, she will also learn to turn her feet to point straight because she will not like how it feels with her feet or toes on the outer edges of the board.

*Practice this skill when your child is ready.* If your child is reluctant to walk across the balance beam, let her practice standing on it while you entertain her. You can blow bubbles or sing songs while she practices balancing herself with her feet closer together and pointing straight ahead. She can also practice stepping on and off it. Have her approach the balance beam from the side (board perpendicular to her) and help her step up and down. As she becomes more comfortable playing on the balance beam, she will initiate trying to step across the length of it.

*Leave the balance beam on the floor in the middle of the family room or play area so she can explore it on her own.* With the balance beam in her play space, she will self-initiate walking on it and stepping up and down. She will watch her siblings use it, and she will imitate them. During her playtime, she will be able to choose when and how she wants to play with it.

*When practicing walking across the balance beam without hand support, begin with a couple of steps and increase the distance as tolerated.* At first, she will take small steps, but her steps will get bigger when she is familiar with the activity. After she takes a couple of steps without support, try walking across half the length of the balance beam. When she is ready, encourage her to walk across the full length of the balance beam.

*Practice with a variety of balance beam setups in your community.* Once your child is familiar with and enjoys walking across balance beams, find new ways to practice these activities. You can walk across railroad ties or other wooden borders at playgrounds, parks, and gardens. Since these examples will be raised off the ground, your child may need additional support to learn to walk on them until she is used to the added dimension of the height. She will enjoy playing Follow the Leader with other kids.

Carson enjoyed another way to play with her 10-inch wide balance beam. She loved walking across it and quickly learned to do it without hand support. So we setup the balance beam as an incline. We placed one end on a stair (approximately 8 inches or 20 cm high), and we stabilized the other end. Then Carson would walk up and down the inclined balance beam. By practicing this skill, she combined two post walking skills, walking up and down inclines and across a balance beam.

## Temperament

If your child is an **observer,** she will like doing balance beam activities when she is familiar with them. She will move slowly and carefully and focus on staying within the boundary. She will prefer hand support, so you will need to encourage her to let go and do it by herself. She will need to be motivated by someone or by a favorite toy to take on the challenge of walking across the balance beam without hand support. Once she feels comfortable using the balance beam, she may practice it for fun. Your jobs will be to:

> 1. Assist her until she learns the leg and foot motions and balance needed to walk across the balance beams by herself;

2. Leave the balance beam setup so she can practice it when she wants to.

If your child is **motor driven,** she will want to use her usual fast speed to practice balance beam activities. She will probably learn to walk across the balance beam without hand support at a fast speed. She will take steps and try to adjust her balance as she is stepping on the balance beam or else she will step off. To move quickly, she may choose to step with one foot on the balance beam and one on the ground. Your jobs will be to:

1. Slow down her speed if possible;
2. Focus her attention to look at her feet and the balance beam;
3. Learn the game to keep both feet on the balance beam.

You will need to plan the right time to practice balance beam activities. As the width of the balance beam becomes narrower, it will be more difficult to do and your child may not be interested in practicing it. Try it for brief periods to see when and if she is ready and willing to do it.

---

## Making a Balance Beam

To get lumber to use for a balance beam, it is best if you go to a lumber or hardware store and see what is available. You can cut the lumber to the desired width or use the standard sizes available. Remember to get a piece that is about 6 feet long. Framing lumber is identified by the height, width, and length of the board. The *actual measurement* of the board is different than what the *standard size* says.

1. For the 10-inch wide balance beam, you can use a 10-inch wide shelf, or standard sizes of lumber including 1 x 10 (actual size ¾ x 9¼) or 2 x 10 (actual size 1½ x 9¼).
2. For the 7.5-inch wide balance beam, you can use standard sizes of lumber, including 1 x 8 (actual size ¾ x 7¼) or 2 x 8 (actual size 1½ x 7¼).
3. For the 5.5-inch wide balance beam, you can use standard sizes of lumber, including 1 x 6 (actual size ¾ x 5½) or 2 x 6 (actual size 1½ x 5½). You can also use decking boards, since they are 5½ inches wide and some types are finished.
4. For the 4.5-inch wide balance beam, you can use finished wood pieces for an interior door/window jamb (actual size 11/16 x 4 9/16 x 7 feet long).
5. I have found that the 2 x 4 (actual size 1½ x 3½) and the 1 x 4 (actual size ¾ x 3½) are too narrow for the child to be successful, and that is why a 4- to 4.5-inch wide board is needed.

If a wider balance beam is needed in the beginning, you can use 12-inch wide shelving or foam interlocking squares. You could also use the standard sizes of lumber, including 1 x 12 (actual size ¾ x 11¼) or 2 x 12 (actual size 1½ x 11¼).

## 🏃 ACTIVITY #1: Walking Across a Balance Beam

Follow steps 1-12 using balance beams with the following widths: approximately 10", 7.5", 5.5", and 4.5" (12, 19, 14, and 11 cm). Begin with the widest balance beam. When your child can walk across it without support, with one foot forward of the other, try the next narrower width.

1. Place the balance beam on the floor and test it to make sure it is level and does not wobble as you walk across it. Have someone stand on it to stabilize it from sliding or tilting.

2. Have your child step up on the balance beam. Provide hand support if needed.

3. Stand beside her, with your body facing hers, and have her hold your index finger. (For example, if you are on her left, her left hand holds your left index finger.) Position her hand in front of her chest, at or below her shoulder level. Have her learn to hold your finger and be responsible for balancing herself with this support. If your child prefers two-hand support in the beginning, you can stand in front of her, facing her, and step backwards. Place your feet on the floor, straddling the balance beam.

4. Give her verbal cues ("march," "walk, walk" "two feet on the board"). If she is stepping too fast, you can say "slow" or count to help pace her stepping pattern. Provide visual cues by having a sibling walk in front of her or by taking turns with a sibling. If needed or if you want to be playful, exaggerate the leg movements by marching or stomping your feet while stepping across the balance beam. The verbal and visual cues will help her pay attention.

5. Encourage her to walk across the balance beam. Use motivators if needed.

6. When she walks to the other end of the balance beam, have her step off. Praise her and clap for her.

7. When she can walk across the balance beam holding your finger, decrease the support by having her maintain her balance by propping her hand against the wall. Place the balance beam approximately 8 inches (20 cm) away from the wall. Encourage her to put her hand against the wall for support.

8. When she is ready, encourage her to walk across the balance beam without hand support. Begin with a couple of steps, then half the length of the balance beam, and then increase the distance until she can walk across the full length.

9. While she walks across the balance beam by herself, watch her feet to see what she does to keep her balance. Is she pointing

her feet straight? Is she stepping slowly with her feet side by side and taking small steps? Is she stepping quickly and confidently with one foot forward of the other? When she can step with balance with one foot forward of the other, then she is ready to do the next narrower width board.

10. When your child is ready to do the next narrower size, place the wider board and the narrower board together lengthwise. With this setup, she will confidently walk across one board and then adjust to stepping across the next narrower board.

11. If she is reluctant to walk across the board, have her stand on it with a narrow base and entertain her. Then she can practice stepping on and off it. As she becomes familiar with it, she will become comfortable with stepping across it.

12. When she is comfortable with the balance beam game, let her practice it on her own by leaving the board in her play space to explore on her own. Also practice in the community by walking along curbs or railroad ties at the park.

13. If she loves the balance beam game and wants a challenge, place the balance beam on a stair so it is angled and have her walk up and down.

14. As an alternative, you can setup two mats lengthwise, beside each other with a space in between. Place the mats at the best width for her to practice. Then she can practice walking in between the mats.

## 🏃 MOTOR MILESTONE CHECKLIST

❑ She walks across a 10-inch (25-cm) wide balance beam with one-hand support

❑ She walks across a 10-inch (25-cm) wide balance beam without hand support

❑ She walks across a 7.5-inch (19-cm) wide balance beam with one-hand support

❑ She walks across a 7.5-inch (19-cm) wide balance beam without hand support

❑ She walks across a 5.5-inch (14-cm) wide balance beam with one-hand support

❑ She walks across a 5.5-inch (14-cm) wide balance beam without hand support

❑ She walks across a 4.5-inch (11-cm) wide balance beam with one-hand support

❑ She walks across a 4.5-inch (11-cm) wide balance beam without hand support

# 16

# What's Next?

## Introduction

Congratulations on all of the hard work you have done to arrive at this point. Together you have built the foundation to support exercise and fitness activities throughout your child's life. Now he can do the activities that he likes to do so he is motivated to choose an active lifestyle. He will continue to improve in strength, speed, coordination, endurance, and balance through these recreational and exercise activities.

At this age, he is attending school and spending a large part of the day sitting. Having a variety of fun activities to do for daily exercise will improve his physical skills and will also increase his attention and alertness, social interactions, and confidence. That is why it is so important for him to do the activities that he likes to do. If he likes them, he will establish this winning cycle of:

- self-initiating activities
- challenging himself to improve
- practicing for long periods of time
- having more successful experiences
- being proud of himself and his abilities

He will enjoy being active, using his energy, and having the freedom to express himself through his body. With these experiences, physical exercise will become an integral and enjoyable part of his daily life.

This chapter provides guidelines for choosing *what* activities to do and *how* to do them based on the physical factors and learning style in children with Down syndrome.

## What to Do

Let your child explore activities and choose what he likes to do. At different times in his life, his interests and the goals will change, and he will have the opportunity to practice a wide range of physical activities. The goals of the exercise could be:

1. To have fun and be active with siblings and peers
2. To explore a wide variety of body movements; for example, through creative dance
3. To improve his posture with exercise routines targeting specific areas of his body
4. To do gross motor skills for recreation with his family; for example, riding bikes together
5. To play sports and become competent with the motor skills needed
6. To do exercises for strength training
7. To do exercise routines to improve aerobic conditioning

As he explores various activities, keep focused on doing them in a way that is motivating and fun so he enjoys being active for long periods of time.

When your child is younger, he will want to move and will probably prefer motor activities that engage the whole body (fig. 16.1). By practicing these skills, he will strengthen his trunk, legs, and arms. He will love climbing, running, swimming, dancing, and riding a tricycle. He will enjoy ball skills, which will combine many motor tasks. For example, he may like soccer (running and kicking), basketball (running, dribbling, jumping, and shooting), golf (hitting the ball and running to it), T-ball (hitting the ball and running the bases), and tetherball (standing and hitting the ball). He will practice gross motor skills like running, stairs, jumping,

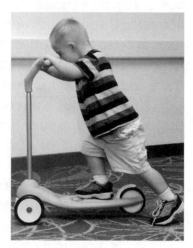

(fig. 16.1)

and riding a bicycle with training wheels, and progress to the advanced performance level. With the combination of all of these skills, his motor performance will improve in all areas.

Keep exploring options for physical activities for your child to see what he likes to do because his preferences may change from year to year. He will enjoy doing what he sees his siblings do or what his family likes to do. These activities will be familiar to him, and they will be valued since his family does them. It is also important to pick activities that are age appropriate for him and that he can do with his peers and children in his neighborhood. By observing what activities your child is exposed to in his daily life at school, in the neighborhood, and with his family, you will discover ideas to try. Look for activities that are easily accessible at home or nearby in the community so your child can do them regularly.

There are many settings for physical activities. In the **preschool years,** your child can participate in motor groups or obstacle courses in his preschool program, or he can attend community programs like My Gym, Little Monkey Bizness, Gymboree, Young Athletes Program through Special Olympics, or at the YMCA. He can go to indoor playgrounds or children's fitness centers. You can also look into the Department of Parks and Recreation and Therapeutic Recreation programs to find classes for all ages.

When he is **school aged,** your child will participate in physical education or adapted physical education classes. Depending on his interests and abilities, he may prefer to be included in community programs like yoga class, dance class, swimming, T-ball, soccer, karate, or gymnastics. He can play sports through community recreation centers, or may have a personal trainer at home or at the gym. Some families use exercise videos or Nintendo Wii games at home. There are also many programs geared specifically for children with disabilities, including:

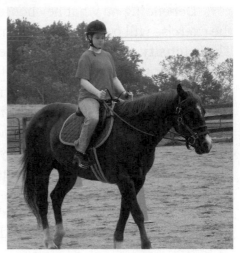

(fig. 16.2)

- Special Olympics, which offers training and competition in summer and winter sports for people with intellectual disabilities aged 8 and up, as well as a Young Athletes program for ages 2 – 7 (www.specialolympics.org)
- Hippotherapy (treatment provided by a PT, OT, or SLP that uses horseback riding as part of a therapeutic intervention program to achieve functional outcomes) or therapeutic riding (any activity on or around a horse specifically geared to people with disabilities) (fig. 16.2). For information about hippotherapy, contact the American Hippotherapy Association (www.americanhippotherapyassociation.org).
- Skiing (there are many programs for children with and without disabilities available depending on age and level of experience)
- The iCan Bike program (see page 456) for people with disabilities who need help learning to ride without training wheels (www.icanshine.org)
- The Golf for Life program (www.golfforlife.org)
- Challenger baseball (www.littleleague.org/learn/about/divisions/challenger.htm)

Look in your community and check with other parents through your local Down syndrome support group to see what programs and camps are offered in your area. For example, in Denver, we have the Be Beautiful Be Yourself Dance program, the Ed McCaffrey Dare to Play Football and Dare to Cheer camps, a Pure Barre program, Dare to Play Soccer, all offered through the Global Down Syndrome Foundation (www.globaldownsyndrome.org) and Adam's Camp (www.adamscamp.org).

Depending on what he chooses to do, the key to achieving benefits from the exercise will be how you design the intensity, duration, and frequency of it. The **intensity** can be low, moderate, or high, and you will determine the number of repetitions based on the difficulty of the activity. The **duration** is how long he does it; for short or long periods. The **frequency** is how often he does it; for example, how many times per day or per week. As your child or adolescent improves, then you can increase the intensity and repetitions, the duration of the practice sessions, the frequency, and the activities. You can use the principles of intensity, duration, and frequency with simple activities like playing on playground equipment, and later, when he is an adolescent, to design strength training or aerobic conditioning programs. By choosing activities he is interested in doing, he will be motivated to practice and cooperate with the design.

# Physical Considerations When Exercising

There are some important physical aspects to consider as your child is participating in his favorite activities and exercise programs. If you think about his **posture, movements,** and **heart rate,** you will be proactive in promoting what he needs and helping to prevent injury and overexertion. It will help you, and his teachers and coaches, to understand the full scope of factors to consider when choosing and implementing exercise programs. The list of postural considerations (below) gives you a framework of areas to monitor as your child is exercising, and as he gets older. If you know the desired posture (fig. 16.3) and areas needing strengthening, you can be strategic in the exercises and activities you choose. You can also provide the support he needs, like foot support, to help him move efficiently with optimal alignment. If you have any questions about any aspects of your child's movements, posture, or heart rate, consult with a physical therapist.

### Posture

As your child is active and exercising, observe his posture, movements, and walking pattern and keep in mind the four critical results to be achieved. With his ligamentous laxity and physical make-up, he may use abnormal patterns of posture and movement as he is exercising. For example, his joints will have extra mobility, and he may move them beyond the safe range of motion and cause injury. Or, he may have "postural habits" like tilting his head or trunk to one side. If you monitor how he does the exercises, you can help him use good mechanics, move within the safe range of motion, and develop strength in the desired muscle groups. You can intervene so he learns to do the exercises efficiently and safely and he does not learn to use problematic compensations that could lead to pain or faulty mechanics if allowed to persist.

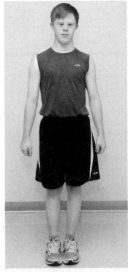

(fig. 16.3)

To help you focus on the potential tendencies and problematic compensations, here are the areas to monitor and suggested tips for interventions:

### Head Posture

**Components to Develop:**
- To hold his head erect and lifted in the midline

**Tendencies:**
- To hold his head tilted to the side (front/back view)
- To tilt his head back on his shoulders, with his chin protruding (side view)

**Interventions:**
- *For Head Tilt:* Talk to the pediatrician to evaluate what is causing this posture (for example, cervical spine abnormalities, scoliosis (curvature of the spine), or a visual impairment). Your pediatrician may recommend an evaluation by an orthopedist or an ophthalmologist. If head tilt is not due to scoliosis, and it tends to be a "postural habit" used periodically throughout the day, do exercises in front of a mirror focusing on increased awareness and improved neck strength to hold the head erect and lifted in the midline.
- *For Head Forward Posture:* Observe when your child uses this position most (for example, in sitting or standing), and then teach the optimal posture in that position. If he uses it mostly in sitting, evaluate the chair he uses and provide the right size and supports (for example, a lumbar support), if needed. Also do neck, arm, and upper trunk strengthening exercises (for example, types of push-ups or plank poses).

---

### Reminder about Atlantoaxial Instability and Atlanto-occipital Instability

Be sure you understand these conditions and are informed of the precautions so you can be proactive. Know the symptoms of spinal cord compression and how to manage it, if present. Notify your child's teachers (especially PE teachers at school, sports coaches, and staff at gymnastics programs) and avoid activities that put stress on the neck or cause forward/backward movements.

---

## Shoulder Posture
### Components to Develop:
- To hold his shoulders fairly even (front/back view)
- To have balanced strength between the front and back shoulder muscles, so his shoulders and arms fall in the middle of the side view, in line with his trunk (side view)

### Tendencies:
- To hold his shoulders uneven, with one consistently higher than the other (front/back view)
- To hold his shoulders rounded (rolled) forward when compared to the line of his trunk (side view)

### Interventions:
- *For Uneven Shoulders:* Talk to the pediatrician to rule out scoliosis. Your pediatrician may refer your child to an orthopedist. If he does not have a scoliosis, do exercises to strengthen both shoulders (and trunk) and do them in front of a mirror, focusing on keeping the shoulders even.
- *For Shoulders Rounded Forward and Arms in Internal Rotation: (Internal rotation: to feel this motion, place your arms at the sides of your trunk and move your arms so your thumbs turn inward and behind. When you exaggerate this motion, you feel your shoulders roll forward.)* Do shoulder exercises that focus on moving the shoulders back (using *external rotation*) so they are in line with the trunk (side view) and strengthen the muscles that pinch the shoulder blades together. *(External rotation: to feel this motion, place your arms at the sides of your trunk and move your arms so your thumbs turn outward and behind. When you exaggerate this motion, you feel your shoulders move back.)* Practice arm exercises and movements that promote stretching out the front of the

chest (from shoulder to shoulder), moving the arms into external rotation, and pinching the shoulder blades together. For example, the arm position for shooting a basket or doing a pull up. Avoid exercises that encourage moving the shoulder blades wide apart and compressing the front of the chest from shoulder to shoulder.

## Trunk Posture
### Components to Develop:
- To hold his trunk erect and straight (front/back view)
- To hold his upper and lower trunk straight, with a balanced posture and balanced strength between his front and back muscles (side view) (fig. 16.4A)

### Tendencies:
- To tilt his trunk to one side (front/back view)
- To have the following tendencies (side view) (fig. 16.4B)
    - Upper back at level of shoulder blades: to hold this area rounded or slouched forward
    - Lower back (at waist level): to hold this area arched forward with his abdomen protruding forward

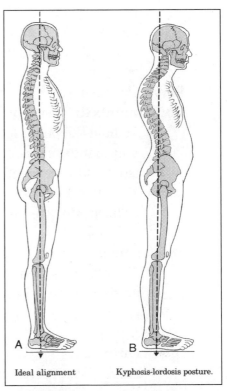

A — Ideal alignment

B — Kyphosis-lordosis posture.

(fig. 16.4) Reprinted with permission from: F.P. Kendall, E.K. McCreary, and P.G. Provance, *Muscles: Testing and Function, with Posture and Pain,* 4th ed. (Baltimore, MD: Williams & Wilkens, 1993), 76.

### Interventions:
- *For Trunk Tilt to One Side:* Talk to the pediatrician to rule out scoliosis. Your pediatrician may refer your child to an orthopedist. If he does not have a scoliosis, do trunk exercises to improve strength and flexibility for both sides of the trunk. Also check his daily routine and sitting posture to see if there is a time when he does it the most. You may find he has a habit of leaning to one side.
- *For Rounding of Upper Trunk:* Do exercises to strengthen his upper and middle trunk. Also make sure that he holds this part

of his trunk up straight when doing other exercises. Observe his sitting posture and if he slouches most of the time, find ways to encourage sitting up straight. (See the box on page 489 for information on proper sitting posture.)

■ *For Excessive Arching of Lower Trunk:* Do abdominal strengthening and gluteal bridge exercises to activate the core and buttock muscles simultaneously. (Consult with a physical therapist if there is low back pain or a more specialized program is needed. The PT can also check range of motion in the low back and hips to determine the best exercise program.)

## Pelvis Posture
### Components to Develop:
■ To hold the pelvis level (front/back view). (To check this, place your hands on the top edge of his pelvis on the right and left sides and note whether your hands are level with each other.)
■ To hold his pelvis in a neutral position, not tilted too far forward or back (side view)

### Tendencies:
■ To hold one side of his pelvis higher (front/back view)
■ To tilt the top of his pelvis significantly forward or backward (side view)

### Interventions:
■ *For Uneven Pelvis:* Talk to the pediatrician to see if your child has scoliosis or if his legs have slightly different lengths.
■ *For Pelvis Tilted Forward:* If his pelvis is tilted forward, his lower trunk is arched, so follow the recommendations above for "lower trunk, excessive arching of."
■ *For Pelvis Tilted Back:* This may be seen when your child is sitting and he will need to learn to sit with an optimal posture. (See page 489 for proper sitting positioning.)

## Hip Posture
### Components to Develop:
■ To stand and walk with his hips in neutral rotation, with his knees and feet pointing straight ahead, and his heels in line with his hips for a narrow base (front view)
■ To move his hips into hyperextension when he walks and runs (side view)

## Proper Sitting Posture

To sit with an optimal posture (fig. 16.5):

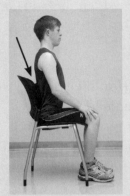

1. The pelvis is up straight and the back of the pelvis is firmly supported against the back of the chair.
2. The trunk is up straight and supported against the back of the chair.
3. If needed, support the low back area (at the waist) with a lumbar cushion so it has a mild curve and the top of the pelvis is tilted slightly forward. (If the pelvis is allowed to tilt backwards, the head and trunk will bend forward and your child will sit with a slouched posture.)
4. The thighs are fully supported on the seat, with the knees about hip width apart, and knees even with the hips.

(fig. 16.5)

5. The feet are flat on the floor, with the feet under the knees.
6. The shoulders are over the hips (side view).
7. The head is lifted, with the ears over the shoulders (side view).
8. The hip, knee, and ankle joints are at a 90 degree angle.
9. The body weight is evenly distributed on both hips and over the sitting bones.

To support the trunk, pelvis, thighs, and feet properly, the length and height of the seat need to fit and can by measured in this way:

1. *Length of the Seat.* There are two measurements to consider: the length of the seat of the chair and your child's seat depth needed for the proper sitting posture.
   a. The length of the seat of the chair is from the forward edge to the seatback.
   b. The child's seat depth is the measurement from the back of the buttocks (with the pelvis up straight) to the crease in the back of the knee (with the knee bent 90 degrees).
   c. For a chair to fit properly, the length of the seat of the chair needs to be the same as your child's seat depth measurement (or 1 inch shorter) so the full length of the thighs are supported by the length of the seat with your child's pelvis up straight against the seatback.
   d. If the length of the seat of the chair is too long, your child will tilt his pelvis back and then his head and trunk will slouch forward.
2. *Height of the Seat.* Measure from the back of the knee to the bottom of the foot. If your child's feet don't rest flat on the floor, try using a footrest or place the right height support under them.

**Tendencies:**
- To stand or walk with his knees and feet turned outward, using a wide base with his heels wider than his hips
- To walk and run with his hips and knees bent, with a short stride
- To have hip flexor tightness

**Interventions:**
- *For a Wide Base and Hips in External Rotation:* See if foot support will improve his posture and reevaluate his posture when he is active and moving quickly (walking, running, and jumping). If a child is provided with the right kind of shoes and foot support and engaged in active exercise, he will narrow his base and point his feet straight ahead.
- *For Learning Hip Hyperextension When Walking and Running:* Practice skills to learn this movement. For example, run fast with his trunk leaning forward, walk up inclines, push a grocery cart or stroller or back of a wagon up a hill, and walk/run on the treadmill.
- *For Muscle Tightness in the Muscles on the Front of the Hip:* Consult with a physical therapist to learn stretching exercises.

## Knee Posture
**Components to Develop:**
- To stand with legs vertical, from his thighs down to his ankles (front/back view)
- To stand with his knees relaxed and unlocked (side view)

**Tendencies:**
- To stand with his knees tilting inward (front/back view)
- To stand with his knees locked and "back-knee" (side view)

**Interventions:**
- *For Knees Tilting Inward:* This is due to ligamentous laxity at his knees, and it frequently occurs in combination with laxity in the ankles. He needs foot support to improve his leg alignment.
- *For Locked Knees:* You want him to learn to stand with his knees unlocked rather than stabilize himself by locking his knees. If he locks his knees and "back-knees," this will injure his knee joints over time so you need to figure out why he is doing it, with what skills, and how often. Foot management will be

helpful because it may provide stability at his ankles so he can relax his knees rather than compensate by locking them.

### Foot Posture
- Observe his foot posture when he is walking rather than standing. (Refer to pages 299-311 for information on foot management.)

### Components to Develop:
- To walk with his heels vertical (back view)
- To activate the muscles of his arches when he is active (e.g., jumping and running) (side view)
- To walk with his feet pointing straight ahead, and with his big toes pointing straight (front view)
- To maintain flexibility in the foot especially along the inside border and at the heel (so the foot can be moved into an arch and the heel can be moved to the vertical position)

### Tendencies:
- To walk with his heels moderately tilted, with a heavy footed pattern (back view)
- To walk with flat arches, bearing weight on the inside borders of his feet (side view)
- To walk with his feet turned outward or inward, or with his big toes turned outward or inward (front view)
- To complain of pain in his feet, or to have a callous. (Pain and callouses are most frequently seen under the ball of his big toe due to excessive rubbing in this area when walking.)
- To lose foot and heel mobility so the foot becomes a rigid flat foot

### Interventions:
- *For Heels Tilting, with Flat Arches and Feet Turned Out-ward:* Provide foot support so he can stand and walk with optimal alignment.
- *For Feet Turning Inward:* Talk to the pediatrician and physical therapist to determine what is causing this problem. Is it due to the posture of his hip, lower leg, or foot? Depending on the cause, the degree and frequency of toeing-in, and how it interferes with his function, the best intervention can be determined.
- *For Callouses under the Ball of the Big Toe:* This happens due to the foot posture, because he is taking weight on the inside border of his foot and then doing toe push-off from the ball of

his big toe when walking and running. Providing foot support and using athletic shoes will be helpful.

## Heart Rate and Cardiovascular Exercise

When your child is exercising, it is important to monitor his heart rate to measure how hard his heart is working and if the intensity level of the exercise is too much for his fitness level. You can do this by measuring his heart rate and then comparing that to his *target heart rate.* You can figure out his target heart rate after calculating his *maximal heart rate.*

For people without Down syndrome, the *maximal heart rate* is generally predicted by subtracting the age of the individual from 220. However, the maximal heart rate of individuals with Down syndrome is lower than that of peers without DS. Using the ACSM (American College of Sports Medicine) guidelines of maximal heart rate significantly over predicts maximal heart rate for individuals with DS.

**A better equation to use for individuals with Down syndrome (Fernhall, 2001) is:**

$$HR_{max} = 210 - [(.56)(age)] - (15.5 \times 2)$$

From this number, you can calculate the *target heart rate.* The generally recommended protocol is training at an intensity of 60 to 80 percent of an individual's maximal heart rate. From the maximal heart rate, you can figure out the target heart rate beginning at 60 percent intensity, progressing to 70 percent, and then to 80 percent.

For example, in an 18 year old with DS:

- His maximal heart rate would be 169. That is, $210 - (.56 \times 18) - (15.5 \times 2) = 210 - 10.08 - 31$. Rounding everything to the nearest whole number, that equals 169.
- His target heart rate at 60 percent would be 101 beats per minute, at 70 percent it would be 118, and at 80 percent, it would be 135 beats per minute.

This is important information to give to PE teachers, sports coaches, and teachers of any exercise classes that your child is involved in. By monitoring his heart rate while he is doing physical exercise, you can set him up to succeed. Otherwise, he may overexert himself and become overheated and fatigued.

## Movement: Gross Motor Problem Areas

There are areas of motor performance that are more challenging for children with Down syndrome. The predominant problem areas are:

- balance (e.g., standing on one foot or riding a bicycle without training wheels)

- response speed, or how quickly the child initiates movement (e.g., standing up quickly from lying on the floor, beginning to run after someone says "Ready, set, go," sitting down quickly as soon as the music stops when playing Musical Chairs, and activating brakes when riding a bike)
- timing of movements (e.g., swinging the bat at a moving ball, kicking a ball that is rolled toward him, hitting the ball in tetherball, catching a ball)
- sequencing of movements (e.g., doing a dance routine, playing hopscotch, doing the hokey pokey)
- coordinating body parts (bilateral coordination) (e.g., doing jumping jacks with simultaneous arm and leg movements, simultaneously pedaling and steering a tricycle, pushing off with one foot and simultaneously steering while riding a scooter)

When your child participates in activities that require these skills, he will be challenged and need practice to become competent and successful. His performance will improve with practice.

# How to Set Your Child Up to Be Successful

Now that you have suggestions about *what* to do and *how* to exercise from a physical perspective, the next consideration is planning how to set your child up to be successful based on his learning style. The main elements are choosing: 1) something he likes to do, 2) the peers or siblings to do it with, and 3) the right teacher to teach him. When he does the activity with others, he will have more fun, do it longer, learn by imitating, and give and receive encouragement and help from the others. You will want to observe the program options and choose instructors who are committed to having your child succeed. The teacher should be skilled in teaching to different learning styles and reading children's cues in order to accommodate their learning style. You want your child to be in a safe and nurturing environment and leave the class feeling confident and loving the activity and the experience.

The teacher will need to focus on the skill and its component parts. He or she should break down the learning process into the following steps:

1. Determine the component parts.
2. Get and keep the child's attention and have him watch you, listen to you, and follow you.
   a. In a group setting, teach him to focus on the leader and model him or her.

      b. Exaggerate movements, facial expressions, and verbal cues to motivate him to stay engaged with you.

3. Teach each part separately, observing your child's tendencies and guiding the desired movements.
      a. Give cues (verbal, visual, and tactile) and provide instructions at his level of comprehension.
      b. Provide props so he understands the setup (for example, a spot to stand on when dancing).
      c. Then practice the part for many repetitions until your child knows it and consolidates it.

4. Put the parts together so he learns the sequence.
      a. Support him through the sequencing of the parts until he can put them together on his own.
      b. Give brief verbal cues at the right time (allowing for his delayed response time) so he is prepared to do the next part.
      c. Provide a video so he can practice on his own at home for many repetitions.

5. Go at the right pace, fast enough to keep him engaged but not too fast that you lose him.

6. Use motivators to make it exciting and fun. For example, use types of music that he responds to, use scarves, or challenge him to race with his friends.

7. Give praise to reward him so he gains confidence and is proud of himself.

8. Once he has mastered the skill, challenge him by adding speed or distance or doing it in a variety of settings.

9. Avoid distractions and pauses in the flow of the activity so he stays focused on what to do and keeps moving.

If your child is having difficulty learning to do a particular activity, imitate what he is doing to identify what is missing. Practice with him so he feels the movements and then see if he can imitate them. By providing tactile cues, he may learn the gross movement and then be able to repeat it. If the skill is too difficult for him right now, you may need to temporarily modify how he performs it.

Below are two examples using the strategies discussed (dance class and exercise video at home):

1. I assist in a weekly dance class (fig. 16.6) and we have learned through experience to focus on the following areas:
      a. To *elicit and maintain each student's attention*: you want him to watch you, listen to you, and follow you, and then to continuously stay focused and engaged. [Step 2]

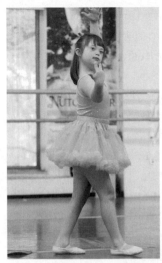

(fig. 16.6)

b. To give *visual cues*, for example to have the students focus on the dance teachers as the models of what to do, and to exaggerate the movements so they clearly see what to do. [Steps 2a, 2b, 3a]

c. To give *verbal cues* using key words that are concise, specific, clear, timely, and continuous. [Steps 3a, 4b]

d. To give *tactile cues* when needed so the student feels the movements and understands what to do. [Step 3a]

e. To provide *cues for organization*, like using spots so the students know where to stand. [Step 3b]

f. To choreograph the music so there are many repetitions of the same movements so the students are familiar with them and competent in doing them. [Step 3c]

g. Provide a *videotape* of the dance routines so the students can *practice* them at home and have the opportunity to consolidate them. [Step 4c]

h. To *sequence the routines* with a *pace* that the students can keep up with. [Step 5]

i. To use *types of music* that the students respond to. [Step 6]

j. To provide *props* for fun and creative expression, like scarves. [Step 6]

k. To *avoid distractions and interruptions*, and to lead all of the students in following the teacher and imitating her movements so that everyone is doing the group activity. [Step 9]

2. The same principles apply if your child is using exercise videos at home. You will need to watch the videos to evaluate which one will work best for your child.

a. Since your child will be exercising with the model(s) in the video, it is essential that the models use the appropriate equipment (mats, athletic shoes, work out clothes), correct form when doing the exercises, and that the models are *motivating role models* to imitate. [Steps 2, 3b, 6]

b. The *instructions* need to be concise and clear, and counting is useful to help him stay focused and anticipate what he needs to do. [Step 3a]

c. It is best to start with *simple movements*, for example focusing on easy arm movements, and then focus on leg movements, and then when both are familiar, they can be combined. It is too difficult for your child to combine arm and leg movements and do them simultaneously. [Steps 3, 4]

d. He will be more successful if the routines have *many repetitions* of the same movements. This will give him time to figure out what to do and then he can do it for many repetitions and really benefit from the intensity of doing the movements for several repetitions. [Steps 3c, 4c]

e. The video needs to be *easy to follow visually*, and the focus needs to be clear. If there are many distractions or if the instructions compete with the music, then it will be hard to follow effectively. [Steps 3a, 9]

f. It needs to be the right *pace* to follow, and slower is better to give him time to process what he needs to do (due to his slower response time when learning new skills). [Step 5]

g. *Music* can be motivating while doing the exercise routine but it needs to complement the routine and not distract from the focus. [Step 6]

## Conclusion

Now you have the general guidelines for exercise. Depending on your child's interests, you can seek the guidance of coaches, personal trainers, physical therapists, or teachers to improve performance in a specific exercise program or sports programs (fig. 16.7). If you provide these guidelines to the teachers, everyone will be setup to succeed. The goal now is for your child to have an active lifestyle, celebrate what he has achieved, and enjoy doing what his body can do! This lifestyle will support him in sustaining a strong and fit body for life.

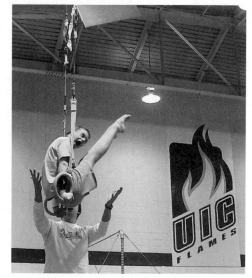

(fig. 16.7)

# References

Adolph, Karen E. "Learning to Keep Balance." *Advances in Child Development and Behavior 30* (2002), 1-40.

American Academy of Pediatrics, Council on Sports Medicine and Fitness. "Policy Statement: Trampoline Safety in Childhood and Adolescence." *Pediatrics 130* (2012), 774-779.

Anson, J. G. "Neuromotor Control and Down Syndrome." In *Approaches to the Study of Motor Control and Learning,* edited by J. J. Summers, 387-412. Amsterdam, the Netherlands: Elsevier Science Publishers, 1992.

Biel, Andrew R., and Dorn, Robin, illustrator. *Trail Guide to the Body: A Hands-on Guide to Locating Muscles, Bones, and More.* Boulder, CO: Books of Discovery, 2010.

Bly, Lois. *Motor Skills Acquisition in the First Year: An Illustrated Guide to Normal Development.* Tucson, AZ: Therapy Skill Builders, 1994, 169.

Bull, Marilyn J. (and the committee on Genetics). "Clinical Report—Health Supervision for Children with Down Syndrome." *Pediatrics* 128 (2011): 393-406. (http://pediatrics.aappublications.org/content/128/2/393.full.pdf).

Calais-Germain, Blandine. *Anatomy of Movement.* Seattle, WA: Eastland Press, 2007.

Fernhall, B., McCubbin, J.A., Pitetti, K.H., Rintala, P., Rimmer, J.H., Millar, A.L., and De Silva, A., "Prediction of Maximal Heart Rate in Individuals with Mental Retardation." *Medicine & Science in Sports & Exercise 33*, no. 10 (2001), 1655-60.

Jobling, A., and Mon-Williams, M. "Motor Development in Down Syndrome: A Longitudinal Perspective." In *Perceptual-Motor Behavior in Down Syndrome,* edited by D. J. Weeks, R. Chua, and D. Elliott, 225-48. Champaign, IL: Human Kinetics, 2000.

Jobling, A., and Virgi-Babul, N. *Motor Development in Down Syndrome: Play, Move and Grow.* Vancouver, BC: Down Syndrome Research Foundation, 2004.

Kendall, F.P., McCreary, E.K., and Provance P.G. *Muscles: Testing and Function, with Posture and Pain,* 4th ed. Baltimore, MD: Williams & Wilkens, 1993, 76.

Latash, M.L. "Motor Control in Down Syndrome: The Role of Adaptation and Practice." *Journal of Developmental and Physical Disabilities* 4 (1992): 227-61.

Latash, M.L. "Motor Coordination in Down Syndrome: The Role of Adaptive Changes." In *Perceptual-Motor Behavior in Down Syndrome,* 199-223. edited by D. J. Weeks, R. Chua, and D. Elliott. Champaign, IL: Human Kinetics, 2000.

Latash, M. L., & Anson, J. G. "Synergies in Health and Disease: Relations to Adaptive Changes in Motor Coordination," *Physical Therapy* 86 (2006): 1151-60.

Leshin, Len. "Medical Concerns in Babies with Down Syndrome." In *Babies with Down Syndrome: A New Parents' Guide,* 3rd ed., edited by Susan J. Skallerup, 75-102. Bethesda, MD: Woodbine House, 2008.

Oelwein, Patrice Logan. *Teaching Reading to Children with Down Syndrome: A Guide for Parents and Teachers.* Bethesda, MD: Woodbine House, 1995.

Pueschel, Siegfried M. *A Parent's Guide to Down Syndrome: Toward a Brighter Future.* Baltimore, MD: Paul H. Brookes Publishing, 2001, 59-73.

Shea, A.M. "Motor Attainments in Down Syndrome." In *Contemporary Management of Motor Control Problems: Proceedings for the II STEP Conference*, 225-36. Alexandria, VA: Foundation for Physical Therapy, 1991.

Sutherland, D.H., Olshen, R.A., Biden, E.N., and Wyatt, M.P. *Clinics in Developmental Medicine No. 104/105: The Development of Mature Walking.* London, England: Mac Keith Press, 1988.

Ulrich, D.A., Burghardt, A.R., Lloyd, M., Tiernan, C., and Hornyak, J.E.. "Physical Activity Benefits of Learning to Ride a Two-Wheel Bicycle for Children with Down Syndrome: A Randomized Trial." *Physical Therapy 91* (2011), 1463-77.

Wishart, J. G.. "Cognitive Abilities in Children with Down Syndrome: Developmental Instability and Motivational Deficits." In *Etiology and Pathogenesis of Down Syndrome,* edited by C. J. Epstein, T. Hassold, I. T. Lott, L. Nadel, & D. Patterson, 57-91. New York, NY: Wiley-Liss, 1995.

Wishart, J. G. "Taking the Initiative in Learning: A Developmental Investigation of Infants with Down Syndrome." *International Journal of Disability, Development and Education* 38 (1991): 27-44.

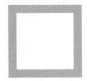

# Resources

**Down Syndrome Education International**
6 Underley Business Centre
Kirkby Lonsdale
Cumbria LA6 2DY
United Kingdom
info@dseinternational.org
www.dseinternational.org

**Down Syndrome Education USA**
1451 Quail Street, Suite 110
Newport Beach, CA 92660
949-757-1877
info@dseusa.org
www.dseusa.org

**Down Syndrome Research Foundation**
1409 Sperling Ave.
Burnaby, British Columbia
Canada V5B 4J9
604-444-3773
info@dsrf.org
www.dsrf.org

**Global Down Syndrome Foundation**
3300 East 1st Ave., Suite 390
Denver, CO 80206
303-321-6277
info@globaldownsyndrome.org
www.globaldownsyndrome.org

**John Langdon Down Foundation (Fundacion John Langdon Down)**
Selva 4, Insurgentes Cuicuilco
Del. Coyoacán, Ciudad de México
Mexico
52-55-5666-8580
www.fjldown.org.mx

**National Center on Health, Physical Activity and Disability**
4000 Ridgeway Dr.
Birmingham, AL 35209
800-900-8086
email@nchpad.org
www.ncpad.org

**National Down Syndrome Congress**
30 Mansell Court, Suite 108
Roswell, GA 30076
770-604-9500; 800-232-NDSC (6372)
info@ndsccenter.org
www.ndsccenter.org

**National Down Syndrome Society**
666 Broadway, 8th Floor
New York, NY 10012
800-221-4602
info@ndss.org
www.ndss.org

# Appendix

# *Evaluation Worksheet*

| Child's Name: | Mom's Name: |
|---|---|
| | Dad's Name: |
| Date: | Sibling or Other: |

| Date of Birth: | STAGE: |
|---|---|
| Current Age: | |
| Home Location: | |
| Brief History: | |

| Strengths | Concerns | Behavior |
|---|---|---|
| | | |

## Background

| Medical History | |
|---|---|
| Early Intervention/School | |
| Current Physical Therapy | |

| Gross Motor Development (Current Abilities) | Posture |
|---|---|
| Trend | |
| Level | |
| Hypotonia | |
| Ligamentous Laxity | |
| Strength | |
| Mobility | |

| Today's Treatment Sequence | Next Session Treatment Sequence |
|---|---|
| | |
| | |
| | |
| | |

## Plan

1. Recommendations:


2. Home program (prioritized order):

# *Follow-Up Treatment Session Worksheet*

| Child's Name: | Mom's Name: |
|---|---|
| | Dad's Name: |
| Date: | Sibling or Other: |

| Date of Birth: | STAGE: |
|---|---|
| Current Age: | |
| Home Location: | |
| Brief History: | |

| Follow-Up | |
|---|---|
| Specific points from last visit or concerns | |
| Medical issues since last visit | |
| Services received, school, and community programs | |
| Notes for setup or motivation | |

| Improvements since last visit | Behavior |
|---|---|
| | |

| Prior Treatment and sequence | Today's Treatment and recommended sequence | Next Session: Treatment/ sequence/ recommendations |
|---|---|---|
| | | |
| | | |
| | | |
| | | |
| | | |

| Plan |
|---|
| 1. Recommendations: |
| 2. Home program (prioritized order): |

# Gross Motor—Stage 1

| Trends | | | | |
|---|---|---|---|---|
| Head Posture (turning more to one side, shape) | | | | |
| Reaching Preference (arm dominance) | | | | |
| Movements (arching, asymmetry, etc.) | | | | |
| **Skill** | **Achieved** | **Notes** | | |
| **Supine** | | **In Lap** | **On Floor** | **Support** |
| Head | | | | |
| Preference (turn to one side) | | | | |
| Holds in midline | | | | |
| Chin tuck | | | | |
| Arms | | | | |
| Hand to mouth | | | | |
| Hands to midline at chest to touch large toy | | | | |
| Reach/bat at suspended toys | | | | |
| Legs | | | | |
| Legs supported | | | | |
| Hip Stretch | | | | |
| **Supported in Side-lying with knee held against abdomen** | | | | |
| Chin tuck | | | | |
| Batting at toy with hand | | | | |
| Hand to mouth | | | | |

| Prone – maximally supported legs and elbows | | |
|---|---|---|
| Head lift to __ degrees | | |
| Prop on elbows __ minutes | | |
| Time: __ seconds/minutes | | |
| **Supported Kneeling at 7" cushion– maximally supported legs, elbows, and trunk** | | |
| Controlled head lift to __ degrees | | |
| Maintain prop on elbows | | |
| Time: __ seconds/minutes | | |
| **Supported Sitting – with maximal support/ posterior support/at chest or in chair** | | |
| Full support in sitting (chest/chair) Holds head up for: | | |
| Time: __ seconds/minutes | | |
| Head lift | | |
| **Rolling – Side-lying to prone with support provided to underneath arm and pelvis/lower leg** | | |
| Head lift | | |
| Roll to prone | | |
| Pause time | | |

# *Gross Motor—Stage 2*

| Trends | | |
|---|---|---|
| **Skill** | **Achieved** | **Notes** |
| **Supine** | | |
| Reaching | | |
| Bridging | | |
| Hand to Foot Play | | |
| **Prone** | | |
| Prop on Elbows | | |
| Prop on Hands | | |
| Reach | | |
| Leg position – address "frog leg" | | |
| **Pull to Sit** | | |
| Shoulder Girdle Support | | |
| Two Hand Support | | |
| Chin Tuck | | |
| Elbow Flexion | | |
| Grip Strength | | |
| **Sitting – Supported** | | |
| Trunk Support – upper/middle | | |
| Time in Sitting | | |

| **Rolling** | | |
|---|---|---|
| Supine to Side-lying | | |
| Side-lying to Prone | | |
| Supine to Prone | | |
| Prone to Supine | | |
| Level of Assistance | | |
| **Supported Kneeling at 8–9" high cushion with legs supported** | | |
| Head Lift | | |
| Prop (Elbows or Hands) | | |
| Reaching | | |
| Trunk position (arching/neutral) | | |

## *Gross Motor—Stage 3*

Trends

| Skill | Achieved | Notes |
|---|---|---|
| **Pivoting in prone** | | |
| Support | | |
| Direction | | |
| Pivots __ degrees | | |
| **Sitting (on the floor with legs in criss-cross sit)** | | |
| Habit or Tendency | | |
| Waist Support | | |
| Pelvic Support | | |
| Independent/How long | | |
| **Moving to Sitting** | | |
| L-Position side-lying / side preferred | | |
| Middle trunk support: prop | | |
| Low trunk support: arm pushes | | |
| **Moving out of Sitting – over which side?** | | |
| Falls laterally to stomach | | |
| Props hands to side, moves to prone | | |
| **Supported Kneeling with Knees Supported Together** | | |
| Low back extension | | |
| Moves kneel to sit / side preference | | |

| 90/90 Sitting | | |
|---|---|---|
| Maintains balance in position | | |
| Rotates trunk to reach | | |
| **Supported Standing – in optimal standing posture with bench behind legs/heels** | | |
| Support: Trunk/hands/edge of surface | | |
| Moves to stand from 90/90 sit | | |
| Lowers from stand to 90/90 sit | | |
| Posture (ideal) | | |
| Feet 2–3" apart, pointing straight, heels at bench | | |
| Knees unlocked/slightly bent | | |
| Trunk (with abdominals activated) | | |
| Bouncing/dancing to music | | |
| Standing at surface/Holding on/Time | | |

## *Gross Motor—Stage 4*

Trends

| Skill | Achieved | Notes |
|-------|----------|-------|
| **Combat Crawling** | | |
| Support | | |
| Method | | |
| Distance/Number of Pulls/Quality | | |
| **Climbing Up** | | |
| Support | | |
| Cushion on floor | | |
| Up top 2 stairs | | |
| On sofa without cushions | | |
| **Climbing down with Support** | | |
| Support | | |
| **Moving into Quadruped** | | |
| With support or independently | | |
| **Creeping** | | |
| Distance and quality | | |
| **Moving into Sitting – over which side?** | | |
| From kneeling | | |
| From prone | | |
| From hands and knees | | |
| With own method | | |

| Moving Out of Sitting—over which side? | | |
|---|---|---|
| To prone with/without control | | |
| To quadruped | | |
| **Pulling to Kneel – over which side?** | | |
| Surface: height | | |
| Surface: edge or flat | | |
| From: sit, quadruped, prone | | |
| **Pulling to Stand** | | |
| Surface: height | | |
| Surface: edge or flat | | |
| From: 90/90 sit | | |
| From kneeling: | | |
| Pops up with both legs | | |
| Through Half-Knee—Right or Left | | |
| **Moving from Standing to Sitting on the Floor** | | |
| Surface: edge or flat | | |
| Lowers to 90/90 sit | | |
| Plops to Sit – knees straight | | |
| Bends knees when lowering / control | | |
| **Standing Holding On** | | |
| Surface: edge or flat | | |
| Hand Support: 2, 1 | | |
| Rises up on tiptoes / bounces | | |

## *Gross Motor—Stage 5*

| Trends | | |
|---|---|---|

| Skill | Achieved | Notes |
|---|---|---|
| **Cruising** | | |
| Height of surface | | |
| Support | | |
| Number of steps/ Direction R/L | | |
| Around corner | | |
| Between adjacent furniture | | |
| Between parallel pieces | | |

| Walking | | Distance | |
|---|---|---|---|
| Support: Trunk/2-hand | | | |
| Lunging to horizontal surface | | | |
| Standing toy/Push-toy/Walker | | | |
| One-hand support – R/L | | | |
| Type of support | | | |
| Independent | | | |
| Symmetry | | | |
| Foot support/Barefoot | | | |

| Climbing | | |
|---|---|---|
| Climbs up stairs: Number | | |
| Method/Side preference | | |
| Climbs off sofa | | |
| Move to prone | | |
| Legs straight/slide | | |
| Push with arms | | |
| Climbs down: Number/Method | | |

| Plantigrade | | |
|---|---|---|
| Assumes plantigrade | | |
| Bear walks | | |
| Modified plantigrade to stand, with posterior support | | |
| 90/90 sit to squat to stand | | |
| Plantigrade to stand: Support | | |
| Plantigrade to stand and walk | | |

| Standing | | |
|---|---|---|
| Hand position | | |
| Props: on or against | | |
| 1 or 2 hands | | |
| Reaches to side/down/behind | | |
| Balances without support | | |
| Time | | |

## *Post Walking Skills*

| Trends | | |
|---|---|---|
| **Basic Gait Analysis** | **Barefoot** | **Foot Support + Shoes** |
| Base: Heel Relative to Hips | | |
| Feet Point | | |
| Pelvic Rotation | | |
| Knee Flexion/Extension | | |
| Trunk Lean | | |
| Hip Hyperextension | | |
| Weight Bearing through foot | | |
| Weight Shift through foot | | |
| Toe Push-Off | | |
| Step Length | | |
| Speed/Endurance | | |
| Asymmetry | | |

| **Walking on Uneven Surfaces** | **Notes** |
|---|---|
| 1. Hand support/Independent: | |
| 2. Surface: | |
| 3. Distance: | |
| 4. Falls: | |
| 5. Walks between surfaces:<br>    With/without hand support surfaces: | |
| 6. Walk over/around obstacles: | |

| **Fast Walking and Running** | **Notes** |
|---|---|
| 1. Hand support: 2, 1, without | |
| 2. Distance: | |
| 3. Speed: | |
| 4. Arm swing: | |
| 5. Trunk: Vertical/lean forward | |
| 6. Hip flexion/ extension/hyperextension | |
| 7. Feet: weight shift/toe push-off | |
| 8. Eye Gaze: | |

| Walking up and down inclines | Walks Up | Walks Down |
|---|---|---|
| Hand support: 2, 1, Without | | |
| Incline (Small, Medium, Large): | | |
| Speed and Control: | | |

| Kicking a ball | | |
|---|---|---|
| Hand support: 2, 1, Without | | |
| Leg Preference: | | |
| Distance kicks the ball: | | |
| Run and Kick: | | |

| Walks up and down curbs | Walks Up | Walks Down |
|---|---|---|
| Hand support: 2, 1, Without | | |
| Curb Height: | | |
| Leads with: | | |
| Control | | |

| Walking up and down stairs | Walks Up | Walks Down |
|---|---|---|
| Stair Size: Toddler, Standard | | |
| Leads with _____: Marking/Alternating | | |
| Hand Support: 2, 1, Without | | |
| Hand: Rail/Wall/Finger | | |
| Control: | | |

| Jumping | Notes |
|---|---|
| Hand support: 2, 1, Without | |
| Surface: mini-trampoline with bar/mat/floor | |
| Bounce: full sole/tiptoe | |
| Liftoff: full sole/ toe push-off | |
| Posture: trunk, hips, knees, feet | |
| Jump: | |
| Lift-off | |
| Forward – Distance | |
| Off step – Height | |
| Variations: march, rock forward/back, rock side to side | |

| Ride-on toy/tricycle/balance bike or bicycle without pedals/no brake bicycle/bicycle with training wheels, bicycle without training wheels | | |
|---|---|---|
| Support: grip liner, footpedal attachments, belt | | |
| Climbs on/off _____ | | |
| Support | | |
| Scoots on _____ | | |
| Support | | |
| Backward/distance: | | |
| Forward/distance: | | |
| Surface: | | |
| Pedaling on the _____ | | |
| Support | | |
| Pushed to learn pedaling | Time/Distance | |
| Independent / Distance | Time/#Pushes | |
| Surface: | | |
| Steering the _____ | | |
| Support | | |
| Participates | | |
| Steers consistently/distance | | |
| Pedals and Steers/Distance | | |
| Support | | |
| Brakes: type | | |
| Support | | |
| Intermittent/consistent use | | |
| **Balance beam skills** | **Notes** | |
| Hand support: 2, 1, Without | | |
| Balance beam width: | | |

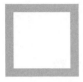

# Index

## *About the author:*

Pat Winders is the Director of Therapies and Senior Physical Therapist at the Anna & John J. Sie Center for Down Syndrome at Children's Hospital Colorado. Prior to this position, she worked at the Kennedy Krieger Institute Down Syndrome Clinic in Baltimore, Maryland. Since 1981 she has specialized in providing physical therapy services to children with Down Syndrome. She is a member of the Down Syndrome Medical Interest Group (DSMIG-USA) and also serves on the Professional Advisory Committee of the National Down Syndrome Congress (NDSC) and the Clinical Advisory Board of the National Down Syndrome Society (NDSS).